1/90

£25. 00

# Disorders of Human Learning, Behavior, and Communication

Ronald L. Taylor and Les Sternberg
Series Editors

Jack A. Stark   Frank J. Menolascino
Michael H. Albarelli   Vincent C. Gray
Editors

# Mental Retardation and Mental Health

## Classification, Diagnosis, Treatment, Services

Springer-Verlag
New York  Berlin  Heidelberg
London  Paris  Tokyo

Jack A. Stark and Frank J. Menolascino, Department of Psychiatry, University of Nebraska Medical Center, Omaha, Nebraska 68105-1065, USA

Michael H. Albarelli, President's Committee on Mental Retardation, Washington, D.C. 20201, USA

Vincent C. Gray, Association for Retarded Citizens, District of Columbia, Washington, D.C. 20011, USA

*Series Editors*: Ronald L. Taylor and Les Sternberg, Exceptional Student Education, Florida Atlantic University, Boca Raton, Florida 33431-0991, USA

Library of Congress Cataloging-in-Publication Data
Mental retardation and mental health.
  (Disorders of human learning, behavior, and communication)
  Based on a National Strategies Conference on Mental Illness in the Mentally Retarded, sponsored by the President's Committee on Mental Retardation (PCMR), held in Washington, D.C. Oct. 30-Nov. 1, 1985.
  Includes bibliographies and index.
  1. Mentally handicapped—Mental health—Congresses. I. Stark, Jack A. II. National Strategies Conference on Mental Illness in the Mentally Retarded (1985 : Washington, D.C.) III. United States. President's Committee on Mental Retardation. IV. Series.
[DNLM: 1. Mental Disorders—etiology—congresses. 2. Mental Retardation—complications—congresses. WM 307.M5 M549]
RC451.4.M47M47    1987        616.85'88        87-16577

former are not especially identified, is not to be taken as a sign that such names, as understood by the Trade Marks and Merchandise Marks Act, may accordingly be used freely by anyone.

While the advice and information in this book are believed to be true and accurate at the date of going to press, neither the authors nor the editors nor the publisher can accept any legal responsibility for any errors or omissions that may be made. The publisher makes no warranty, express or implied, with respect to the material contained herein.

Typeset by Publishers Service, Bozeman, Montana.
Printed and bound by R.R. Donnelley and Sons, Harrisonburg, Virginia.
Printed in the United States of America.

9 8 7 6 5 4 3 2 1

ISBN 0-387-96577-7 Springer-Verlag New York Berlin Heidelberg
ISBN 3-540-96577-7 Springer-Verlag Berlin Heidelberg New York

# Foreword

In late 1985, The President's Committee on Mental Retardation (PCMR) sponsored a National Strategy Conference on Mental Retardation and Mental Health in Washington, D.C. The purpose of this conference was to bring together our nation's leadership in the fields of mental retardation and mental health in order to delineate the state of the art relative to the diagnosis, care, and treatment of citizens with mental retardation/mental illness, as well as to chart a national course for the support and integration of citizens with these challenging needs into the confluence of family and community life.

The President's Committee on Mental Retardation recognized that citizens with these needs constitute one of the most underserved and, at times, forgotten segments of the population. With this in mind, the PCMR called together governmental, professional, and parental representatives from across the nation to define the nature and extent of the problem, programs, and services that promise hope for substantive improvement in the quality of life of citizens with mental retardation/mental illness.

The conference focused on several major themes: epidemiology, prevention, training, research, clinical diagnosis and treatment challenges, issues centering on the family system, community treatment-management alternatives, model service programs, and legal and legislative barriers and supports. To analyze these critical issues, the PCMR invited academic, governmental, and parental experts from across the nation for this national conference. Each of the major themes was reviewed, analyzed, and critically questioned through individual presentations, panel discussions, and audience participation. The range of discussion resulted in a significant amount of consensus relative to basic issues and needed change strategies. A few of the issues created more controversial debate and the stated need for further study and analysis. As such, the views expressed in these chapters are those of the authors. Although the PCMR has taken no position on these works, it presents them as a contribution to the research, study, thinking, and planning required to address the major issues associated with meeting the needs of the nation's citizens with mental retardation and mental illness.

Albert L. Anderson, D.D.S.
Vice-Chairman, President's Committee on
Mental Retardation

# Preface

The strength of this edited volume lies in its comprehensive contribution by some 50 authors representing numerous professional disciplines. One potential weakness, however, is agreeing on and using a common set of definitions given the use of terms unique to each discipline. It becomes a truly challenging task agreeing on a set of terms when individuals from such areas as medicine, law, psychology, social work, human services, administration, and social/policy analysis come together to write (both collectively and individually) on a common topic.

This semantic phenomena is particularly evident in the use of the term "dual diagnosis." When referring to the mental health aspects of persons who are mentally retarded, each discipline tends to use their own set of terms familiar to them. For example, psychologists use the term "behavioral problems" or "emotional disorders," lawyers and social workers use the terms "mental health aspects," and psychiatrists use "psychiatric disorders" or refer to the psychopathology and specific diagnostic issues.

One contributor (Baumeister) noted that definitions and classifications may be more directly driven by political, social, and economic considerations than by scientific or professional concerns. Szymanski has cogently argued against the use of the term "dual diagnosis" as an imprecise and possibly inappropriate label (i.e., would a retarded person be viewed as "quadrally diagnosed" if they also displayed epilepsy, cerebral palsy, and a major auditory disorder). Still others point out that this term is increasingly being used to describe individuals with the "dual problem" of alcoholism and mental illness.

Despite these concerns, the term "dual diagnosis" remains immensely popular in the field of mental retardation, particularly among the direct services providers. It serves as a label that quickly describes who they serve and what their services are about. Indeed, the National Association for the Dually Diagnosed (NADD) now has some 2,000(+) members in just the few years since its founding. The founders of this national organization, Menolascino and Fletcher, feel that the term "dual diagnosis" serves to draw national attention to the issues concerning a special group of mentally retarded individuals who have the coexistence of mental illness/mental retardation. The rationale for the usage of the term is to bring attention to both the complexity of the needs and multiplicity of services necessary for this underserved population. Hopefully, this explanation will help the reader better understand the terminology issues as they progress through the various sections written by the top professionals in their respective disciplines on this common topic.

Lastly, the issue of style requires a brief comment. The contributors to this book are sensitive about the possible pejorative use of labels—having served as advocates on behalf of the rights of persons with mental retardation for a good portion of our professional careers. The linguistic use of "persons who are mentally retarded" is most appropriate and was used as frequently as possible. However, for readability and space considerations, the use of "mentally ill/mentally retarded" or "mentally retarded person," "citizen," or "individual" was sometimes substituted. This literary style is not intended to deprecate this population of fellow citizens whom we are proud to serve.

# Acknowledgments

In planning the national conference and the subsequent publication of this book, the President's Committee on Mental Retardation established an Interagency Planning Group comprised of representatives from five other federal agencies. Together, these six federal agencies and assembled professionals from across several disciplines were brought together to identify research needs and strategies necessary for the delivery of effective mental health services to persons with mental retardation. The six sponsoring agencies were:

Office of Special Education and Rehabilitative Services, U.S. Department of Education

National Institute of Child Health and Human Development, National Institute of Health, Department of Health and Human Services

National Institute of Mental Health, Alcohol, Drug Abuse and Mental Health Administration, Department of Health and Human Services

Assistant Secretary for Planning and Evaluation, Department of Health and Human Services

Administration on Developmental Disabilities, Office of Human Development Services, Department of Health and Human Services

President's Committee on Mental Retardation, Office of Human Development Services, Department of Health and Human Services

The President's Committee on Mental Retardation appreciates the opportunity to present this book to the field of mental retardation and mental health. Listed on the following page are members of the Committee and staff whose efforts helped to bring about this final product.

## Members of PCMR

The Honorable Otis R. Bowen, M.D.
  Chairperson
Lucia L. Abell
Martin S. Appel
James Bopp, Jr.
Lee A. Christoferson, M.D.
Dorothy Corbin Clark, R.N.
Margaret Ann Depaoli
Lois Eargle
Thomas J. Farrell*
Vincent C. Gray*
Jean G. Gumerson
Matthew J. Guglielmo
Madeline B. Harwood
Elsie D. Helsel, Ph.D.*

Albert L. Anderson, D.D.S.
  Vice Chairperson
William Kerby Hummer, M.D.
Roger Stanley Johnson, M.D.
Richard J. Kogan*
D. Beth Macy*
J. Alfred Rider, M.D., Ph.D.
Fred J. Rose*
U. Yun Ryo, M.D., Ph.D.
Dwight Schuster, M.D.
Anne C. Seggerman
Marguerite T. Shine*
Virginia J. Thornburgh
Martin Ulan
Ruth A. Warson, R.N.

### PCMR Staff

Susan Gleeson, R.N., M.S.N.
  Executive Director
Jim F. Young
  Deputy Executive Director
Janet T. Bolt
Nancy O. Borders
George Bouthilet, Ph.D.

Ashot Mnatzakanian
Essie Norkin (deceased May 1987)
Laverdia T. Roach
Rosa Singletary
Bena Smith
David Touch
Terry Visek

*Term expired in June 1986

Special appreciation is also extended to Dr. Jean K. Elder, Former Acting Assistant Secretary, Office of Human Development Services, Jim F. Young, Deputy Executive Director, PCMR, Vincent C. Gray, former PCMR member, and Michael Albarelli, former PCMR staff member, with special thanks to Susan Gleeson, R.N., M.S.N., Executive Director, PCMR, Dr. Frank Menolascino, and Judy Moore for their invaluable contributions and support to this project. Recognition is due to Vicki Morrison, Tammi Goldsbury, and Earl Faulkner for their assistance in the preparation of this manuscript.

The Committee is thoroughly committed to identifying and addressing those dynamics that weaken rather than strengthen the emotional fiber of families with a member who has mental retardation. When a family is strong, so too is its ability to cope with unusual and unexpected situations.

# Executive Summary

The editors present this executive summary as a prelude to the book to provide the reader with a synopsis of the major tenets of each section of this comprehensive text. This encapsulated summary is intended both as a guide to the book and as a section that can be reread from time to time in one's efforts to better understand and care for this group of individuals.

## Epidemiology

There is no doubt as to the tremendous human needs and challenges presented by persons with the diagnosis of both mental retardation and mental illness. Although there is some question as to the precise incidence rate of mental illness in the mentally retarded, it was unanimously agreed that the incidence rate is dramatically higher than in the nonretarded population and that there are psychiatric syndromes that are unique to the mentally retarded. A number of panelists cited studies of mental illness in the mentally retarded that encompassed the entire spectrum of psychiatric diagnoses.

The past studies concerning the incidence and prevalence of mental retardation are in need of current replication. More recent data are needed so as to study further the special subpopulation of the mentally ill/mentally retarded. It is clearly known that neurological and major language disorders place persons with mental retardation in an at-risk group to develop an allied mental illness. The current state of key research developments in this topical area was also reviewed by a number of the contributors. The focus is clearly on the psychobiological and behavioral mechanisms that interrupt and/or interfere with the appropriate modulation of central nervous system functions. The recent availability of highly sophisticated laboratory technology now permits the direct study of human behavior that, until recently, could only be conjectured. Promising areas of current and future research on this topic are clearly presented and reviewed in this book.

Further clarification of the epidemiology of mental illness in persons with mental retardation and of the mechanisms by which they are produced holds great promise for prevention (e.g., techniques for actively decreasing the mental health "at-risk" status of retarded citizens via special parental supports and psychoeducational approaches).

## Diagnostic Issues

In this section, special attention is focused on the diagnostic issues related to mental illness in the mentally retarded. It is clear that psychiatric diagnoses are relatively easy to make in the mildly retarded, but diagnostic formulation becomes much more of a challenge in the more severely retarded owing to the communication and cognitive problems related to this level of functioning. This diagnostic formulation challenge was repeatedly cited in relation to the entire range of psychiatric disorders. For example, the diagnosis of depression in a mildly retarded person is a rather straightforward process similar to that of depression in the nonretarded. However, such a diagnosis in the severely retarded individual requires significantly more astute sensitivity and skills on the part of the mental health practitioner. The same holds true for the full spectrum of diagnoses of mental illness in persons at all levels of mental retardation.

A much-debated issue is the common practice of attributing mental illness to mere behavior problems and the concurrent problem of dealing with observable behaviors alone, rather than underlying mental illness. Conference participants underscored the need for appropriate diagnoses as a prelude to adequate treatment.

Emphasis was also placed on the range of other allied developmental and medical needs (e.g., seizures) that make the diagnosis and treatment of mental illness in the mentally retarded more difficult. Many persons with mental retardation have other needs that compound the diagnostic and treatment challenges. Some of these are related to allied disabilities such as seizures, communication deficits, and developmental deficits. Others are related to environmental deprivation and societal prejudice. Conference participants emphasized the need to develop diagnostic pressures to treat the whole person.

Another major diagnostic issue was the fact that some behavioral patterns observed in the mentally retarded appear to be unique. Sometimes there is no symptomatological equivalent of these behavioral patterns in the nonretarded population. For example, much attention was given to the phenomenon of persistent and oftentimes entrenched patterns of self-injurious behavior seen in more severely retarded persons. Some panelists believed that this phenomenon was the result of years of environmental deprivation as often seen in substandard institutional settings. Others believed that these behavioral patterns were due to biological or metabolic disorders such as Lesch-Nyhan syndrome, Cornelia de Lange's syndrome, and phenylketonuria. Some panelists focused on the learned nature of such self-destructive behaviors, and still others cited the possible existence of unique psychiatric disorders that are not yet well researched and defined. It became evident that all these etiological factors might play a role in such unique behavioral patterns and that, indeed, perhaps new psychiatric syndromes need to be defined.

Major consensus centered around the need to develop practical diagnostic tools and to apply such tools in the diagnostic and treatment process. It was agreed that most mental health and mental retardation professionals woefully lack the training and experience to make appropriate diagnoses of mental illness in the mentally retarded. A major conference recommendation emphasized the need to provide training experiences for mental health and mental retardation professionals in the diagnosis and treatment of mental illness in the mentally retarded. It was agreed that very few institutions of higher learning have focused on this training need.

## Treatment Issues

This book presents and deals with a range of treatment issues. Major themes centered on the use of psychoactive drugs, behavioral analysis, and various psychotherapies. A large number of panelists at the conference debated the often seemingly contradictory issue of the use of psychopharmacy versus the use of the principles of applied behavioral analysis. Although these two issues were often presented as a dichotomy, a more in-depth debate resulted in consensus that each has a role to play in the treatment process; one was not regarded as necessarily more restrictive than the other. Intense debate revolved around this misapplication, as many participants pointed out the misuse of each of these treatment modalities. However, conference participants agreed that each can play a dramatically helpful role in the treatment process if used appropriately. It appears that national attention needs to be given to the inappropriate use of psychoactive drugs such as their use as a chemical restraint that is unrelated to any psychiatric diagnosis or treatment process. Similarly, the misuse of behavioral techniques as a systematic tool for restraint and punishment was heatedly debated. Some attributed this to inadequate training; others held that entirely new treatment strategies need to be developed and researched to preclude the use of punishment as an accepted treatment modality.

As conference participants debated these issues, a consensus emerged as reflected in this book that current research efforts tend to focus on singular treatment mechanisms such as the use of punishment to control aggressive or self-injurious behaviors rather than more creative and holistic approaches. Some participants defended their singular treatment modality to the end. The majority of participants agreed, however, that there is a national need to embark on more balanced and humanizing treatment approaches. A strong need was defined to move away from historical assumptions on which much research has been based, and move toward the analysis and delineation of new treatment approaches.

## Programmatic Issues

Two themes were immediately discussed relative to the types of programs and services available to the mentally retarded/mentally ill. The first theme was that the mentally retarded/mentally ill are the most at-risk population to be placed in long-term institutional settings, oftentimes for lifelong custodial care. The second theme dealt with the issue of the paucity or unavailability of the programs and services needed to meet the needs of this complex group of retarded citizens within the mainstream of community life. The agreed-upon challenge was to define and develop programmatic mechanisms to prevent the institutionalization of the mentally retarded/mentally ill and to find ways to bring those tens of thousands who are currently institutionalized back into the confluence of family and community life. Although a few participants held that long-term institutionalization might be necessary, the large majority of participants agreed on the need to develop and support a range of community-based alternatives for the mentally retarded/mentally ill. Panelists cited several state and community initiatives that could serve as national models. The array of programs and services that states and communities need to develop included models for acute psychiatric care and treatment, specialized educational and vocational programs, community residential alternatives such as group homes, and a number of supportive services such as day hospitals, counseling services, and family support programs.

There was consensus that there is a national need to have various tertiary care centers that specialize in the care and treatment of the more acutely mentally ill. These centers would provide highly specialized diagnostic and treatment services as well as conduct state-of-the-art research and training for larger population bases. The few already existing centers that provide these specialized services would then serve as backup programs for the more complex and difficult-to-treat mentally retarded individuals. In these short-term, acute care settings, more complex persons receive appropriate diagnostic and treatment interventions, plus special focus is placed on basic and applied research and intensive professional-level training. It was highly recommended that the availability of tertiary care centers be expanded and that they serve a three-part role of treatment, training, and research.

In the description of other state-of-the-art programs and services, it was clearly pointed out that states and communities, with the assistance of local and federal government support, need to include the mentally retarded/mentally ill in the entire range of programs and services available to mentally retarded and mentally ill individuals. These need not be separate programs and services, but programs and services that individualize the care and treatment of the mentally retarded/mentally ill. Much discussion throughout both the conference and this book centers on the wisdom of avoiding separate services just for this population. The group consensus was to integrate the mentally retarded/mentally ill into existing programs for the mentally retarded and mentally ill. For example, it was suggested that a mildly retarded person with schizophrenia could live in a group home with other nonpsychiatrically involved mentally retarded persons as long as there was community-based backup support for the treatment and management of the person's mental illness. This approach is in contrast to the now widespread practice of establishing separate programs and services for just the mentally retarded/mentally ill. On the other hand, panelists, discussants, and authors urge that more generic mental health services be made accessible and immediately available for the psychiatric needs of the mentally retarded. For example, many communities now use local mental health centers for the mental health needs of the mentally retarded, although these are often extended only to the less severely retarded. A strong need was cited to make such community mental health services available to the more severely retarded. The trend accepted by conference participants was that mental health centers should engage in acute and follow-along care, while mental retardation programs should focus on the living, schooling, and vocational needs of the mentally retarded/mentally ill.

Discussion also centered on certain groups of mentally retarded/mentally ill persons who present unique service challenges, such as those with personality disorders with resultant criminal justice system involvement. It was pointed out that even this population could be served in the community given highly specialized and supervised programs and services.

There was agreement at the conference that programs and services for the mentally retarded need to adopt nonrejection policies. It was often cited that the mentally retarded/mentally ill are the last to be served and the first to be rejected from community-based programs for persons with mental retardation. Conference participants and contributors to this book were unanimous in their desire to change this practice.

The high number of mentally retarded/mentally ill persons in state institutions was an often-cited national problem. A corollary problem dealt with the mentally retarded/mentally ill being shuffled from institutions for the mentally retarded to institutions for the mentally ill in a lifelong cycle of nontreatment. Conference participants agreed that this cycle of despair needs to be halted. The best approach advocated was to treat the acute psychiatric needs of the mentally retarded in psychiatric settings and to meet their long-term needs in community programs for the mentally retarded with secondary support provided by mental health systems.

## Legal and Legislative Issues

It was emphasized that the mentally retarded/mentally ill have the same rights and privileges as other citizens of the United States—the right to be free from harm, the right to minimally adequate treatment, the right to live in settings that least restrict their freedoms, and so on. The current law and legislative mandates for the mentally retarded and developmentally disabled apply equally to the mentally retarded/mentally ill. It was pointed out that these rights are often obscured by the Catch-22 of having this combined diagnosis. That is, the "dual diagnosis" often results in interagency shuffles that leave the mentally retarded/mentally ill poorly served by both systems. Conference panelists, as reflected in their chapters, strongly stated the need to apply the same legal, legislative, and regulatory standards to the mentally retarded/mentally ill individual as to persons with mental retardation, that is, the Developmental Disabilities Act and the Bill of Rights, Public Law 94-142 (Right to Education Act).

Authors in this section of the manuscript described the most common legal challenges that confront the mentally retarded/mentally ill. The two most common themes were the lack of treatment services for this population and the concomitant range of excessively restrictive and even punitive intervention strategies resulting from the lack of adequate and appropriate treatment and programmatic interventions. Related legal issues were major and substantive concerns, such as the misuse of psychoactive medications and the systematic use of restraint and punishment in lieu of active and positive developmental intervention strategies.

The authors in this section reviewed a wide range of legal and legislative issues besides the above and encouraged further systematic analysis of the legal status of persons with mental illness and mental retardation in whatever settings they are served.

## Parental and Family Issues

The broader dimension of the family was also a major theme of both the conference and its final product—this book. Families with members who have both mental retardation and mental illness are often left without adequate support from either system. Often their sons and daughters remain unserved or underserved or are sent to long-term institutional settings with little hope for amelioration or return to family and community life. These families are more at risk to institutionalize their children for they often have nowhere else to turn for assistance.

Parents with sons and daughters with these exceptional needs require a range of in-home and supportive services such as parent training and respite care to support rather than supplant the family. Communities need to be ready and able to provide a range of residential, educational, and vocational services if institutionalization is to be prevented. The lack of such services clearly represents a profound national challenge to parents, professionals, and persons with mental retardation.

Discussions also centered on the need to prevent mental illness in the mentally retarded through intervention programs with the mentally retarded and their parents, through the provision of supportive services as early in life as possible. Parent training and respite care for families were the two most cited prevention strategies.

## Recommendations

A fundamental purpose of this book is to develop a series of action strategies that might help to ameliorate the needs of the mentally retarded/mentally ill in the United States. Conference participants and chapter authors developed recommendations related to new and improved services, more relevant and in-depth training, and more innovative basic and applied research. It was agreed that major strides have been made in many respects over the past 20 years, especially in regard to the application of the principles of applied behavioral analysis, the use of psychoactive drugs, the evolution of models of care, and the application of a number of psychotherapeutic intervention techniques. It was also debated that some intervention strategies have brought some negative effects owing to their misuse, such as the use of psychoactive drugs as chemical restraint and the practice of punishment in many behavioral change programs. Conference participants and chapter authors concurred that past gains need to be developed if this population is to take its rightful place in the confluence of family and community life. Parents, professionals, researchers, and government entities have major roles to play in these recommendations.

The area of innovative services elicited several recommendations:

1. To create regional acute treatment centers for the diagnosis and treatment of complex cases of mental illness in the mentally retarded. These centers would also have allied research and training thrusts.
2. To encourage University Affiliated Facilities in general to assume the responsibility for model program development throughout the establishment or support of services such as acute care, outpatient mental health clinics, day hospitals, prevocational and vocational services, parent training, medication and program monitoring, and diagnostic and treatment clarification.
3. To include the specialized area of mental illness in the mentally retarded in all University Affiliated Programs vis-a-vis interdisciplinary training and practicum experiences.

This area of research brought a number of important recommendations. It was felt that the innovative services outlined above should also serve as a vehicle for a range of applied research projects. Conference participants cited a spectrum of research questions:

1. To conduct research relative to similarities and dissimilarities of mental illness in the mentally retarded as compared to the nonretarded population.
2. To develop easy-to-administer assessment instruments that can be used by both mental health and mental retardation professionals, especially in such diagnostic areas as schizophrenia, affective disorders, and personality disorders.
3. To create a national data bank on research and programmatic mechanisms so that state-of-the-art information might be available as effectively and as efficiently as possible.
4. To conduct basic research related to neurochemistry, neuroendocrinology, and neurophysiology, so as to enhance scientific understanding and to create new intervention strategies.
5. To establish a separate governmental review mechanism for research projects that deal with mental illness in the mentally retarded.

The area of training was cited time after time as a major national need. It was felt that, with few exceptions, mental retardation and mental health professionals are unprepared to meet the acute and chronic needs of this population. It was recommended that institutions of higher education focus attention on training:

1. To increase competencies in the diagnosis and treatment of mental illness in the mentally retarded through continuing education experiences as well as more formal training through fellowships, residencies, and so on.
2. To integrate the area of the dual diagnosis in all interdisciplinary training programs.
3. To develop curricula and media packages for training in this area.

## Conclusion

In this book, the authors review the presentations and discussions of the National Strategies Conference on Mental Illness in the Mentally Retarded. It is hoped that this book will point out the major issues that confront parents and professionals as the nation centers its attention on this problem. More importantly, a critical analysis of these chapters will hopefully enable parents, professionals, and advocates to develop viable and integrative intervention programs and services for our nation's mentally retarded/mentally ill citizens.

In summary, the purpose of the conference was to bring together the complete spectrum of disciplines and points of view that are prevalent in the United States relative to the dual diagnosis. In this book, the authors review the presentations and discussions of the National Strategies Conference on Mental Illness in the Mentally Retarded as well as specific recommendations developed by each panel. The proceedings of the conference clearly demonstrate the major issues that mental illness in the mentally retarded bring to the fields of mental retardation and mental health.

The ultimate challenge is for the reader to analyze the proceedings and synthesize areas of consensus and areas of disagreement in the hope that new and creative research, training, and service interventions may be created as a result of this focus.

Jack A. Stark
Michael H. Albarelli

Frank J. Menolascino
Vincent C. Gray

# Contents

## Section IV: Clinical Treatment Issues

## Section V: Program Models

## Section VI:  Legal Issues

### Section VII:  Service Systems

# Contributors

*Robert B. Allin, Jr.*, M.A., Chesterfield Mental Health and Mental Retardation Services, Lucy-Corr Court, Chesterfield, Virginia 23832

*Alfred A. Baumeister*, Ph.D., Director, John F. Kennedy Center for Research on Education and Human Development, Peabody College, Vanderbilt University, Nashville, Tennessee 37203

*Lenore Behar*, Ph.D., Special Assistant for Child and Family Services, Division of Mental Health, Mental Retardation, and Substance Abuse Services, North Carolina Department of Human Resources, Raleigh, North Carolina 27611

*Sidney W. Bijou*, Ph.D., Professor of Psychology and Special Education and Rehabilitation, College of Education, University of Arizona, Tucson, Arizona 85721

*Elizabeth Monroe Boggs*, Ph.D., Association for Retarded Citizens of the United States, Hampton, New Jersey 08827

*Sharon A. Borthwick*, Ph.D., University of California Research Group at Lanterman Developmental Center, Pomona, California 91768

*Robert H. Bruininks*, Ph.D., Director, Minnesota University Affiliated Program on Developmental Disabilities, Department of Educational Psychology, College of Education, University of Minnesota, Minneapolis, Minnesota 55455

*Frederic B. Chanteau*, Executive Director, The Rock Creek Foundation, Silver Spring, Maryland 20910

*Donald J. Cohen*, Vanderbilt Child and Adolescent Psychiatric Hospital, Nashville, Tennessee 37212

*Joseph T. Coyle*, M.D., Director, Division of Child Psychiatry, School of Medicine, The Johns Hopkins University, Baltimore, Maryland 21205

*Paul R. Dokecki*, Ph.D., Professor of Psychology, Associate Director, John F. Kennedy Center for Research on Education and Human Development, Peabody College, Vanderbilt University, Nashville, Tennessee 37203

*James W. Ellis*, J.D., Professor of Law, University of New Mexico, School of Law, Albuquerque, New Mexico 87131

*Lilia A. Evangelista*, M.D., Medical Director, Lincoln Children's Evaluation and Rehabilitation Center Satellite, Lincoln Hospital, Bronx, New York 10451

*Robert J. Fletcher*, A.C.S.W., Executive Director, National Association for the Dually Diagnosed, Beacon House, Kingston, New York 12401

*William I. Gardner*, Ph.D., Professor of Rehabilitation Psychology, Waisman Center on Mental Retardation and Human Development, University of Wisconsin, Madison, Wisconsin 53705

*Robert M. Gettings*, Executive Director, National Association of State Mental Retardation Program Directors, Inc., Alexandria, Virginia 22314

*Tammi Goldsbury*, M.A. Department of Psychiatry, University of Nebraska Medical Center, Omaha, Nebraska 68105

*C. Thomas Gualtieri*, M.D., Neuropsychiatric Research Program, Biological Sciences Research Center, University of North Carolina, Chapel Hill, North Carolina 27514

*Craig Anne Heflinger*, M.A., John F. Kennedy Center for Research on Education and Human Development, Peabody College, Vanderbilt University, Nashville, Tennessee 37203

*Stanley S. Herr*, J.D., Ph.D., Associate Professor of Law, University of Maryland School of Law, Clinical Law Office, Baltimore, Maryland 21201

*Bradley K. Hill*, M.A., Assistant to the Director, Minnesota University Affilated Program on Developmental Disabilities, University of Minnesota, Minneapolis, Minnesota 55455

*Peter A. Holmes*, Ph.D., Director, Clinical Behavioral Program, Department of Psychology, Eastern Michigan University, Ypsilanti, Michigan 48197

*Robert D. Hunt*, M.D., Vanderbilt Child and Adolescent Psychiatric Hospital, Nashville, Tennessee 37212

*William E. Kiernan*, Ph.D., Director, Rehabilitation Development and Evaluation, The Children's Hospital Medical Center, Boston, Massachusetts 02115

*Richard A. Kunin*, M.D., Orthomolecular Medical Society, San Francisco, California 94115

*Earl A. Loomis, Jr.*, M.D., Professor of Psychiatry, Head, Section of Child, Adolescents and Family Psychiatry, Department of Psychiatry and Health Behavior, Medical College of Georgia, School of Medicine, Augusta, Georgia 30912-7300

*Ruth Luckasson*, J.D., Associate Professor of Special Education, University of New Mexico, School of Law, Albuquerque, New Mexico 87131

*Ronald W. Manderscheid*, Ph.D., Chief, Survey and Reports Branch, National Institute of Mental Health, Rockville, Maryland 20857

*Johnny L. Matson*, Ph.D., Professor, Department of Psychology, Louisiana State University, Baton Rouge, Louisiana 70803

*John J. McGee*, Ph.D., Associate Professor, Creighton University, Omaha, Nebraska 68105

*Frank J. Menolascino*, M.D., Chairman and Professor of Psychiatry, Creighton University–University of Nebraska Medical Center, Omaha, Nebraska 68105

*Lanny E. Morreau*, Ph.D., Professor, Department of Special Education, Illinois State University, Bloomington-Normal, Illinois 61761

*Steven Reiss*, Ph.D., Professor of Psychology, Psychology Department, University of Illinois at Chicago, Behavioral Sciences Building, Chicago, Illinois 60680

*Norman S. Rosenberg*, J.D., Director, Mental Health Law Project, Washington, D.C. 20036-4909

*Marilyn J. Rosenstein*, B.A., Supervisory Survey Statistician, Survey and Reports Branch, National Institute of Mental Health, Rockville, Maryland 20857

*Andrew T. Russell*, M.D., Associate Professor, Mental Retardation and Child Psychiatry Division, Neuropsychiatric Institute, University of California–Los Angeles, Los Angeles, California 90024

*Richard C. Scheerenberger*, Ph.D., Director, Wisconsin Center for the Developmentally Disabled, Madison, Wisconsin 53694

*Keith G. Scott*, Ph.D., Professor of Psychology and Pediatrics, Mailman Center for Child Development, Miami, Florida 33101

*Michael W. Smull*, Ph.D., Deputy Director, Developmental Disabilities Program, University of Maryland, Baltimore, Maryland 21201

*Robert Sovner*, M.D., Medical Director, Lutheran Center for Mental Health and Mental Retardation, Brighton, Massachusetts 02138

*Jack A. Stark*, Ph.D., Associate Professor of Medical Psychology, University of Nebraska Medical Center, Omaha, Nebraska 68105

*Ludwik S. Szymanski*, M.D., Assistant Professor of Psychiatry, Harvard Medical School, Director of Psychiatry, Developmental Evaluation Clinic, The Children's Hospital Medical Center, Boston, Massachusetts 02115

*Donald Taylor*, Deputy Director, Division of MH/MR–SAS, North Carolina Department of Human Resources, Raleigh, North Carolina 27611

*Travis Thompson*, Ph.D., Professor, Department of Psychology, University of Minnesota, Elliott Hall, Minneapolis, Minnesota 55455

*Matthew A. Timm*, Director, The Regional Intervention Program for Preschoolers and Parents, Nashville, Tennessee 37204

*H. Rutherford Turnbull, III*, Ll.B., Ll.M., Professor of Special Education and Law, University of Kansas, Lawrence, Kansas 66045

*David L. White*, M.A., Co-Director, Office of Special Offenders Services, Lancaster, Pennsylvania 17603-1881

*Michael J. Witkin*, M.A., Supervisory Statistician, Survey and Reports Branch, National Institute of Mental Health, Rockville, Maryland 20857

*Hubert Wood*, M.A., Office of Special Offenders. Courthouse, Lancaster, Pennsylvania 17603-1881

*Cecil R. Wurster*, B.A., Associate Director, Division of Biometry and Applied Sciences, National Institute of Mental Health, Rockville, Maryland 20857

# Section I: Epidemiology
# Introduction

SHARON A. BORTHWICK

The objective of this section is to focus on issues related to the epidemiology of mental health problems among mentally retarded people. Epidemiology involves the study of the distribution of disease (descriptive epidemiology) as well as the search for the determinants or causes of the distribution (analytical epidemiology). Not surprisingly, the majority of discussions in this section are centered on description rather than analysis. We realize that description without causal implication does not fulfill the objective of epidemiology. However, unless we have good, reliable data on which to base the study of causal mechanisms, it is impossible to draw meaningful conclusions.

Two issues emerge repeatedly in this section. First, there is a lack of consensus regarding the *measurement and classification* of mental illness and mental retardation. To examine the prevalence of a health problem, that problem must be well defined and reliably measured. For example, if adaptive behavior deficiencies are included in the criteria defining mental retardation, there are likely to be more retarded people identified who also have behavior problems than if people were labeled retarded on the basis of IQ alone. In the most widely cited British epidemiology study of mental retardation and mental illness, adaptive behavior was not included in the criteria for intellectual retardation, yet the accepted definition of mental retardation in the United States requires that an individual be deficient in both cognitive and behavioral domains. The controversy over this issue is currently being rekindled, potentially affecting prevalence rates as well as the analysis of causes. Similarly, the diagnosis of mental health problems among mentally retarded people is far from being clear-cut and ranges from the formal psychiatric diagnosis of mental disorders to the measurement of observable maladaptive behaviors. Some individuals who are not formally diagnosed as having a psychiatric disorder are still considered to have mental health problems, evidenced by maladaptive behavior. Are these people to be included in the epidemiology? Problems of classification and measurement are compounded in attempts to determine whether individuals are mentally retarded *and* mentally ill, given the effects of both of these disorders on behavior and performance. The authors of this section discuss classification and measurement from several perspectives, highlighting the issues and identifying areas in need of improvement.

The second theme of this section revolves around the practical issues of *data reporting and management of data bases*. The perfect classification system would be useless without representative data from the population being studied. In this age of computer technology, it would seem a relatively easy task to obtain descriptive information from data systems around the country and from federal reporting systems. However, concomitant emphasis on human rights and confidentiality have affected both the quality and accessibility of individualized data. Moreover, unique to the particular group of people of interest in this book is the fact that they can be served by more than one service system, that is mental health and mental retardation agencies. The reasons why individuals will be served by one or both types of agencies and the implications of this situation are discussed elsewhere in this volume. In this section, the authors discuss the consequences of a lack of coordination between agencies, problems associated with volunteer reporting systems, and the need for uniform reporting.

As noted earlier, the analytic epidemiology of mental retardation and mental health is only as good as the data at hand. In light of the data-related problems outlined above, causal implications should be viewed as tentative. The relationship between the two disorders — mental retardation and mental illness — is of particular interest to the epidemiology of persons with both developmental disabilities and psychiatric disorders and is discussed in this section. The authors also discuss possible predictors of mental retardation and mental illness, as well as the effects of these conditions on other aspects of the individual's life.

The authors of this section on epidemiology represent a variety of backgrounds and professional interests, ranging from medicine and psychiatry to psychology and biostatistics. It is therefore somewhat surprising that there is considerable overlap among the concerns of these individuals who view mental health and mental retardation from such different perspectives. On the other hand, their insights and recommendations clearly reflect a wide range of viewpoints.

# 1
# Prevalence and Implications of Maladaptive Behaviors and Dual Diagnosis in Residential and Other Service Programs

Robert H. Bruininks, Bradley K. Hill, and Lanny E. Morreau

Maladaptive behaviors among mentally retarded people present service problems that act a serious barriers to their personal development and to opportunities for social integration. Given the seriousness of this issue, there is clearly a need to describe the extent and nature of problems or maladaptive behaviors, including the incidence of dual diagnosis of mental retardation and mental illness, among retarded individuals. This concern has often been expressed by service personnel in studies that assess their training needs (Bruininks, Thurlow, Nelson, & Davis, 1984). It is also evident from numerous research reports over a 50-year period that serious maladaptive behaviors among mentally retarded people limit their development of adaptive skills and their integration into schools, families, residential placements, employment, and social settings.

Problem behaviors should be viewed within the total context of competence and personal and social adjustment. Foster and Ritchey (1979) define social competence as "those responses which, within a given situation, prove effective or, in other words, maximize the probability of producing, maintaining, or enhancing positive effects for the interactor" (p. 626). Therefore, a behavior should be considered a problem from a social perspective if its presence reduces the probability that an individual would derive positive consequences from it or if it increases the probability that the individual will receive negative consequences from social interactions with others. From a behavioral perspective, a person's actions become a problem when they adversely affect the individual, the physical environment, or others.

Behaviors that result in harm to the individual, to others, or to the environment are more likely to result in negative sanctions than behaviors that are simply disruptive. At the same time, disruptive behaviors would more likely have negative consequences than behaviors that are only perceived negatively. In a study conducted by Ho and Morreau (1985), direct-service employees in a public institution rated 242 problem behaviors on a five-point scale from least to most severe. Destructive behaviors posing a threat to the individual, to other people, or to property were considered the most serious. Behaviors that elicited inappropriate attention from others or that were disruptive to others were considered to be somewhat less severe.

The definitions and strategies for assessing problem behaviors among retarded individuals are quite varied and frequently ambiguous. Careful definitions and descriptions of such behaviors are essential antecedents to the more complex diagnoses of mental health problems and to the development of effective intervention strategies. The purpose of this chapter is to discuss available evidence on the prevalence of problem behaviors among mentally retarded people and the implications of such findings for diagnosis, research, and services.

## Impact of Problem Behaviors

Throughout the past 40 years numerous studies have documented the fact that problem behavior and antisocial acts are among the leading reasons cited for institutionalization and reinstitutionalization (Eagle, 1967; Eyman & Borthwick, 1980; Eyman, Borthwick, & Miller, 1981; Eyman, O'Connor, Tarjan, & Justice, 1972; McCarver & Craig, 1974; Moen, Bogen, & Aanes, 1975; Pagel & Whitling, 1978; Schalock, Harper, & Genung, 1981; Windle, 1962). While many other factors, including measured intelligence, age, and physical disabilities, are related to out-of-home placement, the presence of problem behaviors is a major factor in decisions related to the residential situations of mentally retarded persons. In fact, next to the overall severity of mental retardation, problem behaviors appear to be the most significant factor influencing initial placements in institutions (Maney, Pace, & Morrison, 1964; Saenger, 1960; Spencer, 1976).

The presence of problem behaviors also acts as a serious barrier to integration and adjustment of mentally retarded people in community settings (Bruininks, 1982; Conley, 1973; Eyman & Borthwick, 1980; Eyman et al., 1981; Hill, Bruininks, & Lakin, 1983; McCarver & Craig, 1974; Morreau, 1985; Sternlicht & Deutsch, 1972; Windle, 1962). Behavior problems, for example, are consistently cited as a major factor influencing the readmission of mentally retarded persons to state institutions (Lakin, Hill, Hauber, Bruininks, & Heal, 1983; Landesman-Dwyer & Sulzbacher, 1981). As observed by Pagel and Whitling(1978), maladaptive behavior was the primary cause of failure in community placements across all levels of disability; 45% of the individuals in their study were readmitted to institutions for reasons of maladaptive behavior. Similarly, Keys, Boroskin, and Ross (1973) reported that of 126 readmissions, 35% directly resulted from the presence of behavior problems. These findings are supported by those of Sutter, Mayeda, Call, Yanagi, and Yee (1980), who reported that mentally retarded persons who were unsuccessfully placed in community programs displayed a variety of maladaptive behaviors significantly more frequently than their successfully placed peers. Of equal importance, the authors reported that these behaviors precipitated the requests that individuals be removed from community-based facilities.

It is clear that serious problem behaviors limit the opportunities for mentally retarded people to reside in community settings. A survey conducted by Hill and Bruininks (1981) with personnel of residential facilities for developmentally disabled persons illustrates the pervasive impact of behavior problems on community integration. Staff members were asked in this study if behavior problems prevented residents from increasing their social integration into the community. Respondents from private residential facilities reported that 47% of their residents with behavior problems (21% of all residents) would have increased opportunities if their behaviors were better controlled, while staff of public residential facilities indicated that 53% of residents with behavior problems (31% of all residents) were limited in community participation by their problem behaviors (Hill and Bruininks, 1984).

Results from employment studies seem to parallel those found in residential facilities and family environments regarding the adverse effects of maladaptive behaviors. Problem behaviors are reported in many studies as contributors to job loss and lowered job status (McCarver & Craig, 1974; Schalock, Harper, & Garver, 1981; Sternlicht & Deutsch, 1972). Poor interpersonal skills were reported by Niziol and DeBlassie (1972) as the major source of problems related to securing and retaining employment among mentally retarded persons; and Schalock and Harper (1978) found that inappropriate behavior was one of the major reasons mentally retarded individuals were returned to employment training from a job placement. Foss and Peterson (1981), in their survey of job placement personnel, reported that a great number of respondents indicated that "refraining from exhibiting bizarre or irritating behavior" and "controlling aggressive behavior" were most relevant to job tenure.

## Prevalence Studies: Problem Behaviors and Dual Diagnosis

The prevalence of behavior problems and the dual diagnosis of mental retardation and mental illness or emotional disturbances among mentally retarded people have been researched in a number of studies (Balthazar & Stevens, 1975; Beier, 1964; Lewis & MacLean, 1982; Menolascino, 1970). In reviewing many of the available studies, Lewis and MacLean (1982) reached the following conclusion:

The available studies lead to the inescapable conclusion that emotional disorders are much more common among mentally retarded persons than in the general population. This conclusion is based on investigations using very different patient samples and very different methodologies. (p. 7)

Tables 1.1 and 1.2 present brief summaries of selected studies on extent of behavior problems and dual diagnosis found in various samples of mentally retarded children and adults. Table 1.1 indicates that maladaptive behaviors are reported with relatively high rates in a number of the samples. The rates appear somewhat higher among referred samples and among those being served in specialized programs.

Table 1.2 presents selected studies on dual diagnosis. Rates reported in these studies vary across a wide range. The most comprehensive assessment with a

TABLE 1.1. Selected studies reporting the prevalence of problem behaviors.

| Study | Sample | Method | Results |
|---|---|---|---|
| Groden, Domingue, Pueschel, & Deignan (1982) | 1,114 mentally retarded children and adolescents at community evaluation clinic | Computer search of records | 25% of sample with serious behavioral/emotional problems |
| Jacobson & Janicki (1985) | 22,256 developmentally disabled clients in New York state mental retardation/developmental disabilities service system | One or more mentions of behavior problems on standard survey form | Community Programs<br><br>Severely retarded / Profoundly retarded: 57%<br>Severely retarded: 60%<br><br>Institutions<br>79% / 74% |
| Koller, Richardson, Katz, & McLaren (1983) | Total population of children born between 1951 and 1952 in a city of Great Britain, with follow-up of 221 retarded young adults at 22 years | Extensive interviews with structured behavior classifications of behavior disturbances | 59% with behavior disturbances in childhood, 59% in postschool years, 27% rate for moderately/severely retarded as children and 20% rate as adults |
| Lindberg & Putnam (1979) | 11,303 noninstitutionalized, developmentally disabled children and adults in West Virginia | Household survey of 67 census districts; Adaptive Behavior Scale (ABS), interviews | 28 to 41% depending on age, with significant maladaptive behaviors (≥ 80th percentile on ABS maladaptive section) |
| Richardson, Koller, & Katz (1985) | 143 mildly retarded children and a matched random sample of nonhandicapped children all from the same city in Great Britain and born between 1951 and 1955, with follow-up at the age of 22 years | Comprehensive life history interviews, study of school, social service, and court records | 45% of retarded subjects experienced high degrees of unstable conditions of upbringing whereas only 5% of the comparison group did—with unstable upbringing associated with increased behavior disturbance |

TABLE 1.2. Selected studies reporting on prevalence of dual diagnosis.

| Study | Sample | Method | Results |
|---|---|---|---|
| Heaton-Ward (1977) | 1,251 mentally retarded residents in institutions | Survey of client records (characteristics, histories, and treatment) | 5.4% total—serious psychiatric conditions |
| Jacobson (1982) | 30,578 mentally retarded clients in various service settings in New York State | Extracted frequently occurring behavior problems and presence of psychiatric impairment from New York data base (DDIS) | 11.6% with formally classified psychiatric disturbances |
| Rutter, Tizard, Yule, Graham, & Whitmore (1976); Rutter, Tizard, & Whitmore (1970); Rutter (1971) (see Russell in this volume for more extensive discussion of these studies | 9–11-year-old cohort ($N=2,199$) in Isle of Wight, Great Britain | Extensive interviews and clinical assessments with parents and/or teachers | 30% rated as seriously disturbed by parent information, and 42% from teacher information versus 5.4% for control peers |
| Wright (1982) | 1,507 mentally retarded residents in an institution (75% considered severely retarded) | Survey using nonverbal and verbal criteria to identify various conditions; longitudinal follow-up on 110 with probable mental illness | 2.8% affective disorders; 1.8% schizophrenic; 2.7% early childhood psychosis; 7.3% total—serious psychiatric conditions |

control group was reported by Rutter and his colleagues in the Isle of Wight studies (Rutter, 1971; Rutter, Tizard, & Whitmore, 1970; Rutter, Tizard, Yule, Graham, & Whitmore, 1976). This extensive study is discussed in detail by Russell in Chapter 3 of this book.

It is not an easy task to synthesize findings from extant studies on the prevalence of problem behaviors or dual diagnosis among mentally retarded children and adults. At considerable risk of oversimplification, it would appear that 20 to 40% of mentally retarded people in various samples and service programs consistently exhibit behaviors that are perceived by others in their environment as serious problems. Rates for such behavior problems generally run higher among those in licensed residential facilities and among clinically referred samples than among more randomly distributed people in community settings. Rates of more serious behavioral and emotional disturbances that might lead to a clinical diagnosis of mental retardation and mental illness appear to be much lower than those reported for problem behaviors. Depending on the sample and procedures used, rates of dual diagnosis among samples of mentally retarded people generally range between 5 and 13%. Studies relying on case records for diagnostic data of large samples of people in service programs report a prevalence of around 12% (Hill & Bruininks, 1981; Jacobson, 1982).

While there may be some confusion regarding the precise meaning of terms such as "problem behaviors," "maladaptive behaviors," "dual diagnosis," or "mental illness" among mentally retarded children or adults, there is little doubt that successful identification and treatment of these behaviors is essential to their development and social integration. Despite some inadequacy in our current information, the evidence from many studies indicates that maladaptive behaviors among mentally retarded people are strongly related to life outcomes such as (1) initial out-of-home placement and reinstitutionalization, (2) failure in community placements and readmission to supervised residential placements, (3) increased probability of transmitting certain diseases and health problems, (4) reduced opportunity for social integration and leisure in community settings, and (5) reduced prospects for employment.

## Prevalence of Behavior Problems and Dual Diagnosis in Residential Facilities

Nearly all the studies that report statistics on maladaptive or problem behaviors, emotional disturbances, or dual diagnosis are based on referrals or on samples being served in various programs. Hill and Bruininks (1981) conducted an extensive analysis on the prevalence and frequency of occurrence and staff response toward maladaptive behaviors of 2,271 mentally retarded residents in a national sample of 236 residential facilities. Following a probability sampling of facilities, four groups of subjects were selected at random using prescribed sampling procedures: (1) community residential facility (CRF) current residents ($n = 964$), (2) public residential facility (PRF) current residents ($n = 997$), (3) PRF new admissions ($n = 286$), and (4) PRF readmissions ($n = 244$). Definitions of these groups and the sample procedures are presented by Hill and Bruininks (1981).

Demographic and diagnostic information was obtained from resident records. Maladaptive behaviors were assessed through structured interviews with direct-care staff who knew each resident well and had been responsible for providing service over several months. Staff persons were asked which of five types of problem behaviors were exhibited by each sampled resident and to indicate the specific behavior representing the single most significant problem in each of eight selected areas. The most serious problem behavior in each area was then rated for frequency in one of five levels ranging from less than once per month to one or more times per hour. Staff were also asked to indicate how they usually responded when the resident exhibited problem behavior(s). Responses were categorized into five levels: doing nothing, verbal strategies, ignoring the behavior by withholding social reinforcement or reinforcing other more adaptive behaviors, physical responses including restraints, or seeking physical assistance of one or more additional staff members.

TABLE 1.3. Demographic characteristics of residents.

| Characteristic | CRF residents N | CRF residents % | PRF residents N | PRF residents % | PRF new admissions N | PRF new admissions % | PRF readmissions N | PRF readmissions % |
|---|---|---|---|---|---|---|---|---|
| Sex |
| Male | 579 | 60.1 | 552 | 55.4 | 171 | 59.8 | 157 | 64.3 |
| Female | 385 | 39.9 | 445 | 44.6 | 115 | 40.2 | 87 | 35.7 |
| Age in years |
| <6 | 12 | 1.2 | 7 | 0.7 | 15 | 5.2 | 2 | 0.8 |
| 6–10 | 44 | 4.6 | 29 | 2.9 | 40 | 14.0 | 14 | 5.7 |
| 11–15 | 106 | 11.0 | 66 | 6.6 | 30 | 10.5 | 25 | 10.2 |
| 16–20 | 172 | 17.9 | 143 | 14.3 | 55 | 19.2 | 46 | 18.9 |
| 21–30 | 265 | 27.5 | 336 | 33.7 | 68 | 23.6 | 85 | 34.8 |
| 31–40 | 176 | 18.2 | 192 | 19.3 | 45 | 15.7 | 40 | 16.4 |
| 41–50 | 81 | 8.4 | 81 | 8.1 | 22 | 7.7 | 22 | 9.0 |
| 51–61 | 71 | 7.4 | 87 | 8.7 | 8 | 2.8 | 9 | 3.7 |
| 62+ | 37 | 3.9 | 56 | 5.6 | 3 | 1.0 | 1 | 0.4 |
| Race or ethnic background |
| White | 837 | 87.4 | 805 | 81.6 | 206 | 73.0 | 194 | 79.8 |
| Black | 88 | 9.2 | 140 | 14.2 | 58 | 20.7 | 39 | 16.0 |
| Hispanic | 22 | 2.3 | 33 | 3.3 | 16 | 5.7 | 10 | 4.1 |
| Asian or Pacific Islander | 4 | 0.4 | 5 | 0.5 | 2 | 0.7 | 0 | – |
| American Indian or Alaskan Native | 7 | 0.7 | 3 | 0.3 | 0 | – | 0 | – |
| Level of retardation |
| Borderline (IQ 69–84) | 97 | 10.1 | 14 | 1.4 | 10 | 3.5 | 13 | 5.3 |
| Mild (IQ 52–68) | 229 | 23.8 | 78 | 7.8 | 46 | 16.1 | 52 | 21.3 |
| Moderate (IQ 36–51) | 276 | 28.7 | 150 | 15.0 | 62 | 21.7 | 61 | 25.0 |
| Severe (IQ 20–35) | 248 | 25.8 | 287 | 28.8 | 83 | 29.0 | 56 | 23.0 |
| Profound (IQ <20) | 113 | 11.7 | 468 | 46.9 | 85 | 29.7 | 62 | 25.4 |

Table 1.3 presents detailed demographic information and levels of mental retardation for the four sample groups. CRF residents were relatively younger than those in PRFs. Almost 17% of CRF residents were less than 16 years old, compared with only 10.2% of all PRF residents. PRF new admissions and readmissions, however, were relatively younger than PRF current residents; 29.7% of new admissions and 16.7% of readmissions were less than 16 years old.

Nearly every resident's record (98%) contained either an IQ score or a diagnosed level of retardation. The most recent diagnosis or IQ score was used, although neither the source of the evaluation nor the specific test of intelligence was recorded by interviewers. PRF residents were generally more severely retarded than CRF residents. Almost 34% of CRF residents were borderline or mildly retarded, compared with 9.2% of PRF residents; 37.5% of CRF residents were either severely or profoundly retarded. PRF new admissions and readmissions included greater proportions of mildly handicapped individuals than did the PRF current resident sample as a whole. The distribution of intelligence among PRF readmissions was similar to that for CRF residents and paralleled the distribution for residents released from PRFs (Sigford, Bruininks, Lakin, Hill, & Heal, 1982), suggesting that criteria for readmission were not heavily dependent on level of intelligence. Carepersons were asked, "In addition to being mentally retarded, does (resident's name) have any other disabilities?" Carepersons were also asked if each resident was currently receiving a prescribed medication for a psychiatric condition. Finally, each resident's records were reviewed for any mention of autism or mental illness. Table 1.4 summarizes findings from these questions. Although 13% of CRF residents' and 7.8% of PRF residents' records mentioned a mental health problem, only 1.1% of CRF residents and 2.8% of PRF residents were considered by staff to have had a mental health problem at the time interviews took place.

For the purposes of this chapter, residents who had a current diagnosis or a recorded mention of mental illness in addition to mental retardation were analyzed as subgroups of current CRF and PRF samples. The maladaptive behaviors of these subgroups and of PRF new admissions and readmissions are summarized in Table 1.5. The table indicates that most types of maladaptive behavior were reported to be more common among public institution residents than among private facility residents; and, in both public and private facilities, higher among

TABLE 1.4. Percentage of mentally retarded residents with possible dual diagnosis in U.S. residential facilities — 1979.

| | Private facility residents (N = 964) | Public facility residents (N = 997) |
|---|---|---|
| Records mention of mental illness | 13.0% | 7.8% |
| Receive medication for "psychiatric problem" | 6.8% | 4.3% |
| Staff currently cite mental health problems as additional handicap | 1.1% | 2.8% |

TABLE 1.5. Percentage of mentally retarded and mentally ill residents with problem behaviors, U.S. residential facilities – 1979.

| | Private | | | Public | | | | |
| Category | Current residents (N = 839) | Current MR/MI (N = 11) | Previous record MR/MI (N = 125) | Current residents (N = 919) | Current MR/MI (N = 5) | Previous record MR/MI (N = 78) | New admissions (N = 286) | Readmissions (N = 244) |
|---|---|---|---|---|---|---|---|---|
| Hurts self | 9 | 9 | 24 | 22 | 20 | 21 | 22 | 21 |
| Hurts others | 14 | 18 | 31 | 30 | 100 | 35 | 42 | 38 |
| Damages property | 9 | 9 | 22 | 17 | 60 | 18 | 19 | 23 |
| Unusual or disruptive | 26 | 55 | 48 | 33 | 60 | 45 | 38 | 41 |
| Uncooperative | 17 | 18 | 36 | 18 | 60 | 31 | 32 | 33 |

residents with a current and previous dual diagnosis of mental retardation and mental illness. Except for self-injurious behavior, the prevalence of maladaptive behavior was reported to be much higher among public facility new admissions and readmissions than among public facility current residents in general or among private facility current residents. Injuring other residents, damaging property, and various forms of socially unacceptable and uncooperative behaviors were 1.5 times to 6 times more prevalent among public facility new admissions and readmissions than among current residents in smaller, private facilities.

Table 1.6 shows that the frequency of maladaptive behaviors by individual residents ranged from less than monthly to several times per hour. Most behaviors were exhibited several times per week. Staff attempted to manage most problem behaviors with verbal responses. Because nonverbal residents and those with physical limitations were more common in public facilities (19% nonambulatory) than in private facilities (10% nonambulatory), physical responses from public facility staff might have been more likely than other responses. No adjustment for this possibility was made because, from a behavior management perspective, the actual response generally used by staff was hypothesized to be a useful source of information in assessing the impact of maladaptive behaviors on the environment.

## Prevalence of Specific Categories of Problem Behaviors in Residential Facilities

Four categories of maladaptive behavior were investigated in greater detail to describe the precise problem behavior expressed by residents. (The dual diagnosis subgroups were dropped from these analyses because of limited sample sizes.)

TABLE 1.6. Frequency and direct-care staff response to maladaptive behavior of PRF and CRF current residents.

| Frequency/response | Percentage of behaviors |
|---|---|
| Frequency of behaviors | |
| (1) Less than monthly | 11.7 |
| (2) 1–3 per month | 24.3 |
| (3) 1–6 per week | 34.4 |
| (4) 1–16 per day | 25.7 |
| (5) 1 or more per hour | 3.8 |
| Response to behaviors | |
| (1) No response | 2.0 |
| (2) Verbal response | 45.6 |
| (3) Ignore, reinforce other behavior | 17.0 |
| (4) Physical response | 27.6 |
| (5) Get help | 7.8 |

Note: Behaviors include self-injurious, injurious to other people, damage to property, and unusual/disruptive categories. $N = 1638$ behaviors (1–4 categories of behavior exhibited by 928 CRF and PRF current residents).

TABLE 1.7. Prevalence of self-injurious behaviors, frequency, and staff response within residential facilities.

| Behavior/frequency/response | Private current residents | | Public residents | | Public new admissions | | Public read-missions | | F |
|---|---|---|---|---|---|---|---|---|---|
| | N | % | N | % | N | % | N | % | |
| Behavior[a] | | | | | | | | | |
| Bites, picks, scratches self | 57 | 5.9 | 107 | 10.7 | 39 | 13.6 | 26 | 10.7 | 5.60* |
| Bangs head | 36 | 3.7 | 80 | 8.0 | 24 | 8.4 | 18 | 7.3 | 5.47* |
| Hits, slaps, pinches self | 26 | 2.7 | 52 | 5.2 | 15 | 5.2 | 12 | 4.9 | 1.81 |
| Hits self with or throws self against objects | 13 | 1.3 | 40 | 4.0 | 5 | 1.7 | 15 | 6.1 | 6.24* |
| Eats nonedible material | 10 | 1.0 | 44 | 4.4 | 6 | 2.1 | 3 | 1.2 | 9.46** |
| Pokes objects in eyes, ears, and so on | 1 | 0.1 | 3 | 0.3 | 4 | 1.4 | 2 | 0.8 | 1.70 |
| Other | 6 | 0.6 | 10 | 1.0 | 3 | 1.0 | 5 | 2.0 | |
| Total | 107 | 11.1 | 216 | 21.7 | 63 | 22.0 | 52 | 21.3 | 14.31** |
| Frequency[b] | | | | | | | | | 1.34 |
| (1) Less than monthly | 10 | 9.9 | 24 | 11.4 | 7 | 11.7 | 7 | 13.5 | |
| (2) 1–3 per month | 17 | 15.9 | 40 | 19.0 | 12 | 20.0 | 13 | 25.0 | |
| (3) 1–6 per week | 35 | 33.2 | 63 | 30.0 | 16 | 26.7 | 19 | 36.5 | |
| (4) 1–16 per day | 34 | 33.0 | 72 | 34.3 | 18 | 30.0 | 9 | 17.3 | |
| (5) 1 or more per hour | 8 | 8.0 | 11 | 5.2 | 7 | 11.7 | 4 | 7.7 | |
| Staff response[b] | | | | | | | | | 1.67 |
| (1) No response | 3 | 2.8 | 7 | 3.3 | 0 | – | 3 | 5.8 | |
| (2) Ignore, reinforce other behavior | 30 | 28.5 | 44 | 20.5 | 10 | 16.1 | 16 | 30.8 | |
| (3) Verbal response | 40 | 37.4 | 61 | 28.4 | 20 | 32.3 | 11 | 21.2 | |
| (4) Physical response | 27 | 25.7 | 90 | 41.9 | 28 | 45.2 | 16 | 30.8 | |
| (5) Get help | 6 | 5.6 | 13 | 6.0 | 4 | 6.5 | 6 | 11.5 | |

[a] Percentage of all residents. Columns do not sum to total because some residents exhibited more than one type of self-injurious behavior.
[b] Percentage of residents who exhibited self-injurious behavior.
*$p < .001$.
**$p < .0001$.

## SELF-INJURIOUS BEHAVIOR

Table 1.7 indicates specific self-injurious behaviors reported by staff. Up to three self-injurious behaviors were coded for each resident. The rank ordering of various types of self-injurious behavior by prevalence was similar among all resident groups. The proportion of public facility residents exhibiting a particular behavior was consistently almost double the proportion of private facility residents.

Frequency level and level of staff response were reported for the single most prominent self-injurious behavior of each resident. Among self-injurious residents, self-injurious behavior episodes were reported to occur relatively frequently, typically several times a week or more. A one-way analysis of variance, however, indicated that the average frequency level of self-injurious behaviors was not significantly different among resident groups.

The usual staff response to approximately 25% of all residents with self-injurious behavior was to systematically ignore the behavior and reinforce other behaviors that were more desirable. Approximately one-third of self-injurious residents elicited a physical response from staff. The most serious behavior problems were considered to be those that could not be controlled by one staff person. Six percent of self-injurious public facility residents elicited this level of staff responses, as did 5.6% of self-injurious private facility residents. Among readmissions, the proportion of self-injurious behaviors that required more than one staff person (11.5%) was considerably higher than among other resident

TABLE 1.8. Prevalence of behaviors injurious to other people, frequency, and staff response within residential facilities.

| Behavior/frequency/response | Private current residents | | Public residents | | Public new admissions | | Public read-missions | | F |
|---|---|---|---|---|---|---|---|---|---|
| | N | % | N | % | N | % | N | % | |
| Behavior[a] | | | | | | | | | |
| Kicks, slaps, hits | 118 | 12.2 | 232 | 23.3 | 100 | 35.0 | 80 | 32.8 | 28.59*** |
| Scratches, bites | 55 | 5.7 | 144 | 14.4 | 42 | 14.7 | 37 | 15.2 | 14.54*** |
| Pinches, pulls hair | 20 | 2.1 | 56 | 5.6 | 19 | 6.6 | 12 | 4.9 | 6.43** |
| Hurts by pushing or rough-housing | 19 | 2.0 | 51 | 5.1 | 24 | 8.4 | 7 | 2.9 | 6.73** |
| Hits with or throws objects at people | 25 | 2.6 | 38 | 3.8 | 16 | 5.6 | 12 | 4.9 | 2.17 |
| Chokes | 2 | 0.2 | 6 | 0.6 | 3 | 1.0 | 6 | 2.5 | 5.14* |
| Other | 7 | 0.7 | 13 | 1.3 | 5 | 1.7 | 6 | 2.5 | |
| Total | 157 | 16.3 | 302 | 30.3 | 120 | 42.0 | 94 | 38.5 | 32.26*** |
| Frequency[b] | | | | | | | | | 2.58 |
| (1) Less than monthly | 26 | 16.7 | 38 | 12.8 | 8 | 6.8 | 5 | 5.6 | |
| (2) 1–3 per month | 43 | 28.1 | 78 | 26.2 | 25 | 21.2 | 38 | 42.2 | |
| (3) 1–6 per week | 60 | 39.0 | 111 | 37.2 | 50 | 42.4 | 29 | 32.2 | |
| (4) 1–16 per day | 21 | 13.7 | 67 | 22.5 | 33 | 28.0 | 16 | 17.8 | |
| (5) 1 or more per hour | 4 | 2.6 | 4 | 1.3 | 2 | 1.7 | 2 | 2.2 | |
| Staff response[b] | | | | | | | | | 1.48 |
| (1) No response | 1 | 0.6 | 3 | 1.0 | 0 | – | 1 | 1.1 | |
| (2) Ignore, reinforce other behavior | 14 | 8.7 | 31 | 10.2 | 5 | 4.2 | 7 | 7.4 | |
| (3) Verbal response | 83 | 52.9 | 124 | 40.9 | 65 | 54.2 | 39 | 41.5 | |
| (4) Physical response | 50 | 32.0 | 107 | 35.3 | 34 | 28.3 | 28 | 29.8 | |
| (5) Get help | 9 | 5.7 | 38 | 12.5 | 16 | 13.3 | 19 | 20.2 | |

[a] Percentage of all residents. Columns do not sum to total because some residents exhibited more than one type of behavior injurious to other people.
[b] Percentage of residents who exhibited behavior injurious to other people.
*$p < .01$.
**$p < .001$.
***$p < .0001$.

groups. A one-way analysis of variance, however, did not indicate statistically significant differences in average level of staff response to self-injurious behaviors among the four sample groups.

## BEHAVIOR INJURIOUS TO OTHER PEOPLE

Table 1.8 reports on behaviors injurious to other people. Kicking, hitting, or slapping were the most common behaviors in this category. Other types of injurious behaviors included biting, pinching, and throwing things at other people. Some residents caused unintentional injury by pushing or being overly rough. The rank order of the prevalence of various types of behaviors injurious to other people was similar in private and public facilities, although again, the proportion of public facility residents exhibiting each type of behavior was at least twice that of private facility residents.

There was a wide range in the frequency level at which behaviors injurious to other people occurred. In private facilities, 16.7% of the residents who injured other people did so less than once a month, compared to 12.8% of all public facility residents, 6.8% of new admissions, and 5.6% of readmissions who injured other people. Nearly 30% of new admissions who injured other people did so once a day or more often, compared with 23.8% of public facility residents and 16.3% of private facility residents who injured other people. A one-way analysis of variance indicated that the difference was not statistically significant among the groups on average frequency level of behaviors injurious to other people.

Approximately 50% of behaviors injurious to other people elicited a verbal response from staff and approximately 30% elicited a physical response. Compared to self-injurious behaviors, relatively few behaviors injurious to other people were systematically ignored. Among readmissions, 20.2% of behaviors injurious to other people required the intervention of more than one staff person, compared with 13.3% of new admissions, 12.5% of all public facility residents, and only 5.7% of private facility residents. There was no statistically significant difference, however, in average level of staff response among the four resident groups.

## BEHAVIOR THAT DAMAGES PROPERTY

Property damage by residents is summarized in Table 1.9. The most common type of property damage consisted of breaking or damaging toys, furniture, or other objects and materials found within the residential facility. The second most common type of property damage involved the actual building structure with some residents reported to punch holes in walls or doors, break windows or car windshields, or damage light fixtures.

Among residents who damaged property, 5.4% of public facility residents were reported to do so at least hourly, compared with 2.1% of those in private facilities. The average frequency level at which all property damage occurred, however, did not differ among groups.

Relatively few behaviors that damaged property were ignored by staff. Approximately 17% of public facility residents who damaged property required

TABLE 1.9. Prevalence of behaviors that damage property, frequency, and staff response within residential facilities.

| Behavior/frequency/response | Private current residents | | Public residents | | Public new admissions | | Public read-missions | | |
|---|---|---|---|---|---|---|---|---|---|
| | N | % | N | % | N | % | N | % | F |
| Behavior[a] | | | | | | | | | |
| Breaks toys, furnishings, contents of building | 79 | 8.2 | 107 | 10.7 | 29 | 10.1 | 31 | 12.7 | 2.25 |
| Breaks windows, doors, structural parts of building, cars | 43 | 4.5 | 47 | 4.7 | 14 | 4.9 | 23 | 9.4 | 2.53 |
| Tears up or destroys clothing | 21 | 2.2 | 59 | 5.9 | 18 | 6.3 | 11 | 4.5 | 5.77* |
| Throws things, overturns furniture | 11 | 1.1 | 46 | 4.6 | 12 | 4.2 | 20 | 8.2 | 10.50** |
| Stuffs sinks, toilets with paper, and so on | 2 | 0.2 | 4 | 0.4 | 4 | 1.4 | 1 | 0.4 | 0.93 |
| Breaks eyeglasses, hearing aids | 2 | 0.2 | 3 | 0.3 | 2 | 0.7 | 2 | 0.8 | 0.26 |
| Other | 0 | – | 1 | 0.1 | 0 | – | 0 | – | |
| Total | 107 | 11.1 | 175 | 17.6 | 55 | 19.2 | 57 | 23.4 | 8.56** |
| Frequency[b] | | | | | | | | | 3.11 |
| (1) Less than monthly | 23 | 24.1 | 24 | 14.3 | 8 | 15.4 | 11 | 19.3 | |
| (2) 1–3 per month | 34 | 34.7 | 44 | 26.2 | 17 | 32.7 | 23 | 40.4 | |
| (3) 1–6 per week | 22 | 22.3 | 58 | 34.5 | 13 | 25.0 | 12 | 21.1 | |
| (4) 1–16 per day | 16 | 16.9 | 33 | 19.6 | 14 | 26.9 | 10 | 17.5 | |
| (5) 1 or more per hour | 2 | 2.1 | 9 | 5.4 | 0 | – | 1 | 1.8 | |
| Staff response[b] | | | | | | | | | 3.40 |
| (1) No response | 2 | 1.9 | 4 | 2.3 | 1 | 1.8 | 0 | – | |
| (2) Ignore, reinforce other behavior | 13 | 11.9 | 22 | 12.6 | 6 | 10.9 | 3 | 5.3 | |
| (3) Verbal response | 62 | 58.9 | 71 | 40.8 | 24 | 43.6 | 28 | 49.1 | |
| (4) Physical response | 23 | 21.7 | 48 | 27.6 | 15 | 27.3 | 15 | 26.3 | |
| (5) Get help | 6 | 5.7 | 29 | 16.7 | 9 | 16.4 | 11 | 19.3 | |

[a] Percentage of all residents. Columns do not sum to total because some residents exhibited more than one type of behavior that damages property.
[b] Percentage of residents who damaged property.
*$p < .001$.
**$p < .0001$.

the response of at least two staff members, compared with 5.7% of private residents who damaged property. Nevertheless, the average level of staff response did not differ significantly between the two types of facilities.

UNUSUAL OR DISRUPTIVE BEHAVIOR

Unusual or disruptive behaviors are reported in Table 1.10. This category included inappropriate verbal behaviors such as swearing, threatening, yelling, talking too loud, or repeating meaningless phrases. Inappropriate verbal behaviors were more common among private facility current residents and

TABLE 1.10. Prevalence of unusual or disruptive behaviors, frequency, and staff response within residential facilities.

| Behavior/frequency/response | Private current residents | | Public residents | | Public new admissions | | Public read-missions | | F |
|---|---|---|---|---|---|---|---|---|---|
| | N | % | N | % | N | % | N | % | |
| Behavior[a] | | | | | | | | | |
| Inappropriate verbal behavior | 100 | 10.4 | 81 | 8.1 | 30 | 10.5 | 42 | 17.2 | 4.28* |
| Nonverbal, screams, cries, yells | 63 | 6.5 | 101 | 10.1 | 38 | 13.3 | 28 | 11.5 | 3.56 |
| Temper tantrums | 71 | 7.4 | 88 | 8.8 | 21 | 7.3 | 27 | 11.1 | 1.40 |
| Nuisance behavior: slams doors, flicks lights/water faucets | 70 | 7.3 | 48 | 4.8 | 23 | 8.0 | 18 | 7.4 | 2.47 |
| Inappropriate sexual behavior | 41 | 4.3 | 34 | 3.4 | 8 | 2.8 | 11 | 4.5 | 0.45 |
| Throws or overturns things | 22 | 2.3 | 24 | 2.4 | 13 | 4.5 | 8 | 3.3 | 0.79 |
| Strange postures, mannerisms | 19 | 2.0 | 19 | 1.9 | 9 | 3.1 | 3 | 1.2 | 0.54 |
| Pesters, teases, seeks attention | 17 | 1.8 | 13 | 1.3 | 2 | 0.7 | 1 | 0.4 | 0.74 |
| Inappropriate social interaction | 14 | 1.5 | 22 | 2.2 | 7 | 2.4 | 12 | 4.9 | 3.73 |
| Pushes, rough, aggressive | 7 | 0.7 | 15 | 1.5 | 4 | 1.4 | 3 | 1.2 | 1.28 |
| High activity level | 4 | 0.4 | 13 | 1.3 | 8 | 2.8 | 3 | 1.2 | 1.48 |
| Other | 30 | 3.1 | 57 | 5.7 | 17 | 5.9 | 14 | 5.7 | |
| Total | 278 | 28.8 | 342 | 34.3 | 108 | 37.8 | 100 | 41.0 | 4.86* |
| Frequency[b] | | | | | | | | | 6.03** |
| (1) Less than monthly | 28 | 10.6 | 19 | 5.6 | 4 | 3.7 | 1 | 5.1 | |
| (2) 1–3 per month | 68 | 25.6 | 74 | 21.8 | 17 | 15.7 | 19 | 19.2 | |
| (3) 1–6 per week | 99 | 37.0 | 116 | 34.1 | 34 | 31.5 | 41 | 41.4 | |
| (4) 1–16 per day | 61 | 22.7 | 117 | 34.4 | 42 | 38.9 | 32 | 32.3 | |
| (5) 1 or more per hour | 11 | 4.1 | 14 | 4.1 | 11 | 10.2 | 2 | 2.0 | |
| Staff response[b] | | | | | | | | | 1.40 |
| (1) No response | 6 | 2.2 | 7 | 2.1 | 5 | 4.6 | 1 | 1.0 | |
| (2) Ignore, reinforce other behavior | 54 | 19.7 | 76 | 22.6 | 15 | 13.9 | 25 | 25.0 | |
| (3) Verbal response | 162 | 59.1 | 159 | 47.2 | 54 | 50.0 | 53 | 53.0 | |
| (4) Physical response | 46 | 16.8 | 71 | 21.1 | 30 | 27.8 | 16 | 16.0 | |
| (5) Get help | 6 | 2.3 | 24 | 7.1 | 4 | 3.7 | 5 | 5.0 | |

[a] Percentage of all residents. Columns do not sum to total because some residents exhibited more than one type of unusual or disruptive behavior.
[b] Percentage of residents who exhibited unusual or disruptive behavior.
 *$p < .01$.
**$p < .001$.

among PFR readmissions than among PRF current residents in general, no doubt partially because less than half of all PRF residents could talk. Public facility residents were more likely to scream, cry, or make nonverbal noises than were private facility residents. Temper tantrums were the third most common type of disruptive behavior. As with other major categories of maladaptive behavior, the rank order by prevalence for various types of disruptive behavior was similar for the facility groups. Few residents were reported to be disruptive because of a general high activity level, although many were reported to receive medication for overactive behavior (15.7% of private facility residents; 29.9% of public facility residents).

Most disruptive residents engaged in this behavior less frequently than once per day; 22.7% of disruptive private facility residents and 34.4% of disruptive public facility residents were reported to be disruptive daily; and approximately 4% of each group were reported to be disruptive at least hourly. Overall, the average frequency level of disruptive behaviors was higher for public facility residents and new admissions than for private facility residents ($p < .001$). Most disruptive behaviors were ignored or given a verbal response by staff. The average level of staff response did not significantly differ among resident groups.

The specific behaviors most frequently found among mentally retarded persons in an institution were also reported by Ho, Morreau, and Repp (1985) from a sample of 500 residents. The *Prescriptive Inventory of Problem Behaviors* (Morreau, 1981) was administered to direct-care workers who had one or more years experience with members of the sample. Staff were asked to check the behaviors that were exhibited most frequently by the recipients. The results are summarized in Table 1.11. These studies and others (cf. Eyman & Call, 1977) have reported a relatively high prevalence of maladaptive behavior among mentally retarded people in residential facilities.

It is important to avoid overgeneralizing from these studies, however, to prevent what might be an exaggerated estimate of emotional disorders among mentally retarded children and adults. Most available studies report sample data on either referred or service populations. This perspective likely distorts conclusions regarding children and adults with retardation in general, especially those who receive little or no structured services.

Postschool follow-up studies of mildly retarded adults, for example, have reported higher-than-normal rates of problem behaviors (Baller, 1936; Deno, 1965; Kennedy, 1948; Peterson & Smith, 1960), without benefits of adequate control groups of nonhandicapped subjects. Even in these samples, however, the rates of deviant behavior appear to decline substantially with age (Baller, Charles, & Miller, 1967; Kennedy, 1966).

The literature is also mixed and inconclusive regarding rates of problem behaviors in community service programs. Halpern, Close, and Nelson (1985), for example, found very low rates of deviant behavior among approximately 300 mildly and moderately retarded persons in semi-independent living programs in four western states. The clients registered few problems in a specially devised problem behavior scale. Furthermore, their rates of violent crimes, arrests, and use of alcohol, marijuana, and tobacco were extremely low. Although the authors acknowledge the possible effects of careful selection and supervision on rates of problem behavior, their data strongly suggest that serious deviant behaviors are probably quite low among mentally retarded citizens living independently or with minimal support. Important ethnographic studies by Edgerton seem to corroborate these findings for individuals living in relatively independent circumstances (Edgerton, 1981).

TABLE 1.11. Summary of specific problem behaviors in an institution sample.

| Category | Behavior problems | Percentage |
|---|---|---|
| Maladaptive | Urinates in clothes | 65 |
| | Defecates in clothes | 57 |
| | Urinates in inappropriate places | 47 |
| | Ignores requests/directions | 45 |
| | Places hands/fingers in body orifices | 43 |
| | Stares at people/into space | 42 |
| | Laughs without reason | 41 |
| | Makes strange noises | 40 |
| | Nods/rolls/shakes head | 40 |
| | Wipes nose on hand or clothes | 40 |
| Disruptive | Takes objects from others | 32 |
| | Screams | 31 |
| | Tears objects (eg, books, clothes) | 25 |
| | Grabs/holds others | 23 |
| | Scoots chair | 23 |
| | Grabs others' food | 23 |
| | Throws self to floor | 23 |
| | Masturbates publicly | 21 |
| | Smears objectional material on self | 19 |
| | Undresses publicly | 19 |
| Destructive | Hits others | 33 |
| | Bites self | 26 |
| | Hits self | 22 |
| | Pushes others | 20 |
| | Bangs head | 19 |
| | Throws objects | 17 |
| | Kicks others | 16 |
| | Scratches others | 16 |
| | Kicks objects | 16 |
| | Scratches self | 12 |

The relative basis by which society determines what behavior is considered to be unacceptable makes it difficult to judge the severity of maladaptive behavior among mentally retarded people. Goroff (1967) used a critical incident technique to identify specific behavioral events that had precipitated readmission of a sample of reinstitutionalized residents. An important finding was that the majority of critical incidents that included behavior problems would have been considered inconsequential if they had been performed by a nonretarded person (e.g., a nonretarded person would not be institutionalized for missing work). Another frequently cited study (Nihira & Nihira, 1975) indicated that of 1252 incidents of problem behavior among 424 retarded residents of community residential facilities (i.e., problems that were considered to be bothersome, unacceptable, or beyond the threshold of community acceptance), only 16% were considered to jeopardize the health, safety, general welfare, or legal status of residents.

In the Hill and Bruininks (1981) study of severely handicapped people in residential facilities, private facility staff reported that 30% of their residents exhibited at least one of four categories of maladaptive behavior. Half of these behaviors, however, never elicited more than a verbal response from staff and never occurred more than once daily. If such behaviors were excluded, only about 19% of private facility residents would be considered to have behavior management problems. Using the same criteria (i.e., either more than once per day or more than a verbal response), however, 36% of all PRF residents, 42% of PRF new admissions, and 44% of PRF readmissions would still be considered to exhibit significant behavior management problems. Private facility staff reported that 8.4% of their residents with behavior problems (3.8% of all current residents) were in danger of being demitted, compared with 2.5% of public facility residents with behavior problems (1.5% of all residents). In response to a general question, staff reported that 88% of private facility current residents, 85% of PRF current residents, 83% of PRF new admissions, and 81% of PRF readmissions "got along" with other residents very well or generally well with few problems. This finding suggests that perhaps, while the rates of problem behaviors were high, service personnel felt most of them were manageable within current environments.

## Observations and Needed Research

### Assessment and Diagnosis

When reviewing available research literature on behavior and emotional disorders among mentally retarded people, it is important to emphasize that generalizations regarding the nature and extent of such problems must be considered tenuous at best. The first observation is that the literature is generally limited in this area, especially studies using instruments and procedures of known reliability and validity. Published reports involve a variety of measurement techniques and occasionally clinical diagnostic procedures. Little consistency exists in terminology and procedures across studies (e.g., few studies on dual diagnosis use any of the various DSM versions).

One obvious impediment to synthesizing information on the extent of problem behaviors or dual diagnosis among mentally retarded persons is the absence of clearly defined descriptions and procedures of assessing maladaptive behavior. Bruininks, Woodcock, Weatherman, and Hill (1985) addressed this issue by designing an empirically derived taxonomy and maladaptive behavior indexes as part of the *Scales of Independent Behavior*. The model was derived using a critical incident procedure with a national sample of retarded children and adults in public and private residential facilities, a variety of samples in service programs, and through data reported by Morreau (1985) from information provided by about

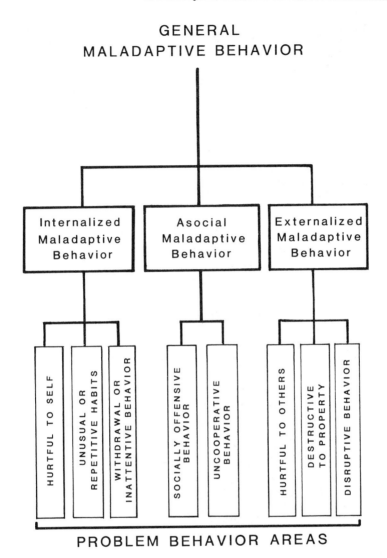

FIGURE 1.1. Model of maladaptive behavior.

1500 teachers and direct-care personnel. Over 150 discrete serious problems or maladaptive behaviors were organized into eight broader categories and then scaled and normed on a nationally representative sample of people from infancy to about 45 years old in 40 communities throughout the United States. Figure 1.1 presents the model of maladaptive behavior and empirically derived clusters or indexes of maladaptive behaviors. This model illustrates a hypothetical continuum of maladaptive functioning, ranging from internally directed to externally directed expressions of behavior. At the base of the figure are categories for describing problem behaviors. The maladaptive indexes combine ratings of problem behaviors within these categories into broader measures. These broader indexes quite closely resemble factors derived from the maladaptive behavior section of the *Adaptive Behavior Scale* in a series of studies by Eyman, Meyers, and Nihira (cf. Meyers, Nihira, & Zetlin, 1979). This model and measurement procedure has been used extensively to describe and evaluate the seriousness of problem behaviors in a wide range of samples and settings. It represents one approach to a difficult problem in assessing the need for service and planning effective treatments for individuals exhibiting serious problem behaviors and mental health disorders. Carefully delineated behavioral referents are critical for future research in estimating the nature and prevalence of problem behaviors (or dual diagnosis), in the development of services, or in the design of effective client-based treatment programs.

It would be helpful in assessing service needs and planning more appropriate treatment strategies if the research process proceeded in three stages. The first stage would present a survey of behavior problems using four criteria: (1) precise description of critical behavior incidents, (2) the frequency of significant behavior problems, (3) the perceived severity of significant behavior problems, and (4) the types of response from others to deviant behaviors. Following a description of the critical behaviors, detailed observations using time sampling procedures in different environments should be conducted to assess consistency of problem behaviors over time and across settings. Finally, further procedures and criteria could be employed to derive clinical diagnoses using standardized classification models such as DSM-III (American Psychiatric Association, 1980). Importantly, the process of research and diagnosis would begin with precisely describing and assessing critical dimensions of problem behaviors. Without specific behavioral descriptions, the synthesis of literature or assessment of service needs of mentally retarded people cannot be achieved.

## Programming and Environmental Considerations

Related to a need for more precise assessment of behavior disorders is the importance of considering environmental factors. From a number of studies it is becoming clearer that behavior problems among mentally retarded people are evaluated differently by parents and teachers (Bruininks et al., 1985; Rutter, 1971), and their significance may vary across environments and evaluators. To identify environmental differences in expression of problem behaviors, Morreau and Rittenhouse (1984) assessed the behavior of 68 severely and profoundly retarded persons residing in a community residence and attending school programs. The behavior of the residents was assessed by two different staff members who worked with them in either a residential or an educational environment. The behaviors were first assessed through staff ratings using the Behavior Problem Scale of the *Scales of Independent Behavior* (Bruininks et al., 1985) and *The Prescriptive Inventory of Problem Behaviors* (Morreau, 1981). Behaviors identified on both instruments were then selected as target behaviors for observation during a 3 to 5 day period. The agreement was 100% between the actual occurrence or nonoccurrence of behaviors and staff ratings on the structured scales. These data showed remarkable consistency between ratings on the scales and actual occurrence of problem behaviors. According to the ratings, a large proportion (nearly 75%) of the problem behaviors occurred in both environments; however, 25% of the problem behaviors occurred in only one of the two environmental settings. Clearly, problem behaviors expressed by retarded individuals are related to environmental factors that deserve serious consideration in assessment, diagnosis, placement, and treatment strategies.

## Psychopharmacological Approaches

Despite improvement in assessment and programming, and despite the fact that community settings rather than public institutions have become the locus of service for handicapped people, psychotropic drugs are still widely prescribed for mentally retarded people with problem behaviors. Sprague and Baxley (1978) reported that psychotropic drugs (i.e., drugs that affect mood, cognition, or behavior) have been used to treat behavior in four broad categories: (1) acting out, (2) impulse control, (3) self-abuse, and (4) stereotypes. Lipman (1970) found that 50% of the residents in state and private facilities had, at some point, been given psychotropic drugs. Consistent with these data, Sprague (1977) found that 66% of the moderately/profoundly retarded residents of a large institution and 65% of the residents of a new, smaller community-based residence were receiving drug treatment programs. Sprague and Baxley (1978) concluded that the frequency of drug usage in the average institution had not declined over the past 10 years and that this usage of large doses was substantial. Hill, Balow, and Bruininks (1985), Intagliata and Rinck (1985), and Agran and Martin (1985) reported that from 26 to 48% of mentally retarded people in community residential or vocational settings and from 38 to 76% of institutionalized mentally retarded people receive psychotropic medication.

Gualtieri and Keppel (1985) explained this phenomenon as follows:

The wide use of neuroleptic drugs in this population is not difficult to understand. Neuroleptics appear to possess, for many brain-damaged patients, reliable acute calming or sedating effects. This is in contrast to traditional sedatives like the barbiturates, benzodiazepines, or antihistamines which frequently exercise paradoxical effects and cause agitation, confusion, or disinhibition. The wide use of neuroleptics in elderly demented patients is probably attributable to this acute tranquilizing action also (Ray et al., 1980). Thus, in the acute management of agitation, hyperactive, assaultive, destructive, or self-injurious behavior, a short course of neuroleptic treatment may afford at least some measure of symptom relief, and a window of time to introduce a behavior management program....

The major problem around neuroleptics in the retarded is over long-term treatment. There is a widespread concern that too many retarded people are on chronic neuroleptic therapy (Cohen & Sprague, 1977; Hill et al., 1983; Lipman, 1970; Sprague, 1982) in the absence of good scientific data to support the efficacy of the practice (Sprague & Werry,

1971); that very serious side effects may, indeed, occur in retarded patients on neuroleptic drugs (Gualtieri et al., 1982a,b); that neuroleptic polypharmacy is a frequent occurrence (Ellenor, 1977); that high doses of the most sedating neuroleptics tend to be preferred (Lipman, 1970); and that toxic effects like corneal opacities and tardive dyskinesia may be dose-related (Gualtieri et al., 1982a,b). Further, there is concern that neuroleptic treatment may, in some circumstances, impair learning and compromise a retarded person's ability to profit from behavioral or habilitative programming (Hartlage, 1965). p. 304

In the same issue of the *Psychopharmacology Bulletin*, Schroeder (1985) stated the following in a summary paper:

Although the widespread use of psychotropic drugs (Lipman, 1970) and the questionable validity of and applicability of psychotropic drug research to the mentally retarded population (Sprague & Werry, 1971) have been noted repeatedly for nearly 15 years, little research progress has been made on the many issues relating to mentally retarded people who are emotionally or behaviorally disturbed. In fact, so little has been done that the level of advancement of research in this area relative to other problems of mental illness appears to be in the Stone Age. (p. 323)

The use of psychotropic agents may create a Catch-22 situation in the assessment, reporting, and management of problem behaviors. Data on prevalence and severity may be distorted by the suppression of problem behaviors and by reduction in the potential of retarded individuals to acquire alternative and more adaptive behaviors. The development of greater adaptive skills would likely act to reduce the prevalence of problem behaviors (Glaser & Morreau, 1986).

Because the prevalence of drug prescription almost exceeds the reported prevalence rates of the maladaptive behaviors that these drugs are purported to treat, it behooves researchers as well as practitioners to examine this issue closely.

## Labeling Effects

There is some concern whether the diagnosis and assigned label "mental retardation" acts to change the perceptions of behavior disorders among mentally retarded people. Reiss and his colleagues have documented, through a number of studies, that the diagnosis of mental retardation increases the likelihood that professionals will evaluate emotional problems among mentally retarded people differently than they would in the absence of the diagnosis (Reiss, Levitan, & Szysko, 1982; Reiss & Szysko, 1983). This finding has also been documented by Alford and Locke (1984) with a sample of doctoral-level clinical psychologists. This process may operate simultaneously in two contradictory directions. On one hand, this "diagnostic overshadowing" phenomenon may act to underestimate the clinical significance of behavior disorders among retarded people. On the other hand, behavior disorders in combination with mental retardation may reduce the normal tolerance of people toward any deviant behaviors. The evidence regarding the impact of behavior problems on employment and community living as well as the overshadowing phenomenon documented by Reiss and his colleagues suggests that there is a need to research the effects of labeling on clinical diagnosis and environmental tolerance for problem behaviors among mentally retarded people.

The existing research literature provides some useful information to assess the extent and significance of behavior disorders among mentally retarded children and adults. There is need for more methodologically sensitive studies in this area to guide the planning of investment for research and development, the design of intervention programs, and the development of useful information, training, and technical assistance. Except for self-injurious behaviors, behavior problems in the study by Hill and Bruininks (1981) were highest among residents currently and previously identified as dually diagnosed in both public and private residential facilities and new admissions and readmissions to public residential facilities. Many years ago, Guskin (1963) summarized a number of studies that indicate an often inappropriate tendency among the general public to link conditions of mental illness with mental retardation. Exploring the association between these conditions may advance research and treatment; but it is also imperative that strategies be used that avoid the unintended, negative consequences of labeling and diagnosis. It is easy to overgeneralize from the limited evidence on the behavior disorders of mentally retarded citizens. A more prudent course would suggest a cautious interpretation of our information and the development of treatment and service strategies that enhance the development of appropriate social behaviors of retarded citizens and increase their assimilation in normal environments.

## References

Agran, M., & Martin, J. (1985). Establishing socially validated drug research in community settings. *Psychopharmacology Bulletin, 21*(2), 285–290.

Alford, J., & Locke, B. (1984). Clinical responses to psychopathology of mentally retarded persons. *American Journal of Mental Deficiency, 89*(2), 195–197.

American Psychiatric Association. (1980). *Diagnostic and statistical manual of mental disorders* (3rd ed.). Washington, DC: Author.

Baller, W. (1936). A study of the present social status of a group of adults who, when they were in elementary school, were classified as mentally deficient. *Genetic Psychology Monographs, 18*, 165–244.

Baller, W., Charles, D., & Miller, E. (1967). Mid-life attainment of the mentally retarded: A longitudinal study. *Genetic Psychology Monographs, 75*, 235–329.

Balthazar, E., & Stevens, H. (1975). *The emotionally disturbed, mentally retarded: A historical and contemporary perspective*. Englewood Cliffs, NJ: Prentice-Hall.

Beier, D. (1964). Behavioral disturbances in the mentally retarded. In H. Stevens & R. Heber (Eds.), *Mental retardation: A review of research*. Chicago, IL: University of Chicago Press.

Breuning, S.E., & Davidson, N.A. (1981). Effects of psychotropic drugs on intelligence test performance of institutionalized mentally retarded adults. *American Journal on Mental Deficiency, 85*, 575–579.

Bruininks, R. (1982). Deinstitutionalization of the handicapped. In H. Mitzel, J. Best, W. Rabinowitz, & A. Landy (Eds.), *Encyclopedia of education research*, (5th ed.). Washington, DC: American Educational Research Association.

Bruininks, R., Thurlow, M., Nelson, R., & Davis, E. (1984). *Feasibility study report on establishing a UAF Satellite Center in Minnesota*. Minneapolis, MN: University of Minnesota, Department of Educational Psychology.

Bruininks, R., Woodcock, R., Weatherman, R., & Hill, B. (1985). *Scales of Independent Behavior*. Allen, TX: DLM Teaching Resources.

Conley, R. (1973). *The economics of mental retardation*. Baltimore, MD: Johns Hopkins University Press.

Deno, E. (1965). *Retarded youth: Their school rehabilitation needs*. Minneapolis, MN: Minneapolis Public Schools.

Eagle, C. (1967). Prognosis and outcome of community placement of institutionalized retardates. *American Journal of Mental Deficiency, 72*, 232–243.

Edgerton, R. (1981). Crime, deviance, and normalization: Reconsidered. In R. Bruininks, C. Meyers, B. Sigford, & K. Lakin (Eds.), *Deinstitutionalization and community adjustments of mentally retarded people*. Washington, DC: American Association on Mental Deficiency.

Eyman, R., & Borthwick, S. (1980). Patterns of care for mentally retarded persons. *American Journal of Mental Deficiency, 18*, 63–66.

Eyman, R., Borthwick, S., & Miller, C. (1981). Trends in maladaptive behavior of mentally retarded persons placed in community and institutional settings. *American Journal of Mental Deficiency, 85*, 473–477.

Eyman, R., & Call, T. (1977). Maladaptive behavior and community placement of mentally retarded persons. *American Journal of Mental Deficiency, 82*, 137–144.

Eyman, R., O'Connor, G., Tarjan, G., & Justice R. (1972). Factors determining residential placement of mentally retarded children. *American Journal of Mental Deficiency, 76*, 692–698.

Foss, G., & Peterson, S. (1981). Social–interpersonal skills relevant to job tenure for mentally retarded adults. *Mental Retardation, 19*, 103–106.

Foster, S., & Ritchey, W. (1979). Issues in the assessment of social competence in children. *Journal of Applied Behavior Analysis, 12*, 625–638.

Glaser, B., & Morreau, L.E. (1986). Effects of interdisciplinary team review on the use of antipsychotic agents with severely and profoundly mentally retarded persons. *American Journal of Mental Deficiency, 90*, 371–379.

Goroff, N. (1967). Research and community placement—an exploratory approach. *Mental Retardation, 5*(4), 17–19.

Groden, G., Domingue, D., Pueschel, S.M., & Deignan, L. (1982). Behavioral/emotional problems in mentally retarded children and youth. *Psychological Reports, 51*(1), 143–146.

Gualtieri, C., & Keppel, J. (1985). Psychopharmacology in the mentally retarded and a few related issues. *Psychopharmacology Bulletin, 21*(2), 304–309.

Guskin, S. (1963). Social psychologies of mental deficiency. In N. Ellis (Ed.), *Handbook of mental deficiency: Psychological theory and research*. New York: McGraw-Hill.

Halpern, A., Close, D., & Nelson, D. (1985). *On my own: The impact of semi-independent living programs for adults with mental retardation*. Baltimore, MD: Paul H. Brookes Publishing Company.

Heaton-Ward, A. (1977). Psychosis in mental handicap. *British Journal of Psychiatry, 130*, 525–533.

Hill, B., Balow, E., & Bruininks, R. (1985). A national study of prescribed drugs in institutions and community residential facilities for mentally retarded people. *Psychopharmacology Bulletin, 21*(2), 279–284.

Hill, B. & Bruininks, R. (1981). *Physical and behavioral characteristics and maladaptive behavior of mentally retarded people in residential facilities.* Minneapolis, MN: University of Minnesota, Department of Psychoeducational Studies.

Hill, B., & Bruininks, R. (1984). Maladaptive behavior of mentally retarded people in residential facilities. *American Journal of Mental Deficiency, 88*, 380–387.

Hill, B., Bruininks, R., & Lakin, K. (1983). Characteristics of mentally retarded people in residential facilities. *Health and Social Work, 8*, 85–95.

Ho, D., & Morreau, L. (1985). *Perceptions by the severity of problem behaviors held by institutional staff.* Normal, IL: Illinois State University (unpublished manuscript).

Ho, D., Morreau, L., & Repp, A. (1985). *Prevalence of problem behavior in an institution for mentally retarded people.* Normal, IL: Illinois State University (unpublished manuscript).

Intagliata, J., & Rinck, C. (1985). Psychoactive drug use in public and community residential facilities for mentally retarded persons. *Psychopharmacology Bulletin, 21*(2), 268–278.

Jacobson, J. (1982). Problem behavior and psychiatric impairment within a developmentally disabled population. I: Behavior frequency. *Applied Research in Mental Retardation, 3*, 121–139.

Jacobson, J., & Janicki, M. (1985). Functional and health status characteristics of persons with severe handicaps in New York State. *The Journal of the Association for Persons with Severe Handicaps, 10*(1), 51–60.

Kennedy, R.F. (1966). *A Connecticut community revisited: A study of the social adjustment of a group of mentally deficient adults in 1948 and 1960.* Hartford, CT: Connecticut State Department of Health, Office of Mental Retardation.

Kennedy, R.J. (1948). *The social adjustment of morons in a Connecticut city.* Hartford, CT: Mansfield-Southbury Training Schools.

Keys, V., Boroskin, A., & Ross, R. (1973). The revolving door in an MR hospital: A study of returns from leave. *Mental Retardation, 11*(1), 55–56.

Koller, H., Richardson, S.A., Katz, M., & McLaren J. (1983). Behavior disturbances since childhood among a 5-year birth cohort of all mentally retarded young adults in a city. *American Journal of Mental Deficiency, 87*, 386–395.

Lakin, K., Hill, B., Hauber, F., Bruininks, R., & Heal, L. (1983). New admissions and readmissions to a national sample of public residential facilities. *American Journal of Mental Deficiency, 88*, 13–20.

Landesman-Dwyer, A., & Sulzbacher, F. (1981). Residential placement and adaptation of severely and profoundly retarded individuals. In R. Bruininks, C. Meyers, B. Sigford, & K. Lakin (Eds.), *Deinstitutionalization and community adjustment of mentally retarded people.* Washington, DC: American Association on Mental Deficiency.

Lewis, M., & MacLean, W. (1982). Issues in treating emotional disorders. In J. Matson & R. Barrett (Eds.), *Psychopathology in the mentally retarded.* New York: Grune & Stratton.

Lindberg, D., & Putnam, J. (1979). *The developmentally disabled of West Virginia: A profile of the substantially handicapped who are not in institutions.* Elkins, WV: Davis and Elkins College.

Lipman, R. (1970). The use of psychopharmacological agents in residential facilities for the retarded. In F. Menolascino (Ed.), *Psychiatric approaches to mental retardation.* New York: Basic Books.

Maney, A., Pace, R., & Morrison, D. (1964). A factor analytic study of the need for institutionalization: Problems and populations for program development. *American Journal of Mental Deficiency, 69,* 372–384.

McCarver, R., & Craig, E. (1974). Placement of the retarded in the community: Prognosis and outcome. In N.R. Ellis (Ed.), *International review of research in mental retardation* (Vol. 7). New York: Academic Press.

Menolascino, F. (1970). *Psychiatric approaches to mental retardation.* New York: Basic Books.

Meyers, C., Nihira, K., & Zetlin, A. (1979). The measurement of adaptive behavior. In N.R. Ellis (Ed.), *Handbook of mental deficiency: Psychological theory and research* (2nd ed.). Hillsdale, NJ: Lawrence Erlbaum Associates.

Moen, M., Bogen, D., & Aanes, D. (1975). Follow-up of mentally retarded adults successfully and unsuccessfully placed in community group homes. *Hospital and Community Psychiatry, 26,* 754–756.

Morreau, L. (1981). *Prescriptive inventory of problem behaviors.* Normal, IL: Illinois State University.

Morreau, L. (1985). Assessing and managing problem behaviors. In K. Lakin & R. Bruininks (Eds.), *Strategies for achieving community integration of developmentally disabled citizens.* Baltimore, MD: Paul H. Brookes Publishing Company.

Morreau, L., & Rittenhouse, R. (1984). *Influence of settings, time and rater characteristics on the assessment of adaptive behavior.* Paper presented at the 108th Annual Meeting of the American Association on Mental Deficiency, Minneapolis, MN.

Nihira, L., & Nihira, K. (1975). Jeopardy in community placement. *American Journal of Mental Deficiency, 79,* 538–544.

Niziol, O., & DeBlassie, R. (1972). Work adjustment and the educable mentally retarded adolescent. *Journal of Employment Counseling, 9,* 158–166.

Pagel, S., & Whitling, C. (1978). Readmissions to a state hospital for mentally retarded persons: Reasons for community placement failure. *Mental Retardation, 16,* 164–166.

Peterson, L., & Smith, L. (1960). A comparison of the post-school adjustment of educable mentally retarded adults with that of adults of normal intelligence. *Exceptional Children, 26,* 404–408.

Reiss, S., Levitan, G.W., & Szysko, J. (1982). Emotional disturbance and mental retardation: Diagnostic overshadowing. *American Journal of Mental Deficiency, 86,* 567–574.

Reiss, S., & Szysko, J. (1983). Diagnostic overshadowing and professional experience with mentally retarded persons. *American Journal of Mental Deficiency, 87,* 396–402.

Richardson, S., Koller, H., & Katz, M. (1985). Continuities and change in behavior disturbances: A follow-up study of mildly retarded young people. *American Journal of Orthopsychiatry, 55*(2), 220–229.

Rutter, M. (1971). Psychiatry. In J. Wortis (Ed.), *Mental retardation: An annual review* (Vol. 3). New York: Grune & Stratton.

Rutter, M., Tizard, J., & Whitmore, K. (1970). *Education, health and behavior.* New York: Wiley.

Rutter, M., Tizard, J., Yule, W., Graham, & Whitmore. (1976). Isle of Wight studies, 1964–1974. *Psychological Medicine, 6,* 313–332.

Saenger, G. (1960). *Factors influencing the institutionalization of mentally retarded individuals in New York City.* Albany, NY: New York State Interdepartmental Health Resources Board.

Schalock, R., & Harper, R. (1978). Placement from community-based mental retardation programs: How well do clients do? *American Journal of Mental Deficiency, 83,* 240–247.

Schalock, R.L., Harper, R.S., & Garver, G. (1981). Independent living placement: Five years later. *American Journal of Mental Deficiency, 86*(2), 170–177.

Schalock, R.L., Harper, R.S., & Genung, T. (1981). Community integration of mentally retarded adults. *American Journal of Mental Deficiency, 85*(5), 478–488.

Schroeder, S. (1985). Issues and future research directions of pharmacotherapy in mental retardation. *Psychopharmacology Bulletin, 21*(2), 323–326.

Sigford, B., Bruininks, R., Lakin, K., Hill, B., & Heal, L. (1982). Resident release patterns in a national sample of public residential facilities. *American Journal of Mental Deficiency, 87,* 130–140.

Spencer, D. (1976). New long-stay patients in a hospital for mental handicap. *British Journal of Psychiatry, 128,* 467–470.

Sprague, R. (1977). Overview of psychopharmacology for the retarded in the United States. In P. Mittler (Ed.), *Research to practice in mental retardation* (Vol. 3). Baltimore, MD: University Park Press.

Sprague, R., & Baxley, G. (1978). Drugs for behavior management. In J. Wortis (Ed.), *Mental retardation* (Vol. 10). New York: Brunner/Mazel.

Sternlicht, M., & Deutsch, M. (1972). *Personality development and social behavior in the mentally retarded.* Lexington, MA: D.C. Heath & Co.

Sutter, P., Mayeda, T., Call, T., Yanagi, G., & Yee, S. (1980). Comparison of successful and unsuccessful community placed mentally retarded persons. *American Journal of Mental Deficiency, 85,* 262–267.

Windle, C. (1962). Prognosis of mental subnormals. *American Journal of Mental Deficiency* (monograph suppl.) *66*(5), 180.

Wright, E.C. (1982). The presentation of mental illness in mentally retarded adults. *British Journal of Psychiatry, 141,* 496–502.

# 2
# Maladaptive Behavior Among the Mentally Retarded: The Need for Reliable Data

Sharon A. Borthwick

Considerations of the mental health of mentally retarded individuals should not be limited to aspects of diagnosed mental illness. It is well established in the literature that mentally retarded individuals are especially vulnerable to emotional problems that often promote the display of various kinds of maladaptive behavior (Chess, 1970; Reiss, Levitan, & McNally, 1982; Szymanski & Grossman, 1984). However, the fact that many persons who are referred for psychiatric assessment are *not* determined to be mentally ill suggests that a significant proportion of people who do not suffer from mental illness still evidence problem behaviors that impact the quality of their lives. Moreover, maladaptive behavior has been repeatedly cited as a leading cause of out-of-home placement for a substantial number of clients living in institutions and community care facilities. The majority of these people are unlikely to be referred for psychiatric assessment. Their behavior problems are attributed to the presence of mental retardation and are tolerated as such.

Since maladaptive behaviors are not unique to retarded persons with diagnosed mental illness, the monitoring of and dealing with problem behaviors among the entire population of retarded individuals are important issues to consider. Even for those clients who have been diagnosed as having a mental illness and have been treated by special training programs, drugs, therapies, or residential environments, evaluation of the intervention is most always dependent on an examination of *observed behaviors* (e.g., temper outbursts, aggression, self-injurious behavior) rather than on psychiatric classifications. The purpose of this chapter is to discuss some of the issues related to the identification of mental illness in mentally retarded people, to review the recent literature with regard to maladaptive behavior among the retarded, and to suggest areas in which data from state mental retardation systems can become more reliable and more useful to persons involved in research and policy decisions.

## Mental Illness and Mental Retardation

There are a number of problems associated with the identification of mental illness in mentally retarded individuals. The American Association on Mental

Deficiency definition of mental retardation states that a person will be both subaverage in intelligence and deficient in adaptive behavior. Hence, failure to perform appropriate social roles *identify* mentally retarded individuals (Stein & Susser, 1974). Schroeder, Mulick, and Schroeder (1979) concluded from a review of the literature that the relationship between behavior disturbance and retardation becomes even more obscured with the severely retarded because of their multiple handicaps. For example, communication skills are lacking in a significant proportion of the severely and profoundly retarded, making it extremely difficult to determine whether problem behaviors in their repertoire are due to a mental disorder, to the brain injury associated with the retardation, or to environmental influences. The confounding between mental illness and performance on an IQ test further complicates the diagnosis of mental retardation, particularly among the mild and borderline retarded (Padd & Eyman, 1985).

Tarjan concluded in 1977 that the mental health care of the retarded was an early casualty of the separation of mental health and mental retardation bureaucracies. Retarded people with emotional and personality disturbances have recently been identified as an undeserved population by professionals in the field (Reiss, Levitan, & McNally, 1982). As a consequence, initial screening and diagnosis of retarded people in residential facilities and parental homes have become the responsibility of persons who may not be qualified to determine whether or not an observed behavior might be the result of mental illness in this group of people.

Rutter and Graham (1970) found that while teachers and parents could adequately describe childrens' behaviors, they were likely to misinterpret the *source* of behavior problems they observed, and that they were also not good at providing an adequate description of the child's emotional responsiveness and interpersonal relationships. Reiss, Levitan, and Szyskzo (1982), as well as Alford and Locke (1984), found that the presence of mental retardation tends to decrease the diagnostic significance of abnormal behavior. This suggests that the likelihood of a person being referred for psychiatric assessment might be affected by his or her[*] intelligence level. These limitations underscore the complexity of both screening and diagnosis, as well as the importance of involving qualified psychiatric professionals in the mental health care of the retarded.

In addition to problems associated with the diagnosis of mental illness, prevalence estimates are affected by the selection of the target population to be studied (Chess, 1970; Jacobson, 1981; Reiss, Levitan, & McNally, 1982; Schroeder et al., 1979; Stein & Susser, 1974). The majority of prevalence studies have reported data only on individuals referred to clinics for psychiatric assessment. They are not identified unless they are referred for assessment; hence, they underrepresent the population of retarded people as a whole. These studies have reported prevalence rates of mental illness among the retarded ranging from 31 to 100% (Jacobson, 1981). The wide range in results is likely due to differences in sampling and in criteria for referral and diagnosis (Reiss, Levitan, & McNally, 1982). Jacobson reported a prevalence rate of only 15% for psychiatric disorders among the mentally retarded who were receiving residential or other services from the State of New York. This lower rate, at least in part, was due to the broader sample, which extended beyond those referred for psychiatric assessment to all persons receiving state services.

Target populations are also restricted by characteristics of the people studied. Rutter found that more than one-fifth of the intellectually retarded children he studied had a psychiatric disability; however, the restricted IQ range of his retarded sample and the fact that adaptive behavior was not included in his criteria for intellectual retardation limit the generalizations of his results to his definitional criteria (Schroeder et al., 1979).

From the standpoint of researchers in the field investigating the prevalence of maladaptive behavior among the mentally retarded in state mental retardation systems, efforts to unravel the issues related to the identification of mental illness have not been successful. The value of studying diagnosed mental illness among a population of mentally retarded people is not challenged. However, at this point we have not discovered how to overcome the complexities of diagnosis, complications brought on by the multiple handicaps of the retarded, and restricted sampling procedures used in prevalence studies that require a psychiatric diagnosis.

## Maladaptive Behavior Among the Mentally Retarded

There is a soft epidemiology of behavior problems among the retarded. The literature has established that mentally retarded individuals are at significant risk of developing emotional behavioral disorders (Chess, 1970; Eyman & Call, 1977; Hill & Bruininks, 1984; Padd & Eyman, 1985; Reiss, Levitan, & McNally, 1982). While it is unclear whether or not all these behavior disorders are associated with psychiatric impairment, a number of professionals have suggested that it is more important to identify the behavioral characteristics of a retarded individual than to be concerned with particular diagnostic categories (Bialer, 1970; Schroeder et al., 1979; Szymanski & Grossman, 1984). For the most meaningful interpretation of data, we can best deal with operational definitions of observed behavior and report in that context.

It is apparent that maladaptive behavior is more prevalent among retarded residents living in institutions than in community settings (Borthwick, Meyers, & Eyman, 1981; Eyman & Borthwick, 1980; Eyman, Borthwick, & Miller, 1981; Eyman & Call, 1977). Eyman and Call, for example, found that over 50% of the institutionalized residents in their study were involved in physical violence, as compared to only 25% of individuals with similar IQs living at home or in a community facility. Similarly, Eyman and Borthwick (1980) and Hill and Bruininks (1981) found that over 60% of the institutionalized residents they studied exhibited frequent and severe maladaptive behaviors, regardless of the level of mental retardation.

Although most studies suggest that behavior problems of retarded individuals *led* to their institutionalization (Craig & McCarver, 1984; Eyman, O'Connor, Tarjan, & Justice, 1972; Keys, Boroskin, & Ross, 1973; Lakin, Krantz, Bruininks, Clumpner, & Hill, 1982; Pagel & Whitling, 1978; Schalock, Harper, & Carver, 1981; Scheerenberger, 1980; Sternlicht & Deutsch, 1972), some investigators have argued that institutions encourage the development of maladaptive behavior (Ingalls, 1978; MacMillan, 1982). In litigation involving lawsuits against institutions, expert witnesses have testified that institutional life produces maladaptive behavior (e.g., *Garrity v. Gallen*, 1979; *Parisi v. Rockefeller*, 1973; *Welsch v. Noot*, 1985). Empirical evidence does not support these claims, however. Since it is well documented that maladaptive behavior is a factor often leading to institutionalization, it is difficult to show that institutions produce maladaptive behavior over and above behavior changes that would occur in another setting (Eyman et al., 1981; Schroeder et al., 1979). Both Kushlick (1974) and Weinstock, Wulkan, Colon, Coleman, and Goncalves (1979) found no differences in rates of inappropriate behaviors for clients who had been moved from large institutions to smaller facilities. Hemming, Lavender, and Pill (1981) found that initial increases in maladaptive behavior after transfer to smaller facilities were reduced to baseline levels after four months, with the exception of self-abusive behavior, which remained at significantly higher levels for the two years of follow-up. A number of investigators have attempted to compare behavior change of clients who have been deinstitutionalized with a matched group of clients who remain in the institution; however, these studies suffer from methodological problems unless clients have randomly been assigned to placement groups (Butterfield, 1985; Conroy, Efthimiou, & Lemanowicz, 1982).

Eyman et al. (1981) statistically controlled for the preplacement maladaptive behavior of 426 retarded people admitted to institutions and community facilities in California. The results clearly indicated that no significant time trend was present for either the institutionalized or community groups, regardless of age or level of retardation. Whatever maladaptive behavior was present at the time of placement did not significantly change over a two-year period for any of the subgroups studied.

Behavior problems have also been found to discriminate among clients living in the various community settings. Borthwick, Eyman, and White (1985) recently examined the residential placements and personal characteristics of approximately 68,000 people receiving services for the retarded in California. Among a host of characteristics included in the analysis, maladaptive behavior was the variable best able to distinguish among clients in community care facilities of different sizes, institutions, foster family care, independent living, and parental homes. It was also determined that an overall score of maladaptive behavior was a more powerful predictor of placement than any single behavior problem. These findings support the earlier results of cross-sectional evaluations of clients placed in the various residential setting types in the western states (Borthwick et al., 1981; Eyman & Borthwick, 1980).

We recently reported the results of a 25-year natural history study, in which we found that behavior problems were consistently shown to be related to membership in movement groups in the residential service system (Eyman, Borthwick, & Tarjan, 1984). In a separate study, we again found that the presence of maladaptive behavior was a primary indicator of population movement groups who had been admitted and readmitted to institutions and who had been referred or released to community settings from 1982 to 1984 (Borthwick, McGuire, & Ray, 1985). The literature continues to restate the importance of reducing behavior problems to promote adjustment in less restrictive residential placements (Hill & Bruininks, 1984; Keys et al., 1973; Lakin, Hill, Hauber, Bruininks, & Heal, 1983; Landesman-Dwyer & Sulzbacher, 1981; Padd & Eyman, 1985; Pagel & Whitling, 1978; Sternlicht & Deutsch, 1972). Scheerenberger (1980) found that, regardless of level of retardation, behavior problems were ranked first among obstacles to the community placement of hospital residents, as well as first among problems causing a return to the residential facility. Jacobson and Schwartz (1983) also identified maladaptive behavior as characteristic of clients who were in jeopardy of failure in community group home facilities.

The relationship between behavior problems and level of retardation has not been clearly established. Ross (1972), and later Eyman and Call (1977) in a study of approximately 7,000 people, found that severely retarded individuals, unless handicapped by not being able to move around, exhibited more behavior problems than moderately and mildly retarded persons in institutions and community placements. Among the clients studied by Hill and Bruininks (1984), however, it was the moderately retarded group that displayed more maladaptive behavior. Hill and Bruininks further found that their results were dramatically different when certain behaviors were excluded from the data analysis. These differences illustrate the importance of taking into account the specific behaviors being examined, the severity of behaviors, sampling biases, and setting differences when interpreting results and comparing findings across studies.

## Requirements for Uniform Data Reporting Among States

I have attempted to highlight some of the ways in which behavior problem data have been useful to clinicians, researchers, and policymakers in the field of mental retardation. The importance of establishing a reliable data base with this information is generally unquestioned. However, an epidemiology of behavior problems is dependent on (1) standardized, reliable measurements, (2) comparability of prevalence rates across studies and states, and (3) availability of data on mentally retarded people.

Currently, comparisons across states and even within states are difficult to interpret because of varying operational definitions. The criteria on which society determines the behavior to be unacceptable vary considerably, making it difficult to operationalize the definitions of many problem behaviors (Hill & Bruininks, 1984). Moreover, assessment of maladaptive behavior in institutional and community settings might be confounded by the caregivers' tolerance of problem behavior, which is affected by exposure to behaviors, and by the relative severity of behaviors evinced by retarded and nonretarded peers. Critics of behavior rating scales have repeatedly stressed the importance of describing maladaptive behavior in terms of both severity and frequency of occurrence. A number of investigators have suggested that weighted scores might effectively account for the interactions of the various response components (McDevitt, McDevitt, & Rosen, 1977; Spreat, 1982; Taylor, Warren, & Slocumb, 1979), although the efficacy of weighted behavior scores has not yet been demonstrated. In any case, standardized, operational definitions are a prerequisite to meaningful prevalence data, and continued efforts to identify adequate definitions should be encouraged.

Reliability estimates of reported behavior problems are usually acceptable, yet they have been consistently lower for maladaptive than for adaptive behaviors, because of the interpretation of operational definitions, seriousness of behavior relative to peers and environment, and the subjective nature of inappropriate behavior (McDevitt et al., 1977; Nihira, Foster, Shellhaas, & Leland, 1975; Taylor et al., 1979). The quality of routine data reporting by residential care staff has also been questioned with some justification. In California, funding and staffing allocations are partly based on maladaptive behavior ratings; hence, the state recognizes the importance of staff training and audit procedures, and we are reasonably confident of the data because of this. It is imperative that rating scales undergo rigorous evaluations of reliability, as well as continuous monitoring of reporting quality.

Considerable attention has been directed toward the identification of dimensions or factors of maladaptive behavior. Widaman, Gibbs, and Geary (1987), for example, recently found that two dimensions of behavior problems (personal and social) emerged from multisample factor analyses for the severe, moderate, and mildly retarded, while only one stable dimension was meaningful for the profoundly retarded. Others have preassigned behavior items to categories (Hill & Bruininks, 1984; Taylor et al., 1979). Clearly, there are times when global scores provide more useful and reliable information than single behaviors. The identification of stable, meaningful factors of maladaptive behavior are critical to this aspect of measurement.

Meyers, Nihira, and Zetlin (1979) reported the existence of over 100 adaptive behavior scales in 1979. There are likely to be half again as many new ones developed since then. Meyers et al. (1979) suggested the marketplace should settle down eventually with the continued use of only a few of the better scales, though not just of one, since there is too great a variety in the functioning levels and applications to be covered. Our recent comparisons of factor analytic results of some of the more widely used scales lend optimistic support to the hope that the results of studies using different adaptive behavior instruments can be compared when we become sure of the relationship of these factors to one another. Considering the wide variety of scales being used in the different states, some attention will be given to this issue. Until there are standard definitions of behavior problems and comparable factors, there can be no classification of maladaptive behavior for the mentally retarded.

The few computerized state data bases that contain individualized behavior data are limited to people who are receiving services for the retarded from the state. They provide what Kushlick (1974) referred to as "administrative prevalences" rather than "true" prevalences. Administrative and true rates will be relatively similar for the more severely handicapped who most always require services from the state; however, the true prevalence of maladaptive behavior among the mildly retarded is likely to be different since a significant proportion of these people make no contact with service agencies. Nevertheless, data bases containing information on all clients receiving services from a state are a notable improvement over those that depend on referrals to clinics for psychiatric or psychological services.

Accepting these limitations as inevitable for the moment, we turn our attention to the status of data bases of served populations across the country. We recently surveyed the state mental retardation directors and learned that a very small percentage of states have computerized data bases containing comprehensive information on all retarded clients whom they serve. Schroeder et al. (1979) concluded that the prevalence of maladaptive behavior was largely unknown in community settings. Similarly, we learned from our survey that several states have been unable to collect reliable data for clients in community facilities or for those living at home. This situation will have a significant impact on studies of prevalence or other topics related to maladaptive behavior. In California, for example, 35% of retarded people served by the state live in community facilities and over 50% live with their parents or relatives. No longer can studies of client behavior rely on data from institutionalized samples or on groups of retarded people who are receiving psychiatric or psychological assistance from clinics. A significant proportion of those who live outside the institution may never be referred for any kind of psychiatric assessment, yet the problem behaviors they manifest should not be overlooked in examinations of observed behavior that can seriously affect a person's chances of living in a less restrictive environment, as well as affecting his or her overall quality of life.

We also learned from our survey that a number of states either do not include adaptive and maladaptive behavior information in their computerized systems or are using checklists that have not been tested for reliability and validity. Instruments that have not been examined for these properties are essentially of no use to agencies using the data, although they may not realize or acknowledge the limitations involved. Furthermore, it is extremely important to identify the measures that are currently used in the different states and to establish a comparability of nomenclature and classification across states.

In the 1970s, there appeared to be a commitment by the federal government to improve and make compatible the reporting of client information by state mental retardation departments. For example, during the funding period for the Individualized Data Base (IDB) Project (Grossman & Eyman, 1980), 11 states annually reported scores on a version of the AAMD Adaptive Behavior Scale (as well as demographic, diagnostic, and service data), demonstrating the feasibility and usefulness of a computerized, standardized reporting system. Experience with the IDB Project revealed a number of issues related to the coordination of data collection. Overall, it became clear that the challenge was to make data compatible across states and agencies by modifying ongoing systems without mandating specialized procedures and instruments that were required *in addition* to existing state reporting systems.

The funding for the IDB Project was terminated once it had been demonstrated that states could collect and report client information and once a core set of variables for uniform reporting had been identified. It was never the intent of the IDB Project to become a data processing service for the 50 states. However, it would seem that the next step might be a federal coordination of state efforts to monitor and assist in the development of computerized reporting systems among the states and to establish a standard nomenclature of behaviors and other variables to ensure consistency of reporting to nationally sponsored projects and agencies.

Federal agencies have continued to express interest in knowing the prevalence of maladaptive behaviors and the relationship of problem behavior to other variables by supporting such projects as the Developmental Disabilities Project on Residential Services and Community Adjustments at the University of Minnesota and Scheerenberger's (1977, 1980, 1982) surveys of clients living in communities and public residential facilities. The kind of information reported by states for these studies should be easily accessible and compatible with operational definitions required by national surveys.

More than half of the states in our 1985 survey reported that their computerized data bases had been implemented since 1980. This recent activity is encouraging and underscores the importance and timeliness of addressing issues of measurement and comparability in these developing systems.

Russell (Chapter 3) suggests we move away from the simple measurement of behavior problems to include the diagnosis of specific psychiatric disorders. Currently, however, psychiatric assessments of all persons identified by state mental retardation systems are not done, for very practical reasons, and screening by direct-care staff or other trained persons may not be adequate. If at some point in the future these data could become available, the knowledge of relationships among diagnostic categories of mental illness, maladaptive behaviors, and other characteristics of individual and environment would contribute significantly to the treatment and care of the mentally retarded. This would, of course, depend on reliable identification of psychiatric disorders, even among the severely and profoundly retarded with their confounding handicaps and disabilities.

The definitional and other problems associated with measuring maladaptive behavior must be resolved. The work of Bruininks, Hill, and Morreau (Chapter 1) and others (e.g., Widaman et al., 1987) represent positive steps in this direction. With continued research and administrative support, as suggested by Mandersheid, Wurster, Rosenstein, and Witkin (Chapter 5), the epidemiology of behavior problems among the mentally retarded can be improved significantly in the not too distant future. Moreover, with proper planning, reliable and compatible data on observed behaviors can become available at a national level.

## References

Alford, J.D., & Locke, B.J. (1984). Clinical responses to psychopathology of mentally retarded persons. *American Journal of Mental Deficiency, 89*(2), 195–197.

Bialer, I. (1970). Emotional disturbance and mental retardation: Etiologic and conceptual relationships. In F.J. Menolascino (Ed.), *Psychiatric approaches to mental retardation.* New York: Basic Books.

Borthwick, S.A., Eyman, R.K., & White, J.F. (1985). *Client characteristics and residential placement patterns.* Paper presented at the annual meeting of the American Association on Mental Deficiency, Philadelphia.

Borthwick, S.A., McGuire, M., & Ray, E. (1985). Factors that affect deinstitutionalization of the mentally retarded. In A.B. Silverstein & A. Fluharty (Eds.), *Pacific State archives* (Vol. X). Pomona, CA: UCLA-MRRC Lanterman Developmental Center Research Group.

Borthwick, S.A., Meyers, C.E., & Eyman, R.K. (1981). Comparative adaptive and maladaptive behavior of mentally retarded clients of five residential settings in three western states. In R.H. Bruininks, C.E. Meyers, B.B. Sigford, & K.C. Lakin, (Eds.), *Deinstitutionalization and community adjustment of mentally retarded people* (Monograph #4). Washington, DC: American Association on Mental Deficiency.

Butterfield, E.C. (1985). The consequence of bias in studies of living arrangements for the mentally retarded adult. In D. Bricker & J. Filler (Eds.), *Severe mental retardation: From theory to practice.* Lancaster, PA: Lancaster Press.

Chess, S. (1970). Emotional problems in mentally retarded children. In F.J. Menolascino (Ed.), *Psychiatric approaches to mental retardation.* New York: Basic Books.

Conroy, J. Efthimiou, J., & Lemanowicz, J. (1982). A matched comparison of the developmental growth of institutionalized and deinstitutionalized mentally retarded adults. *American Journal of Mental Deficiency, 86,* 581–587.

Craig, E.M., & McCarver, R.B. (1984). Community placement and adjustment of deinstitutionalized clients: Issues and findings. In N.R. Ellis & N. Bray (Eds.), *International review of research in mental retardation* (Vol. 12). Orlando, FL: Academic Press.

Eyman, R.K., & Borthwick, S.A. (1980). Patterns of care for mentally retarded persons. *Mental Retardation, 18,* 63–66.

Eyman, R.K., Borthwick, S.A., & Miller, C. (1981). Trends in maladaptive behavior of mentally retarded persons placed in community and institutional settings. *American Journal of Mental Deficiency, 85,* 473–477.

Eyman, R.K., Borthwick, S.A., & Tarjan, G. (1984). Current trends and changes in institutions for the mentally retarded. In N. Ellis & N. Bray (Eds.), *International review of research in mental retardation* (Vol. 12). Orlando, FL: Academic Press.

Eyman, R.K., & Call, T. (1977). Maladaptive behavior and community placement of mentally retarded persons. *American Journal of Mental Deficiency, 82,* 137–144.

Eyman, R.K., O'Connor, G., Tarjan, G., & Justice, R.S. (1972). Factors determining residential placement of mentally retarded children. *American Journal of Mental Deficiency, 76,* 692–698.

*Garrity v. Gallen* (1979). State of New Hampshire.

Grossman, H.G., & Eyman, R.K. (1980). *Individualized data base project.* Washington, DC: Administration on Developmental Disabilities, DHHS Office of Human Development, Grant No. 54-P-71117/9, Final Project Report.

Hemming, H., Lavender, T., & Pill, R. (1981). Quality of life of mentally retarded adults transferred from large institutions to new small units. *American Journal of Mental Deficiency, 86,* 157–169.

Hill, B.K., & Bruininks, R.H. (1981). *Physical and behavioral characteristics and maladaptive behavior of mentally retarded people in residential facilities.* Minneapolis, MN: University of Minnesota, Department of Psychoeducational Studies.

Hill, B.K., & Bruininks, R.H. (1984). Maladaptive behavior of mentally retarded individuals in residential facilities. *American Journal of Mental Deficiency, 88*, 380–387.

Ingalls, R.P. (1978). *Mental retardation: The changing outlook.* New York: Wiley.

Jacobson, J.W. (1981). *Problem behavior and psychiatric impairment within a developmentally disabled population* (OMRDD Technical Monograph #81-02). New York: Office of Mental Retardation and Developmental Disabilities.

Jacobson, J.W., & Schwartz, A.A. (1983). Personal and service characteristics affecting group home placement success: A prospective analysis. *Mental Retardation, 21*, 1–17.

Keys, V., Boroskin, A., & Ross, R. (1973). The revolving door in an MR hospital: A study of returns from leave. *Mental Retardation, 11*, 55–56.

Kushlick, A. (1974). Epidemiology and evaluation of services for the mentally handicapped. In M.J. Begab & S.A. Richardson (Eds.), *The mentally retarded and society: A social science perspective.* Baltimore, MD: University Park Press.

Lakin, K., Hill, B., Hauber, F., Bruininks, R., & Heal, L. (1983). New admissions and readmissions to a national sample of public residential facilities. *American Journal of Mental Deficiency, 88*, 13–20.

Lakin, K.C., Krantz, G.C., Bruininks, R.H., Clumpner, J.L., & Hill, B.K. (1982). One hundred years of data on populations of public residential facilities for mentally retarded people. *American Journal of Mental Deficiency, 87*, 1–8.

Landesman-Dwyer, S., & Sulzbacher, F. (1981). Residential placement and adaptation of severely and profoundly retarded individuals. In R.H. Bruininks, C.E. Meyers, B.B. Sigford, & K.C. Lakin (Eds.), *Deinstitutionalization and community adjustment of mentally retarded people.* Washington, DC: American Association on Mental Deficiency.

MacMillan, D.L. (1982). *Mental retardation in school and society.* Boston, MA: Little, Brown & Co.

McDevitt, S., McDevitt, S., & Rosen, M. (1977). Adaptive Behavior Scale Part II: A cautionary note and some suggestions for revision. *American Journal of Mental Deficiency, 82*, 210–212.

Meyers, C.E., Nihira, D., & Zetlin, A. (1979). The measurement of adaptive behavior. In N.R. Ellis (Ed.), *Handbook of mental deficiency, psychological theory and research.* Hillsdale, NJ: Lawrence Erlbaum Associates.

Nihira, K., Foster, R., Shellhaas, M., & Leland, H. (1975). *Manual for AAMD adaptive behavior scale.* Washington, DC: American Journal on Mental Deficiency.

Padd, W.S., & Eyman, R.K. (1985). Mental retardation aggression: Epidemiologic concerns and implications for deinstitutionalization. In A.F. Ashman & R.S. Laura (Eds.), *The education and training of the mentally retarded.* New York: Nichols Publishing Company.

Pagel, S.E., & Whitling, C.A. (1978). Readmissions to a state hospital for mentally retarded persons: Reasons for community placement failure. *Mental Retardation, 16*, 164–166.

*Parisi v. Rockefeller.* (1973). New York State.

Reiss, S., Levitan, G.W., & McNally, R.J. (1982). Emotionally disturbed mentally retarded people: An undeserved population. *American Psychologist, 37*, 361–367.

Reiss, S., Levitan, G.W., & Szyszko, J. (1982). Emotional disturbance and mental retardation: Diagnostic overshadowing. *American Journal of Mental Deficiency, 86*, 567–574.

Ross, R.T. (1972). Behavioral correlates of levels of intelligence. *American Journal of Mental Deficiency, 76*, 545–549.

Rutter, M., & Graham, P. (1970). Epidemiology of psychiatric disorder. In M. Rutter, J. Tizard, & K. Whitmore (Eds.), *Education, health and behavior.* London: Longman Group Ltd.

Schalock, R., Harper, R.S., & Carver, G. (1981). Independent living placement: Five years later. *American Journal of Mental Deficiency, 85*, 170–177.

Scheerenberger, R.C. (1977). *Current trends and status of public residential facilities for the mentally retarded, 1976.* Madison, WI: National Association of Superintendents of Public Residential Facilities for the Mentally Retarded.

Scheerenberger, R.C. (1980). *Community programs and services.* Madison, WI: National Association of Superintendents of Public Residential Facilities for the Mentally Retarded.

Scheerenberger, R.C. (1982). *Public residential services for the mentally retarded, 1981.* Minneapolis, MN: University of Minnesota, Department of Psychoeducational Studies.

Schroeder, S.R., Mulick, J.A., & Schroeder, C.S. (1979). Management of severe behavior problems of the retarded. In N.R. Ellis (Ed.), *Handbook of mental deficiency, psychological theory and research.* Hillsdale, NJ: Lawrence Erlbaum Associates.

Spreat, S. (1982). An empirical analysis of item weighting on the Adaptive Behavior Scale. *American Journal of Mental Deficiency, 87*, 159–163.

Stein, Z., & Susser, M. (1974). Public health and mental retardation: New power and new problems. In M.J. Begab & S.A. Richardson (Eds.), *The mentally retarded and society: A social science perspective.* Baltimore, MD: University Park Press.

Sternlicht, M., & Deutsch, M.R. (1972). *Personality development and social behavior in the mentally retarded.* Lexington, MA: D.C. Heath & Co.

Szymanski, L., & Grossman, H. (1984). Dual implications of "dual diagnosis." *Mental Retardation, 22*, 155–156.

Tarjan, G. (1977). Mental retardation and clinical psychiatry. In P. Mittler (Ed.), *Research to practice in mental retardation: Care and intervention* (Vol. I). Baltimore, MD: University Park Press.

Taylor, R.L., Warren, S.A., & Slocumb, P.R. (1979). Categorizing behavior in terms of severity: Considerations for Part II of the Adaptive Behavior Scale. *American Journal of Mental Deficiency, 83*, 411–413.

Weinstock, A., Wulkan, P., Colon, C.J., Coleman, J., & Goncalves, S. (1979). Stress inoculation and interinstitutional transfer of mentally retarded individuals. *American Journal of Mental Deficiency, 83*, 385–390.

*Welsh v. Noot.* (1985). State of Wisconsin.

Widaman, K.F., Gibbs, K.W., & Geary, D. (1987). The structure of adaptive behavior: I. Replication across 14 samples of mildly, moderately, and severely retarded people. *American Journal of Mental Deficiency, 91*, 348–360.

# 3

# The Association Between Mental Retardation and Psychiatric Disorder: Epidemiological Issues

ANDREW T. RUSSELL

It is well known that mentally retarded individuals are at risk for the development of a wide variety of emotional and behavioral disorders (Matson & Barrett, 1982; Sigman, 1985; Szymanski & Tanguay, 1980). The magnitude and importance of this problem have been emphasized by two relatively recent trends. The first has been the deinstitutionalization and "mainstreaming" of retarded persons. The second has been the development of separate service delivery systems for the developmentally disabled and mentally ill. These two trends in health care have contributed to the growing realization that a significant proportion of developmentally disabled individuals have coexisting psychiatric disorders. Besides "falling between the cracks" of the separate health care systems, these individuals have exposed the fact that many professionals in both systems have serious gaps in their training and skills (Cushna, Szymanski, & Tanguay, 1980).

In the last two decades, it has also become clear that carefully designed epidemiological research addressing this strong association between mental illness and mental retardation has been limited in quality and that many studies have been plagued with major methodological problems.

One such problem is how to define mental retardation. The criteria used to make the diagnosis of mental retardation can produce dramatic differences in the measured prevalence (Mercer, 1973; Tarjan, Wright, Eyman, & Keeran, 1973). For example, it is critical whether mental retardation is defined in purely psychometric terms or includes a dimension of adaptive behavior. Rutter (1970) has gently argued that using adaptive behavior criteria to select a retarded population will produce spuriously high rates for behavioral and psychiatric disorder. Other important variables related to the measured prevalence of mental retardation are age, socioeconomic status, degree of handicap, and the mutability of tested intelligence (Russell, 1985). Much epidemiological research has failed to account properly for these variables.

A second major issue is the tremendous heterogeneity of the retarded population. Many studies have simply lumped together all individuals with an IQ less than 70 as their research population. The fact that two individuals (one mildly retarded and one severely retarded) are dramatically different in almost every dimension is often not appropriately dealt with in research designs.

A third problem has been that most research has dealt with institutionalized or referred subjects, samples that are hardly representative of the general population of retarded individuals. This is particularly true of research examining psychiatric disorders.

Finally, and perhaps most important of all, is the issue of psychiatric diagnosis itself. Diagnostic criteria, of known or unknown reliability, have varied dramatically from study to study. This is over and above the issue of whether standardized assessment was part of the research design and the very real clinical and research problems of identifying symptoms and disorders within this population.

Keeping these four major problem areas in mind (and the fact that there are many others), we examine three basic epidemiological questions, summarize what we do know about the answers to each question, and relate the above problems to what differing results have been obtained. Finally, some recommendations for future epidemiological research are presented.

The three basic epidemiological questions to be considered are deceptively simple.

1. What is the prevalence of psychiatric disorder in mentally handicapped individuals?
2. Are specific *types* of psychiatric disorders associated with mental retardation?
3. What are some of the mechanisms that may underlie the association between retardation and psychiatric disorders?

This selective review focuses on studies involving children and adolescents and refers frequently to a series of studies conducted by Rutter and his colleagues on the Isle of Wight in England (Rutter, Graham, & Yule, 1970; Rutter, Tizard, & Whitmore, 1970; Rutter, Tizard, Yule, Graham, & Whitmore, 1976).

The Isle of Wight study, although conducted more than 20 years ago, deserves a brief description. It probably remains our single best source of information on the association between mental illness and mental retardation in childhood and attempts to address and actually study some of the methodological problems referred to previously. The Isle of Wight study avoided some of the problems of sampling bias by studying an entire age cohort—that of 9, 10, and 11 year olds. The age cohort design allowed comparisons between retarded children and the nonhandicapped peers. The study of psychiatric disorder was a two-stage design, employing in the first stage screening questionnaires when obtaining psychiatric symptom ratings from both teachers and parents. In the second stage, an intensive psychiatric assessment was conducted with direct interviews and the collection of other measures. All assessment techniques were studied for reliability and validity. A comprehensive range of assessments were obtained from a variety of sources including both parents and teachers. The wide range of assessments allowed examination of important associated factors such as neurological and educational handicaps. In regard to cognitive functioning, children were classified on the basis of measured IQ. Thus, the results from the Isle of Wight should not automatically be interpreted as applying to individuals class-

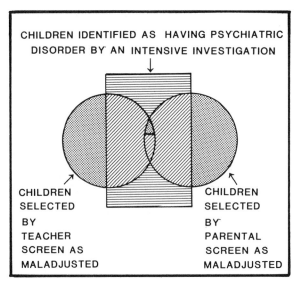

FIGURE 3.1. Representation of the relationship of the teacher screen, parental screen, and intensive investigation in the multistage–multimethod procedure used by Rutter and his colleagues. From "Estimating the Prevalence of Childhood Psychopathology" by M. Schwartz-Gould, et al., 1981, *Journal of the American Academy of Child Psychiatry, 20*, p. 469. Copyright 1981 by the American Academy of Child Psychiatry. Adapted by permission.

ified as mentally retarded using DSM-III or AAMD criteria, which use a dimension of adaptive behavior.

The importance of an epidemiological design using more than one stage and more than one source of information is shown in Figure 3.1. The figure illustrates in graphic form the estimated prevalence of psychiatric disorder among all children in the Isle of Wight study and from a subsequent study in London using a similar methodology. The parental screening questionnaire and the teacher screening questionnaire identified approximately equal numbers of children but they were not the same children! In addition, only about half the children identified by screening were later confirmed by intensive investigation to exhibit a psychiatric disorder. Finally, the screening procedures missed a significant number of children who on direct examination were found to have psychiatric disorder (false negative). These are all important findings that must be kept in mind when evaluating the methodologies of studies reporting prevalence figures for psychiatric disorders among persons with mental retardation.

The prevalence of psychiatric disorders in the total population of 9, 10, and 11 year olds on the Isle of Wight was found to be about 7%. In contrast, the rate of psychiatric disorders in children with IQs less than 70 was 30% based on parental report and 42% based on teacher report with similar rates on direct interviews (Rutter, 1970; Rutter, et al., 1970). Thus, psychiatric disorder was found to be over four times more frequent in intellectually retarded children than in children with normal intelligence. Recently, the Isle of Wight results have been more or less confirmed by a longitudinal birth cohort study by Koller, Richardson, and colleagues, which has followed a sample of all retarded individuals born during a five-year period in a British city (Koller, Richardson, Katz, & McLaren, 1982). Overall rates of behavioral disturbance were 2.5 times greater than a matched control group and severe behavior problems were seven times more frequent. Other studies, generally based on selected or referred samples, including work by Phillips and Williams (1975), Chess (1970), Jacobson 1982), Szymanski (1980), and others, have reported rates of psychiatric disorder varying from 10 to 80%. Rates for adult populations may be comparable or somewhat higher than for children (Reiss, 1985; Lund, 1985). In short, depending on issues of sample selection and definitions of disorder, a population of mentally retarded individuals may exhibit rates of behavioral and emotional disorders averaging between 20 and 40% – all significantly higher than a comparable population of individuals of normal intellect.

A related question is the relationship between differing levels of IQ and psychiatric disorder. An interesting finding from the Isle of Wight studies was that the association between behavioral disturbance (almost all types) and intellectual functioning held for higher as well as lower levels of IQ. For example, Table 3.1 summarizes teacher ratings for the items "miserable," fighting, and poor concentration for boys at five different IQ levels (from Rutter, 1970; Russell, 1985). It can be seen that the frequency of behavioral deviance is inversely related to IQ and this relationship holds at all IQ levels in an almost linear fashion. Studies that have examined similar symptoms at different levels within the retarded range have reached generally similar conclusions (Jacobson, 1982). As IQ level drops, the level of severity of most types of behavioral disturbance increases. However, the pattern of actual symptoms may vary considerably. For example, sterotypies and self-injurious behavior are more common in severely retarded than mildly retarded individuals (Corbett 1977; Jacobson 1982).

This finding leads to the second basic question. Are certain *types* of psychiatric disorder more prevalent in persons with mental retardation as opposed to

TABLE 3.1. Relationship of behavior to IQ in boys (teacher ratings – % of sample).

| | IQ | | | |
|---|---|---|---|---|
| Symptom | <79 | 80–99 | 100–119 | >120 |
| "Miserable" | 20 | 11 | 6 | 3 |
| Fighting | 26 | 17 | 11 | 5 |
| Poor concentration | 76 | 50 | 30 | 11 |

*Note*: The data are from M. Rutter 1970, Psychiatry. In J. Wortis (Ed.), *Mental Retardation, An Annual Review* (Vol. 3). New York: Grune & Stratton. Copyright 1970 by Grune & Stratton. Adapted by permission.

individuals of normal intelligence? Is there a specific psychopathology of mental retardation? The majority of the evidence suggests that the types of psychiatric disorders seen in retarded individuals do not differ in kind from those seen in the general population (Phillips & Williams, 1975; Reid, 1980). While evaluating the research in this area, however, several cautions must be noted. It is difficult to compare the results from different studies because of the lack of consistency in diagnostic criteria between studies. In the United States, earlier studies used DSM-I or DSM-II criteria and only recently have the more specific criteria of DSM-III been applied (American Psychiatric Association, 1980). In Great Britain, recent studies have used criteria developed by Rutter and colleagues for the World Health Organization (Rutter, Shaffer, & Shepherd, 1975). There are many differences between these diagnostic systems and other researchers have developed their own diagnostic categories.

Another important consideration in reviewing research in this area is, once again, the heterogeneity of the retarded population. There is considerable evidence that more severely handicapped individuals (IQs less than 50) may exhibit somewhat different types of psychiatric disorder than individuals in the mild range of mental retardation. Corbett reported findings from a large epidemiological study based on 175,000 residents of the Camberwell district of London (Corbett, Harris, & Robinson, 1975; Corbett, 1977). This study only looked at individuals with IQs less than 50 and used a methodology similar to the Isle of Wight.

In their sample, psychosis (including autism) was diagnosed in 17% of the children, hyperkinetic disorders in 4%, and severe stereotypes in 10%. Only 4% of the sample were diagnosed as having a neurotic disorder and only 4% as having a conduct disorder. This pattern of disorder is considerably different from that found in most studies of children predominantly in the mildly retarded range and in the general population. Of particular note are the high prevalence rates of childhood psychosis, hyperkinetic disorders (as diagnosed in Great Britain), and severe sterotypies in the severely retarded children.

Having established that psychiatric disorder is more common in mentally retarded children and adolescents and that a wide variety of nonspecific disorders is seen in this population (with the exception of the more severely retarded), the third and final basic question is what mechanisms underlie the strong association? The answer to this question is complex and at best the evidence is incomplete. As may be expected from the fact that such a broad spectrum of psychiatric disorders is seen in the retarded and that the retarded themselves are such a heterogeneous group, it is clear that there are multiple factors involved. Figure 3.2 addresses this issue by summarizing some of the epidemiological data relating to psychiatric disorder in children and adolescents.

As described previously, the rate of psychiatric disorder in a mentally retarded population may be four to five times greater than in the general population (Rutter, 1970). Another finding from the Isle of Wight is that children with a chronic physical disorder (e.g., asthma) may be twice as likely to develop behavioral and

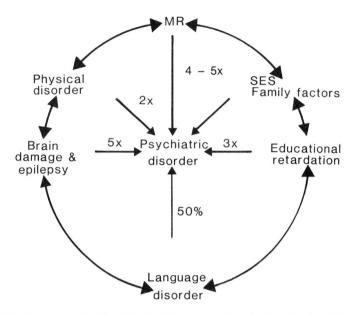

FIGURE 3.2. Summary of epidemiological data on psychiatric disorders in children and adolescents. From "The Mentally Retarded, Emotionally Disturbed Child and Adolescent" by A.T. Russell, 1985. In M. Sigman (Ed.), *Children with Emotional Disorders and Developmental Disabilities: Assessment and Treatment*, p. 130. Orlando, FL: Grune & Stratton. Adapted by permission.

emotional disorder; and, if the central nervous system is involved (e.g., epilepsy), the rate more than doubles (Rutter, Graham, & Yule, 1970). Cantwell and Baker (1980) have found that in an unselected population of children with language disorder half meet DSM-III criteria for a psychiatric disorder. The Isle of Wight and a similar study of London children found that reading retardation (over two years behind on standardized tests, adjusted for IQ) was associated with increased rates of psychiatric disorder, particularly of the conduct type (Rutter et al, 1976). It is well known that socioeconomic and family factors are strongly associated with psychiatric disorders although it is difficult to assign numerical risks to these factors.

Looking at these associations from the other direction, and particularly from the viewpoint of mental retardation, only confirms the importance of all these factors. It is not uncommon that retarded children have other disorders of the central nervous system. Many have language handicaps or learning disabilities beyond their cognitive limitations and are likely to come from lower socioeconomic backgrounds. It is likely that any combination of these factors in a single child greatly increases the risk of development or associated psychiatric disorders.

One implication of these findings is that future epidemiological research, if it is to be helpful in elucidating these (and other) mechanisms, must include measures and methodologies that will allow them to be assessed. For example, an epidemiological study of psychiatric disorder in the retarded could include an independent assessment of language disorder in order to understand this association better.

What lessons can be learned from this brief review in regard to future epidemiological and clinical research? Several issues stand out.

1. Of critical importance is the use of well-defined diagnostic criteria with appropriate measurement of diagnostic reliability. DSM-III with its multiaxial structure is a logical choice and can be applied successfully to the majority of retarded persons. A multiaxial system is probably best able to capture the complexity of these cases. If modification of criteria is required, it should be held to a minimum, be straightforward, and be described clearly. If new and unfamiliar criteria are developed, comparability with other studies of psychopathology will be almost impossible.

2. Hand in hand with the first recommendation is the need to use some of the standardized diagnostic tools (again modified only with great caution) now being used in modern epidemiological research with nonretarded subjects. These include structured or semistructured diagnostic interviews and rating scales. For example, the Beck Depression Inventory has been used successfully in a mildly retarded adolescent population (Beck, Carlson, Russell, & Brownfield, 1987) and in an adult population (Kazdin, Matson, & Senatore, 1983) with considerable success. The use of structured interviews and other similar tools with the retarded need to be evaluated as soon as possible. Examples of recent efforts in this direction are the PIMRA interview (Matson, Kazdin, & Senatore, 1984) and the Aberrant Behavior Checklist (Aman, Singh, Stewart, & Field, 1985).

3. The time has come to move away from just the measurement of behavior problems and toward the ascertainment of the presence or absence of specific psychiatric disorders. Every effort should be made in future research to use methodologies that lead to specific psychiatric diagnoses. It is one thing to describe a subject as sad and withdrawn and another to obtain enough reliable data to make a diagnosis of major affective disorder according to specific diagnostic criteria. It is only with this approach that we will be able to investigate specific treatment interventions for specific disorders.

4. We need to use great care not to confound problems in adaptive behavior with psychiatric disturbance and vice versa. How we do this will affect the selection and diagnosis of a retarded sample.

5. Sample sizes must be large enough to analyze separately data depending on the level of retardation. The developmentally disabled are different in more ways than they are alike, and these differences must be accounted for in any research design.

It is of course not enough, even with improved research designs, simply to add to the quantitative statistics concerning the association of mental retardation and psychiatric disorders. Multidimensional studies are needed to examine such variables as institutional versus home care, risk and protective factors, family factors, and treatment interventions. With an increased knowledge base from such research efforts, we may be better able to meet the complex needs of the underserved population of persons with both developmental disabilities and psychiatric disorders.

## References

Aman, M.G., Singh, N.N., Stewart, A.W., & Field, C.J. (1985). The aberrant behavior checklist: A behavior rating scale for the assessment of treatment effects. *American Journal of Mental Deficiency, 89*,(5), 485–491.

American Psychiatric Association. (1980). *Diagnostic and Statistical Manual of Mental Disorders* (3rd ed.). Washington, DC: Author.

Beck, D., Carlson, G., Russell, A., & Brownfield, F. (1987). Use of depression rating instruments in developmentally and educationally delayed adolescents. *Journal of the American Academy of Child Psychiatry, 26*, 97–100.

Cantwell, D.P., & Baker, L. (1980). Psychiatric and behavioral characteristics of children with communication disorders. *Journal of Pediatric Psychology, 5*, 161–178.

Chess, S. (1970). Emotional problems in mentally retarded children. In F.J. Menolascino (Ed.), *Psychiatric approaches to mental retardation*. New York: Basic Books.

Corbett, J.A. (1977). Populations studies of mental retardation. In P.J. Graham (Ed.), *Epidemiological approaches in child psychiatry*. London: Academic Press.

Corbett, J.A., Harris, E., & Robinson, R. (1975). Epilepsy. In J. Wortis (Ed.), *Retardation and developmental disabilities, VII*. New York: Brunner/Mazel.

Cushna, B., Szymanski, L.S., & Tanguay, P.E. (1980). Professional roles and unmet manpower needs. In L.S. Szymanski & P.E. Tanguay (Eds.), *Emotional disorders of mentally retarded persons*. Baltimore, MD: University Park Press.

Jacobson, J.W. (1982). Problem behavior and psychiatric impairment within a developmentally disabled population: Behavior frequency. *Applied Research in Mental Retardation, 3*, 121–139.

Kazdin, A., Matson, J., & Senatore, V. (1983). Assessment of depression in mentally retarded adults. *American Journal of Psychiatry, 140*, 1040–1043.

Koller, H., Richardson, S.A., Katz, M., & McLaren, J. (1982). Behavior disturbance in childhood and the early adult years in populations who were and were not mentally retarded. *Journal of Preventive Psychiatry, 1*, 453–468.

Lund, J. (1985). The prevalence of psychiatric morbidity in mentally retarded adults. *Acta Psychiatrica Scandinavia, 72*, 563–570.

Matson, J.L., & Barrett, R.P. (1982). *Psychopathology in the mentally retarded*. New York: Grune & Stratton.

Matson, J.L, Kazdin, A.E., & Senatore, V. (1984). Psychometric properties of the psychopathology instrument for mentally retarded adults. *Applied Research in Mental Retardation, 5*, 81–89.

Mercer, J.R. (1973). *Labeling the mentally retarded: Clinical and social systems perspectives on mental retardation*. Berkeley, CA: University of California.

Phillips, I., & Williams, N. (1975). Psychopathology and mental retardation: A study of 100 mentally retarded children: I. Psychopathology. *American Journal of Psychiatry, 132*, 1265–1271.

Reid, A.H. (1980). Psychiatric disorders in mentally handicapped children: A clinical and follow-up study. *Journal of Mental Deficiency Research, 24*, 267–298.

Reiss, S. (1985). The mentally retarded, emotionally disturbed adult. In M. Sigman (Ed.), *Children with emotional disorders and developmental disabilities: Assessment and Treatment*. Orlando, FL: Grune & Stratton.

Russell, A.T. (1985). The mentally retarded, emotionally disturbed child and adolescent. In M. Sigman (Ed.), *Children with emotional disorders and developmental disabilities: Assessment and Treatment* (pp. 111–135). Orlando, FL: Grune & Stratton.

Rutter, M. (1970). Psychiatry. In J. Wortis, (Ed.), *Mental retardation: An annual review* (Vol. 3). New York: Grune & Stratton.

Rutter, M., Graham, P., & Yule, W. (1970). *A neuropsychiatric study in childhood*. London: Spastics International Medical Publications and Heinemann.

Rutter, M., Schaffer, D., & Shepherd, M. (1975). *A multiaxial classification of child psychiatric disorders*. Geneva: World Health Organization.

Rutter, M., Tizard, J., & Whitmore, K. (Eds.). (1970). *Education, health and behavior*. London: Longmans.

Rutter, M., Tizard, J., Yule, W., Graham, P., & Whitmore, K. (1976). Research report: Isle of Wight studies, 1964–74. *Psychological Medicine, 6*, 313–332.

Schwartz-Gould, M., Wunsch-Hitzig, R., & Dohrenwald, B. (1981). Estimating the prevalence of childhood psychopathology. *Journal of the American Academy of Child Psychiatry, 20*, 462–476.

Sigman, M. (Ed.). (1985). *Children with emotional disorders and developmental disabilities: Assessment and Treatment*. Orlando, FL: Grune & Stratton.

Szymanski, L.S. (1980). Psychiatric diagnosis of retarded persons. In L.S. Szymanski & P.E. Tanguay (Eds.), *Emotional disorders of mentally retarded persons*. Baltimore, MD: University Park Press.

Szymanski, L.S., & Tanguay, P.E. (Eds.). (1980). *Emotional disorders of mentally retarded persons*. Baltimore, MD: University Park Press.

Tarjan, G., Wright, S.W., Eyman, R.K., & Keeran, C.V. (1973). Natural history of mental retardation: Some aspects of epidemiology. *American Journal of Mental Deficiency, 77*, 369–379.

# 4
# The Need for a National Epidemiological Study

KEITH G. SCOTT

## Need

In the introduction to this section, Dr. Borthwick succinctly points out that unless we have good, reliable data—via epidemiological studies—we cannot conduct meaningful studies on which we can make astute decisions. It has been demonstrated repeatedly in the previous three chapters of this section that we do not have a universally agreed-upon methodology or data base on both the measurement and classification of either mental retardation or mental illness. Imagine the complexity of the issue when combining these two areas to focus our attention on the epidemiological aspects of this difficult-to-serve subpopulation.

The purpose of this chapter is to highlight briefly the problems we face in conducting these epidemiological studies and to provide a model design on how we can implement an epidemiological analysis of the mentally retarded and mentally ill populations that are demanding of our attention for comprehensive services.

## Problem

The tools of modern epidemiology have not been applied systematically to the problems of mental retardation and coexisting problems of mental health. There are at least two reasons for this. First, those persons who have worked in these areas are either self-taught epidemiologists, like this author, or they have had no formal training in mental retardation. Training in both areas has simply not been readily available and is essential if the field is to mature. Second, as Mausner and Kramer (1985) point out, it is only in the past 20 years that the epidemiological methodology necessary to study chronic disorders such as coronary diseases, cancer, and mental retardation has been developed. The essential point is that the highly prevalent milder forms of mental retardation are not disease entities with single-agent causes as are many infectious diseases. Chronic disorders such as hypertension and mental retardation are defined using arbitrarily assigned scores and may be thought of as treatment categories rather than discrete diseases. As a result, it is necessary to describe individuals who have scores or values that lie both inside and outside the abnormal range so that the consequences of treatment and nontreatment can be determined empirically. At present, the definition of mental retardation contained in the AAMD and DSM-III classification system are an arbitrary set of categories that are the best that could be achieved in the absence of systematic descriptive information.

A similar set of problems has plagued child and adolescent psychopathology. While DSM-III (Diagnostic and Statistical Manual of Mental Disorders III of the American Psychiatric Association) and its revised edition DSM-III-R were prepared with research diagnostic criteria for adults, similar data were not available for children. The reader is referred to Rutter and Shaffer (1980), Achenbach (1980), and Quay (1986) for further discussion of the DSM-III for child populations. Fortunately, Achenbach, Ashikga, Quay, and Conners are currently engaged in a national probability home interview survey using a checklist derived from separate instruments previously developed by Achenbach (1979), Conners (Goyette, Conners, & Ulrich, 1978), and Quay and Peterson (1983). By being based on a national quota sample, this survey will provide a much better basis for the classification of conduct and emotional disorders. In the meantime, estimates of the prevalence of mental retardation and of those who are classified as both mentally retarded and mentally ill can be little better than informed guesses. Russel (1985; and in Chapter 3 of this book) has made an excellent point in that for a person to be classified as mentally retarded and mentally ill (Grossman, 1983), the individual must meet the AAMD criteria (subintellectual functioning, diminished adaptive behaviors, and manifestation during the developmental period) and display maladaptive behavior. Thus, by definition, the mentally retarded population will include more individuals with mental health problems than would a random sample from the general population. In essence, the current estimates of the prevalence of mental retardation and mental health problems are determined via arbitrary definitions using the best information available but conducted in the absence of appropriate descriptive epidemiology.

Most researchers in mental retardation have been concerned that there is no precise data on the prevalence of this developmental disability. This is due not only to the definitional problems outlined above but also to the fact that data have never been collected systematically on a sample of individuals that was a true representation of the U.S. population.

Previous attempts to describe the prevalence of persons with mental retardation have suffered one or both of two serious flaws. First, they have relied on existing case files of persons already diagnosed—thus leaving no objective record of those who have not been diagnosed. Second, the populations studied have been either arbitrary or restricted to a single locale such as an institution. In summary, the existing knowledge is flawed by inadequate sampling from nonrepresentative populations, and the descriptive data are fragmented and partial at best.

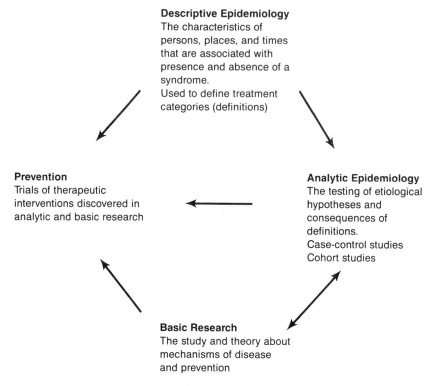

FIGURE 4.1. The epidemiological study cycle.

## Model Design

Valid epidemiological research requires that sound, unbiased descriptive data be collected as the cornerstone of research on the definition, causes, treatment, and basic understanding of mental retardation. In Figure 4.1, this epidemiological process is diagrammatically presented following a model proposed by Mausner and Kramer (1985). It is important to note that the purpose of a national descriptive study extends well beyond the simple estimation of prevalence data and may be seen as central to the overall study of mental retardation and coexisting mental health disorders.

Prevalence figures of persons with mental retardation have not been determined accurately and thus result in a very poor understanding of the etiology of mental retardation. As a result, a proper basis for prevention strategies is currently hampered.

To correct this serious gap in knowledge, a National Epidemiological Study of Mental Retardation (and its subpopulation of dually diagnosed individuals) has been proposed. All definitions would be that of the new descriptive definition of the AAMD as noted previously in this chapter. This would be the sole criterion for a case definition. However, social, personal, and placement data collected on the target population would provide the major descriptive information. The distribution of social–emotional–behavioral problems would be ascertained using a behavioral checklist, such as the ACQ on which national normative data will soon be complete. An adaptive behavior scale would also be administered.

The steps involved in this study might proceed as follows:

1. Based on a representative sample of households, obtain a sample of 30,000 children aged 7 to 12 years of age in seven or eight national sites.
2. Establish a cohort by examining the sample to see that it is representative of all births in the United States.
3. Adjust the sample so that it is representative of the birth cohort for the years in question by using the National Center for Health Statistics Data. The resulting sample would be representative of both households and births.
4. Screen to select those with IQs of less than 80 by using a standardized intelligence screening test.
5. Conduct a full-scale IQ test on all children with scores of less than 80. We estimate this to be about 2,600 cases. The actual cases selected for analysis would be those with full-scale IQ scores below 70.
6. Of the estimated 700 to 800 cases with IQs below 70, collect data on household, personal, and birth record information. Of these, about 200 children will exhibit an IQ of less than 50.
7. Collect identical data from a random comparison sample of 800 cases with IQs of 90 to 110 using the screening test criteria.
8. These samples assume about a 2% prevalence rate and should be robust enough to allow a reasonable descriptive analysis of the subpopulations as defined by SES, ethnicity, maternal age, and parental education.

Several chapters in this book (particularly in Sections IV, V, and VII) have reviewed the tremendous resources needed, both financially and logistically, to serve this dually diagnosed population. There are also many decisions to be made regarding the policy and allocation of these resources. With limited and continually decreasing support, we need to devise innovative approaches and make prudent decisions. Hopefully, the model presented in this chapter will stimulate discussion and result in the implementation of this programmatic epidemiological analysis, which should be a *sene qua non* for the assignment of resources for this population now and in the future.

## References

Achenbach, T.M. (1979). This child behavior profile. *Journal of Consulting and Clinical Psychology, 47*, 223-233.

Achenbach, T.M. (1980). DSM-III in light of empirical research on the classification of child psychopathology. *Journal of the American Academy of Child Psychiatry, 3*, 395-412.

Goyette, C.H., Conners, C.K., & Ulrich, R.F. (1978). Normative data on revised Conners Parent and Teacher Rating Scales. *Journal of Abnormal Child Psychology, 6,* 221–236.

Grossman, H.J. (1983). *Classification in mental retardation.* Washington, DC: American Association of Mental Deficiency.

Mausner, J.S., & Kramer, S. (1985). *Epidemiology: An introductory text.* Philadelphia, PA: W.B. Saunders.

Quay, H.C. (1986). A critical analysis of DSM-III as a taxonomy of psychopathology in childhood and adolescence. In T. Millon and G. Klerman (Eds.), *Contemporary issues in psychopathology.* New York: Guilford Press.

Quay, H.C., & Peterson, D. (1983). *Interim manual for the revised behavior problem checklist.* Available from H.C. Quay, Box 248074, University of Miami, Coral Gables, FL 33124.

Rutter, M., & Shaffer, D. (1980). DSM-III. A step forward or a step backward in terms of the classification of child psychiatric disorders. *Journal of the American Academy of Child Psychiatry, 19,* 371–394.

Russell, A.T. (1985). The mentally retarded, emotionally disturbed child and adolescent. In M. Sigman (Ed.), *Children with emotional disorders and developmental disabilities. Assessment and treatment.* Orlando, FL: Grune & Stratton.

# 5

# Data Collection at the National Institute of Mental Health

RONALD W. MANDERSCHEID, CECIL R. WURSTER,
MARILYN J. ROSENSTEIN, and MICHAEL J. WITKIN

## Historical Background

The National Institute of Mental Health (NIMH) has major responsibility for the collection, analysis, and reporting of national statistics on the caseload, staffing, and financial resources of specialty mental health organizations, as well as the sociodemographic, clinical, and service characteristics of patients served. These data collections are conducted on a voluntary reporting basis through the National Reporting Program for Mental Health Statistics, in close collaboration with the state mental health agencies. Data collection on the combined phenomenon of mental retardation and mental illness is not a focal activity at the Institute. This situation has historical antecedents.

Table 5.1 shows an historical synopsis of the National Reporting Program for Mental Health Statistics (see Manderscheid, Witkin, Rosenstein, & Bass, 1986; Redick, Manderscheid, Witkin, & Rosenstein, 1983). This history can be divided into several eras. In the first period, between 1840 and 1880, national data collections for mental health and mental retardation were under the aegis of the Secretary of State. The coverage of the system included both the community and institutions as they existed at that time, based on 100% enumeration through the decennial census. So, effectively, in the early period of the National Reporting Program, both epidemiological surveys and treatment surveys were conducted simultaneously.

In the second period, the interval between 1880 and 1946, the system underwent a transition. In 1902, Congress made a determination that it was an invasion of privacy to ask some of the questions that had been requested as part of the decennial census. From that time onward, the surveys conducted decennially and later annually were restricted to institutions. However, throughout the entire period between 1840 and 1946, the data collection system included both mental illness and mental retardation (Table 5.1).

The third phase is the period between 1947 and the present, during which the system has been operated by the National Institute of Mental Health. In the early years of this period, the Institute produced reports that included statistics on treated prevalence of both mental illness and mental retardation within organized

TABLE 5.1. History of the National Reporting Program.

| Period | Sponsorship | Coverage |
| --- | --- | --- |
| 1840–1880 | Secretary of State | Community and institutions |
| 1880–1946 | U.S. Bureau of Census | Transition to institutions |
| 1947–present | NIMH/States | Ambulatory and institutional facilities |

institutional and ambulatory facilities. In the 1960s, the data collection system on mental retardation was moved from the National Institute of Mental Health to other federal organizations. In the 1970s, a similar process occurred with respect to data on alcohol abuse and drug abuse, as those institutes were created.

In summary, over the past 25 years at NIMH, attention has not been directed toward collection of statistical information on patients served in facilities for the mentally retarded. However, some data are available from Institute surveys on the treatment of mentally retarded persons within organized institutional and ambulatory facilities for the mentally ill. These data are presented below.

## Current Data

Table 5.2 shows data for mental health organizations that are operated or funded by state mental health agencies. For state psychiatric hospitals, the rates under treatment per 100,000 civilian population range from zero in some states to approximately 22 in other states, for those with mental retardation and developmental disability disorders. For residential programs operated or funded by the state mental health agencies, such as community residential facilities for the mentally ill, the rates range similarly to those for the state psychiatric hospitals, between zero and about 23 per 100,000 civilian population.

The rates vary much more for state operated or funded ambulatory programs in the community. For outpatient programs, the rates vary between zero and approximately 205 per 100,000 civilian population; for partial care programs, between zero and approximately 111 per 100,000 civilian population. It is clear from these data that the treatment rates for individuals within the major disability groups of mental retardation and developmental disability are much higher in state-funded, ambulatory programs than within state psychiatric hospitals.

Table 5.3 shows parallel data for mental health organizations that are not operated or funded by state mental health agencies. Generally, the rates of care are much lower. For example, the rate per 100,000 civilian population for residential programs ranges between 0 and 2 across the states, compared to 0 to 23 for programs that are state operated or funded. This generalization holds true for all types of programs operated by mental health organizations that do not receive state funds. Thus, the private mental health sector generally provides fewer services to the mentally retarded than does the public sector operated or funded by the states.

TABLE 5.2. Patient characteristics by program element: Major disability groups in MHMOs.

| | Residents per 100,000 civilian population | | | | | | | |
|---|---|---|---|---|---|---|---|---|
| | Psychiatric hospitals | | | | Residential programs | | | |
| | Inpatient in state psychiatric hospital[a] | | | | | | | |
| State | Mentally ill | MR/DD | Substance abuse | Other | Mentally ill | MR/DD | Substance abuse | Other |
| Alabama | 52 | 1 | 1 | 0 | 13 | 3 | 1 | 0 |
| Alaska | ** | ** | ** | ** | 4 | 0 | 0 | 0 |
| Arizona | 11 | 1 | 0 | 0 | 38 | 0 | 5 | 0 |
| Arkansas | 11 | 1 | 0 | 0 | 7 | 0 | 1 | 2 |
| California | 17 | 6 | 1 | 0 | 16 | 0 | 1 | 0 |
| Colorado | 27 | 0 | 1 | 0 | 22 | 0 | 1 | 0 |
| Connecticut | 63 | 3 | 9 | 0 | 8 | 0 | 0 | 0 |
| Delaware | 70 | 7 | 6 | 1 | 18 | 3 | 1 | 2 |
| District of Columbia | 251 | 21 | 21 | 0 | 2 | 0 | 0 | 0 |
| Florida | 31 | 2 | 1 | 0 | 16 | 0 | 2 | 0 |
| Georgia | 40 | 22 | 7 | 2 | 18 | 23 | 8 | 0 |
| Hawaii | 25 | 0 | 0 | 0 | 17 | 0 | 1 | 1 |
| Idaho | 17 | 1 | 1 | 0 | 0 | 0 | 0 | 0 |
| Illinois | 28 | 5 | 1 | 0 | 8 | 2 | 1 | 1 |
| Indiana | 35 | 6 | 4 | 0 | 8 | 1 | 1 | 0 |
| Iowa | 23 | 1 | 5 | 1 | 21 | 8 | 1 | 0 |
| Kansas | 42 | 2 | 12 | 0 | 5 | 0 | 3 | 0 |
| Kentucky | 19 | 3 | 1 | 0 | 2 | 7 | 5 | 0 |
| Louisiana | 31 | 3 | 5 | 0 | 3 | 0 | 0 | 0 |
| Maine | 45 | 2 | 3 | 0 | 40 | 0 | 0 | 0 |
| Maryland | 59 | 1 | 4 | 0 | 13 | 0 | 0 | 0 |
| Massachusetts | 42 | 2 | 1 | 1 | 33 | 7 | 1 | 1 |
| Michigan | 42 | 1 | 1 | 1 | 21 | 7 | 2 | 0 |
| Minnesota | 21 | 8 | 4 | 1 | 8 | 1 | 3 | 0 |
| Mississippi | 58 | 5 | 4 | 0 | 0 | 1 | 6 | 0 |
| Missouri | ** | 3 | 4 | 0 | 16 | 0 | 1 | 0 |
| Montana | 43 | 1 | 2 | 0 | 10 | 0 | 0 | 0 |
| Nebraska | 39 | 2 | 2 | 0 | 6 | 0 | 0 | 0 |
| Nevada | 14 | 0 | 2 | 0 | 12 | 0 | 0 | 0 |
| New Hampshire | 23 | 1 | 1 | 0 | 55 | 7 | 1 | 0 |
| New Jersey | 41 | 0 | 0 | 0 | 10 | 0 | 0 | 0 |
| New Mexico | 13 | 0 | 1 | 0 | 31 | 1 | 1 | 0 |
| New York | 132 | 0 | 0 | 0 | 16 | 2 | 0 | 0 |
| North Carolina | 43 | 4 | 2 | 0 | 7 | 9 | 14 | 0 |
| North Dakota | 53 | 6 | 18 | 0 | ** | ** | ** | 0 |
| Ohio | ** | 2 | 1 | ** | 17 | 1 | 0 | 0 |
| Oklahoma | 28 | 1 | 7 | 2 | 2 | 0 | 0 | 0 |
| Oregon | 32 | 0 | 2 | 0 | 8 | 2 | 1 | 0 |
| Pennsylvania | 60 | 3 | 2 | 8 | 25 | 3 | 0 | 0 |
| Rhode Island | 40 | 0 | 0 | 0 | 28 | 0 | 0 | 0 |

TABLE 5.2. *(Continued).*

| | Residents per 100,000 civilian population | | | | | | | |
|---|---|---|---|---|---|---|---|---|
| | Psychiatric hospitals | | | | Residential programs | | | |
| | Inpatient in state psychiatric hospital[a] | | | | | | | |
| State | Mentally ill | MR/DD | Substance abuse | Other | Mentally ill | MR/DD | Substance abuse | Other |
| South Carolina | 71 | 6 | 4 | 7 | 1 | 0 | 0 | 0 |
| South Dakota | 45 | 2 | 7 | 0 | 21 | 2 | 0 | 0 |
| Tennessee | 38 | 3 | 1 | 0 | 2 | 0 | 1 | 0 |
| Texas | 29 | 1 | 4 | 0 | 8 | 3 | 5 | 0 |
| Utah | 17 | 0 | 1 | 0 | 8 | 0 | 2 | 0 |
| Vermont | 31 | 0 | 0 | 0 | 36 | 19 | 6 | 0 |
| Virginia | 58 | 4 | 4 | 0 | 6 | 1 | 1 | 0 |
| Washington | 31 | 0 | 0 | 0 | 8 | 0 | 0 | 0 |
| West Virginia | 36 | 13 | 5 | 0 | 3 | 6 | 3 | 0 |
| Wisconsin | 18 | 1 | 1 | 1 | 15 | 2 | 3 | 0 |
| Wyoming | 38 | 2 | 12 | 0 | 0 | 0 | 0 | 0 |
| Guam | – | – | – | – | 0 | 0 | 0 | 0 |
| Puerto Rico | 25 | 0 | 0 | 0 | 7 | 0 | 0 | 0 |
| Virgin Islands | – | – | – | – | 0 | 0 | 2 | 0 |

| | Number on active roles per 100,000 civilian population | | | | | | | |
|---|---|---|---|---|---|---|---|---|
| | Outpatient programs | | | | Partial care programs | | | |
| State | Mentally ill | MR/DD | Substance abuse | Other | Mentally ill | MR/DD | Substance abuse | Other |
| Alabama | 781 | 24 | 56 | 23 | 26 | 9 | 0 | 0 |
| Alaska | ** | 9 | 59 | ** | 57 | 5 | 1 | 0 |
| Arizona | 685 | 0 | 31 | 0 | 19 | 0 | 0 | 0 |
| Arkansas | ** | 32 | 67 | ** | 23 | 1 | 2 | 2 |
| California | 549 | 2 | 14 | 2 | 65 | 0 | 0 | 0 |
| Colorado | 673 | 10 | 15 | 6 | 51 | 2 | 1 | 0 |
| Connecticut | 500 | 22 | 53 | 71 | 38 | 0 | 0 | 0 |
| Delaware | 644 | 0 | 0 | 0 | 27 | 0 | 0 | 0 |
| District of Columbia | 1,294 | 16 | 83 | 84 | 94 | 1 | 3 | 12 |
| Florida | 575 | 9 | 64 | 84 | 33 | 0 | 0 | 0 |
| Georgia | 532 | 61 | 112 | 9 | 25 | 111 | 3 | 0 |
| Hawaii | 319 | 3 | 31 | 25 | 32 | 1 | 1 | 0 |
| Idaho | 619 | 0 | 0 | 0 | 73 | 0 | 0 | 0 |
| Illinois | 643 | 25 | 69 | 27 | 39 | 13 | 1 | 1 |
| Indiana | 675 | 14 | 123 | 18 | 39 | 0 | 1 | 0 |
| Iowa | 884 | 16 | 25 | 6 | 14 | 0 | 0 | 0 |
| Kansas | 1,085 | 21 | 129 | 27 | 32 | 0 | 0 | 0 |
| Kentucky | 985 | 83 | 183 | 63 | 43 | 19 | 0 | 0 |
| Louisiana | 723 | 39 | 30 | 0 | 12 | 1 | 0 | 0 |
| Maine | 1,243 | 64 | 32 | 22 | 70 | 1 | 1 | 33 |

TABLE 5.2. *(Continued)*.

| | Number on active roles per 100,000 civilian population | | | | | | | |
| | Outpatient programs | | | | Partial care programs | | | |
| State | Mentally ill | MR/DD | Substance abuse | Other | Mentally ill | MR/DD | Substance abuse | Other |
|---|---|---|---|---|---|---|---|---|
| Maryland | 712 | 24 | 86 | 20 | 38 | 0 | 1 | 0 |
| Massachusetts | 1,069 | 41 | 84 | 38 | 97 | 6 | 1 | 2 |
| Michigan | 749 | 73 | 31 | 34 | 75 | 39 | 0 | 0 |
| Minnesota | 1,184 | 32 | 135 | 35 | 54 | 0 | 0 | 0 |
| Mississippi | 620 | 44 | 118 | 71 | 20 | 13 | 0 | 0 |
| Missouri | 720 | 15 | 90 | 2 | 17 | 0 | 0 | 0 |
| Montana | 715 | 27 | 44 | 189 | 72 | 0 | 3 | 0 |
| Nebraska | 567 | 12 | 204 | 5 | 17 | 0 | 0 | 0 |
| Nevada | 830 | 2 | 18 | 5 | 42 | 0 | 0 | 0 |
| New Hampshire | 1,602 | 29 | 136 | 16 | 64 | 1 | 0 | 0 |
| New Jersey | 512 | 7 | 23 | 10 | 46 | 1 | 1 | 0 |
| New Mexico | 1,495 | 123 | 320 | 187 | 17 | 0 | 5 | 0 |
| New York | 763 | 5 | 68 | 5 | 61 | 2 | 2 | 0 |
| North Carolina | 882 | 43 | 144 | 2 | 44 | 61 | 4 | 0 |
| North Dakota | ** | ** | ** | ** | 35 | 4 | 1 | 0 |
| Ohio | 712 | 14 | 49 | 121 | 55 | 1 | 1 | 3 |
| Oklahoma | ** | ** | ** | 3 | 16 | 1 | 1 | 0 |
| Oregon | 651 | 205 | 91 | 13 | 35 | 0 | 0 | 0 |
| Pennsylvania | 583 | 58 | 28 | 13 | 103 | 4 | 1 | 1 |
| Rhode Island | 902 | 3 | 95 | 1 | 128 | 1 | 1 | 9 |
| South Carolina | 801 | 10 | 24 | 25 | 21 | 0 | 0 | 0 |
| South Dakota | ** | ** | ** | 0 | ** | 4 | 3 | 0 |
| Tennessee | 728 | 24 | 73 | 6 | 46 | 3 | 2 | 0 |
| Texas | 432 | 33 | 89 | 14 | 27 | 10 | 2 | 0 |
| Utah | 771 | 20 | 63 | 19 | 79 | 2 | 1 | 0 |
| Vermont | 1,578 | 113 | 402 | 10 | 236 | 39 | 9 | 0 |
| Virginia | 555 | 24 | 57 | 7 | 61 | 0 | 5 | 2 |
| Washington | 708 | 11 | 82 | 2 | 87 | 8 | 2 | 2 |
| West Virginia | 429 | 147 | 116 | 66 | 43 | 55 | 15 | 0 |
| Wisconsin | 1,048 | 47 | 154 | 35 | 36 | 7 | 1 | 3 |
| Wyoming | 685 | 11 | 89 | 269 | 0 | 0 | 0 | 0 |
| Guam | 63 | 2 | 2 | 3 | 19 | 1 | 0 | 0 |
| Puerto Rico | 1,467 | 11 | 4 | 0 | 4 | 0 | 0 | 0 |
| Virgin Islands | 490 | 38 | 164 | 0 | 55 | 4 | 18 | 0 |

[a] Includes ? Psychiatric Hospitals in Wisconsin.
*Note*: −, empty cell; **, value not shown because 75% of the reporting organizations did not supply data for this cell.

TABLE 5.3. Patient characteristics by program element: Major disability groups in MHMOs (non-state-operated-funded).

| | Residents per 100,000 civilian population | | | | | | | |
| --- | --- | --- | --- | --- | --- | --- | --- | --- |
| | Psychiatric hospitals | | | | Residential programs | | | |
| | Inpatient in state psychiatric hospital[a] | | | | | | | |
| State | Mentally ill | MR/DD | Substance abuse | Other | Mentally ill | MR/DD | Substance abuse | Other |
| Alabama | − | − | − | − | 3 | 1 | 0 | 0 |
| Alaska | − | − | − | − | − | − | − | − |
| Arizona | − | − | − | − | 21 | 0 | 2 | 0 |
| Arkansas | − | − | − | − | 4 | 0 | 0 | 2 |
| California | − | − | − | − | 8 | 0 | 0 | 0 |
| Colorado | − | − | − | − | 7 | 0 | 0 | 0 |
| Connecticut | − | − | − | − | 22 | 0 | 2 | 3 |
| Delaware | − | − | − | − | 0 | 0 | 0 | 0 |
| District of Columbia | − | − | − | − | 0 | 0 | 0 | 0 |
| Florida | − | − | − | − | 1 | 0 | 0 | 0 |
| Georgia | − | − | − | − | 12 | 0 | 0 | 1 |
| Hawaii | − | − | − | − | − | − | − | − |
| Idaho | − | − | − | − | 14 | 0 | 0 | 0 |
| Illinois | − | − | − | − | 2 | 0 | 0 | 0 |
| Indiana | − | − | − | − | 7 | 0 | 1 | 1 |
| Iowa | − | − | − | − | 4 | 0 | 0 | 0 |
| Kansas | − | − | − | − | 0 | 0 | 0 | 0 |
| Kentucky | − | − | − | − | 2 | 0 | 0 | 0 |
| Louisiana | − | − | − | − | 0 | 0 | 0 | 0 |
| Maine | − | − | − | − | 0 | 0 | 0 | 0 |
| Maryland | − | − | − | − | 3 | 0 | 0 | 0 |
| Massachusetts | − | − | − | − | 9 | 0 | 0 | 0 |
| Michigan | − | − | − | − | 7 | 0 | 0 | 0 |
| Minnesota | − | − | − | − | 2 | 0 | 0 | 0 |
| Mississippi | − | − | − | − | 0 | 0 | 0 | 0 |
| Missouri | − | − | − | − | 0 | 0 | 0 | 0 |
| Montana | − | − | − | − | 10 | 0 | 0 | 0 |
| Nebraska | − | − | − | − | 0 | 0 | 0 | 0 |
| Nevada | − | − | − | − | 0 | 0 | 0 | 0 |
| New Hampshire | − | − | − | − | 9 | 0 | 0 | 0 |
| New Jersey | − | − | − | − | 2 | 0 | 0 | 0 |
| New Mexico | − | − | − | − | 0 | 0 | 0 | 0 |
| New York | − | − | − | − | 12 | 0 | 0 | 0 |
| North Carolina | − | − | − | − | 0 | 0 | 0 | 0 |
| North Dakota | − | − | − | − | − | − | − | − |
| Ohio | − | − | − | − | 2 | 0 | 0 | 0 |
| Oklahoma | − | − | − | − | 2 | 0 | 0 | 0 |
| Oregon | − | − | − | − | 7 | 0 | 1 | 0 |
| Pennsylvania | − | − | − | − | 3 | 0 | 0 | 0 |
| Rhode Island | − | − | − | − | 0 | 1 | 0 | 0 |

TABLE 5.3.  *(Continued)*.

| State | Residents per 100,000 civilian population | | | | | | | |
| | Psychiatric hospitals | | | | Residential programs | | | |
| | Inpatient in state psychiatric hospital[a] | | | | | | | |
| | Mentally ill | MR/DD | Substance abuse | Other | Mentally ill | MR/DD | Substance abuse | Other |
|---|---|---|---|---|---|---|---|---|
| South Carolina | – | – | – | – | 1 | 1 | 0 | 0 |
| South Dakota | – | – | – | – | 0 | 0 | 0 | 0 |
| Tennessee | – | – | – | – | 7 | 0 | 0 | 0 |
| Texas | – | – | – | – | 6 | 0 | 1 | 0 |
| Utah | – | – | – | – | 10 | 0 | 2 | 1 |
| Vermont | – | – | – | – | 3 | 2 | 2 | 0 |
| Virginia | – | – | – | – | 8 | 0 | 1 | 0 |
| Washington | – | – | – | – | 5 | 0 | 0 | 0 |
| West Virginia | – | – | – | – | 2 | 0 | 0 | 0 |
| Wisconsin | – | – | – | – | 4 | 0 | 1 | 1 |
| Wyoming | – | – | – | – | 20 | 0 | 0 | 0 |
| Guam | – | – | – | – | – | – | – | – |
| Puerto Rico | – | – | – | – | 1 | 0 | 0 | 0 |
| Virgin Islands | – | – | – | – | – | – | – | – |

| State | Number on active roles per 100,000 civilian population | | | | | | | |
| | Outpatient programs | | | | Partial care programs | | | |
| | Mentally ill | MR/DD | Substance abuse | Other | Mentally ill | MR/DD | Substance abuse | Other |
|---|---|---|---|---|---|---|---|---|
| Alabama | 188 | 0 | 27 | 0 | 1 | 0 | 0 | 0 |
| Alaska | – | – | – | – | – | – | – | – |
| Arizona | 124 | 0 | 4 | 0 | 16 | 0 | 0 | 0 |
| Arkansas | ** | ** | ** | ** | 2 | 0 | 0 | 0 |
| California | 314 | 1 | 18 | 2 | 20 | 0 | 0 | 0 |
| Colorado | 185 | 2 | 34 | 14 | 5 | 0 | 0 | 1 |
| Connecticut | 303 | 14 | 22 | 15 | 11 | 0 | 0 | 0 |
| Delaware | 273 | 0 | 0 | 0 | 0 | 0 | 0 | 0 |
| District of Columbia | 378 | 0 | 33 | 0 | 7 | 0 | 0 | 0 |
| Florida | 106 | 6 | 15 | 8 | 7 | 0 | 0 | 0 |
| Georgia | 69 | 4 | 9 | 1 | 0 | 0 | 0 | 0 |
| Hawaii | – | – | – | – | – | – | – | – |
| Idaho | 132 | 0 | 0 | 0 | 0 | 0 | 0 | 0 |
| Illinois | 25 | 0 | 14 | 1 | 0 | 0 | 0 | 0 |
| Indiana | 44 | 0 | 11 | 0 | 0 | 0 | 0 | 0 |
| Iowa | 155 | 0 | 4 | 0 | 7 | 0 | 0 | 0 |
| Kansas | 90 | 0 | 15 | 0 | 5 | 0 | 0 | 0 |
| Kentucky | 70 | 6 | 13 | 5 | 4 | 2 | 0 | 0 |
| Louisiana | 23 | 0 | 6 | 0 | 4 | 0 | 0 | 0 |
| Maine | 1 | 0 | 0 | 0 | 0 | 0 | 0 | 0 |

TABLE 5.3. *(Continued).*

| | Number on active roles per 100,000 civilian population | | | | | | | |
| | Outpatient programs | | | | Partial care programs | | | |
| State | Mentally ill | MR/DD | Substance abuse | Other | Mentally ill | MR/DD | Substance abuse | Other |
|---|---|---|---|---|---|---|---|---|
| Maryland | 83 | 0 | 10 | 15 | 8 | 0 | 0 | 0 |
| Massachusetts | 327 | 2 | 31 | 2 | 15 | 0 | 0 | 0 |
| Michigan | 126 | 3 | 18 | 3 | 2 | 1 | 0 | 0 |
| Minnesota | 232 | 3 | 23 | 11 | 12 | 0 | 0 | 0 |
| Mississippi | 134 | 9 | 25 | 13 | 0 | 0 | 0 | 0 |
| Missouri | 123 | 1 | 7 | 0 | 1 | 0 | 0 | 0 |
| Montana | 0 | 0 | 0 | 0 | 0 | 0 | 0 | 0 |
| Nebraska | 19 | 0 | 7 | 0 | 1 | 0 | 0 | 0 |
| Nevada | 26 | 0 | 7 | 0 | 0 | 0 | 0 | 0 |
| New Hampshire | 47 | 0 | 23 | 0 | 0 | 0 | 0 | 0 |
| New Jersey | 367 | 4 | 19 | 0 | 1 | 0 | 0 | 0 |
| New Mexico | 75 | 0 | 0 | 0 | 3 | 0 | 0 | 0 |
| New York | 288 | 0 | 16 | 1 | 14 | 0 | 0 | 0 |
| North Carolina | 51 | 1 | 2 | 0 | 0 | 0 | 0 | 0 |
| North Dakota | – | – | – | – | – | – | – | – |
| Ohio | 70 | 1 | 26 | 2 | 2 | 0 | 0 | 0 |
| Oklahoma | 500 | 8 | 5 | 9 | 1 | 0 | 0 | 0 |
| Oregon | 91 | 6 | 21 | 4 | 6 | 0 | 0 | 0 |
| Pennsylvania | 203 | 5 | 14 | 15 | 11 | 0 | 0 | 0 |
| Rhode Island | 224 | 0 | 13 | 0 | 46 | 5 | 1 | 0 |
| South Carolina | 87 | 0 | 3 | 0 | 1 | 0 | 0 | 0 |
| South Dakota | 107 | 4 | 9 | 0 | 0 | 0 | 0 | 0 |
| Tennessee | 87 | 0 | 0 | 0 | 4 | 0 | 0 | 0 |
| Texas | 76 | 2 | 12 | 2 | 33 | 11 | 3 | 0 |
| Utah | 62 | 2 | 5 | 2 | 4 | 0 | 0 | 0 |
| Vermont | 228 | 16 | 58 | 1 | 3 | 1 | 0 | 0 |
| Virginia | 164 | 4 | 9 | 1 | 2 | 0 | 0 | 0 |
| Washington | 156 | 1 | 8 | 0 | 17 | 1 | 0 | 0 |
| West Virginia | 133 | 3 | 7 | 1 | 0 | 0 | 0 | 0 |
| Wisconsin | 194 | 3 | 7 | 5 | 0 | 0 | 0 | 0 |
| Wyoming | 356 | 1 | 8 | 25 | 0 | 0 | 0 | 0 |
| Guam | – | – | – | – | – | – | – | – |
| Puerto Rico | 6 | 0 | 0 | 0 | 0 | 0 | 0 | 0 |
| Virgin Islands | – | – | – | – | – | – | – | – |

[a] Includes ? Psychiatric Hospitals in Wisconsin.

*Note*: –, empty cell; **, value not shown because 75% of the reporting organizations did not supply data for this cell.

Recent data from a patient sample survey show that about 10,000 individuals with a principal or primary diagnosis of mental retardation are admitted each year to inpatient care in mental health facilities. Approximately 7,000 of these individuals are admitted to state psychiatric hospitals. Within any given year, approximately 32,000 mentally retarded persons are admitted to ambulatory services, such as outpatient care, partial care, and other types of community programs.

The only data set that contains data on dual diagnosis of mental illness and mental retardation is a sample survey of clients in the Community Support Program for the chronically mentally ill. This program is designed to integrate a range of services for the chronically mentally ill, including psychiatric services, health care services, dental services, case management services, housing, and psychosocial and vocational habilitation and rehabilitation. These services are made available through a case manager, so that functioning of chronically mentally ill persons in the community can be improved.

The Community Support Program has been under evaluation for the last six years. The data show that about 3% of the individuals served in the Community Support Program have a principal diagnosis of mental retardation, and about 9% have a secondary diagnosis of mental retardation. These figures are higher than would generally be assumed.

## Directions for the Future

There are a number of reasons why more comprehensive data are not available on mental retardation. Several of these reasons are historical, as noted above. Also, it is difficult to collect data on dual diagnosis and multiple diagnoses from mental health facilities on a voluntary reporting basis, the principal mechanism by which mental health data are collected. Thus, it is difficult to define stringent criteria for data collections and also extremely difficult to collect a secondary diagnosis or dual diagnosis. Also, on the service system level, the technology is not currently available to measure interorganizational relationships so that the linkages between mental illness and mental retardation facilities can be understood. This will be a high priority in the future.

The data reported in this chapter were derived from a biennial inventory that NIMH has operated for many years and from patient sample surveys of persons served within mental health organizations. The availability and use of uniform data standards in the mental health field make these data collection activities possible. In addition, they facilitate the ability to report comparable data across service provider types and across state mental health service systems and facilitate aggregating state data to produce national statistics.

The mental retardation field suffers from the lack of national data standards and a system for recording and reporting data for national statistics. As a result, only limited data are available on patients who suffer both mental retardation and mental illness. Solutions to similar problems in mental health might serve as a model for solving these data collection problems. The national mental health data collection experience and the Mental Health Statistics Improvement Program (MHSIP) illustrate some of the principles involved in addressing large-scale data collection and analysis problems where many organizations and agencies are involved at all levels of government and the service delivery system. The MHSIP has its conceptual origins in the Model Reporting Area for Mental Hospital Statistics (MRA), which provided the beginning for the federal and state collaboration in setting mental health data standards over the past 35 years. The MRA was organized and supported by the NIMH in the early 1950s to develop definitions for state mental hospital statistical data. It started with 11 states that maintained statistical systems on hospital patients and used automated data processing equipment to store and process individual patient data. As other states incorporated the MRA data standards into their systems, they were admitted into membership, and the MRA grew to 35 states by the early 1960s. As long as state hospitals were the primary setting for the care of the mentally ill, the MRA served well and provided statistics on mental patients and the services they received. However, with the explosion of other types of treatment settings, particularly community outpatient clinics and mental health centers, a need developed to broaden the boundaries of the statistical programs that were operated by the states and NIMH. The MRA was discontinued in the mid-1960s, and the mental health field experienced a period in which national data standards did not exist, except, of course, for the psychiatric diagnostic classification standards. It became difficult, if not impossible, to collect comparable data across systems of mental health services. In an effort to bring order back into the mental health statistics system, the NIMH and the states initiated the MHSIP as a collaborative state/federal program. This was in 1976.

Five major goals were set for MHSIP to accomplish the overall mission of improving mental health information systems. These goals were: (1) develop, maintain, and promulgate standards for data content in mental health information and statistical systems; (2) develop, maintain, and promulgate guidelines for the design of mental health information and statistical systems; (3) achieve implementation of the data standards and design implementation of the data standards and system design guidelines by entities that process or report mental health data; (4) enhance the capacities of mental health agencies in mental health information and statistical systems technologies; and (5) encourage the use of data from mental health information and statistical systems in administration, management, clinical, and research activities. Central to MHSIP has been the development and implementation of standardized national mental health data sets (Patton & Leginski, 1983).

Recommended minimum data sets cover the organizations that comprise the mental health service delivery system, the patients treated and the services they receive, and the characteristics and functions of the staff who provide services in these organizations. The core, uniform data sets, as they relate to larger data

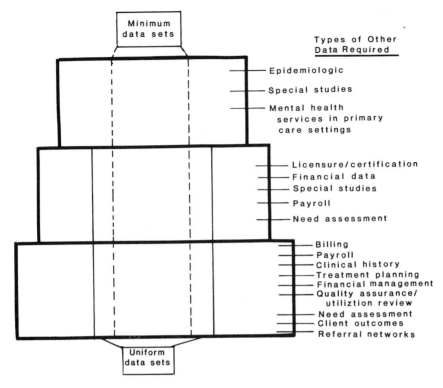

FIGURE 5.1. Core, uniform data sets in relation to the larger data needs at local service provider, substate, state, and federal levels.

needs at local service provider, substate, state, and federal levels, are illustrated in Figure 5.1. The pyramid represents the extent of data needed at all levels, the service provider level needing the most detailed data, the state or substate level needing a subset of that detailed data, and the federal level needing a subset of what is needed at the state level. This conceptual model contains a minimum data set that is needed for the national reporting.

While there is nothing particularly unique about establishing data standards, the fact that these are endorsed by all the state mental health agencies, the NIMH, and the National Council of Community Mental Health Centers is important and is evidence that a true collaborative process is working. Qualities that have contributed to the success of the MHSIP state federal collaboration are described as follows:

First of all, and basic to the program, has been *leadership and continuity*. NIMH has provided the leadership needed by the MHSIP since it was initiated in 1976. Critical to this leadership has been its collegial and unobtrusive nature. A similar effort to develop and implement national data standards for mentally retarded and mentally ill patients will require leadership by some national organization.

A second quality is *advocacy*. Not only is leadership needed, but some prestigious group or groups must advocate for national data standards.

Three, *benefits* must be apparent. For a program of this type to work, all parties must see some direct benefits from participation. In mental health, the states benefit by having comparable data across states for policy, budget, and management decisionmaking. NIMH benefits by having state and organizational data that can be aggregated into national statistics.

Fourth, *commitment, support, and involvement* are important. It is not sufficient for the parties to such a program to provide tacit support. All parties must be involved directly, including executives as well as technical staff.

Fifth, *resources* must be available. Some minimal resources are necessary to support working committees, education and training, and technical assistance.

Sixth, and probably the most important, is *patience*. An effort of this type requires extreme patience. The participatory process, which is critical to the success of the program, is often slow and agonizing and requires negotiation and compromise, but it is essential to full support, endorsement, and ownership of the data sets and the reporting system by all parties involved.

Finally, while the MHSIP is certainly not the only possible approach to meeting the mental retardation/mental illness biostatistical and epidemiological data needs, it is offered as a starting point for a broader collaboration among those in the mental retardation and mental health fields who serve patients with diagnoses in both areas.

## References

Manderscheid, R.W., Witkin, M.J., Rosenstein, M.J., & Bass, R.D. (1986). *The National Reporting Program for Mental Health Statistics: History and findings. Public Health Reports, 101*(5), 532–539.

Patton, R.E., & Leginski, W.A. (1983). *The design and content of a National Mental Health Statistics System*. Rockville, MD: National Institute of Mental Health, DHHS Publication No. (ADM) 83-1095.

Redick, R.W., Manderscheid, R.W., Witkin, M.J., & Rosenstein, M.J. (1983). *A history of the U.S. National Reporting Program for Mental Health Statistics 1840*-1983. Rockville, MD: National Institute of Mental Health, DHHS Publication No. (ADM) 83-1296.

# Conclusion

SHARON A. BORTHWICK

The preceding chapters have presented a rather bleak picture of the state of epidemiology of mentally retarded persons who also have mental health problems. However, the authors have also given some straightforward recommendations for improving the situation. Their suggestions deal primarily with methodological issues. Some of the comments are directed toward researchers, as they design and interpret the results of epidemiological studies. Others reflect broader issues and require coordination at a national or even international level. Each of these is practical and is viewed by the authors as prerequisite to an accurate description of the target population, as well as a meaningful interpretation of the relationships among variables.

1. *Consider the heterogeneity of the people being studied.* Descriptive and analytical epidemiology should take into account such client descriptors as level of retardation, age, etiology of mental retardation, type of psychiatric disorder, specific behavior problems, medication record, socioeconomic background, residential living arrangements, and other handicapping conditions such as language disorders. Studies that generalize to total groups of mentally retarded people without taking individual characteristics into account are of limited use.

2. *Base prevalence estimates and analysis of causes on adequate samples.* Sampling should not be limited to biased groups, such as referred subjects, institutionalized clients, or people served by a single facility or clinic. Sample sizes should be large enough to allow examination of subgroups of clients, based on relevant characteristics such as those cited in Recommendation 1. Encourage national efforts to obtain statewide data and motivate states to collect and report this valuable information. Support large-scale epidemiological studies, obtaining comprehensive information on served and unserved populations and establishing true prevalence rates.

3. *Use valid and reliable methods of assessment.* Consider the context or environment in which assessment occurs. Consider observed behavior problems as well as formal psychiatric diagnosis, using standardized assessment procedures to measure each. Determine efficacy of using instruments previously

standardized with nonretarded subjects. Recognize the limitations of unstandardized rating scales and checklists.

4. *Establish standardized definitions of psychiatric disorders and observable behaviors to ensure comparability across studies.* Determine methods of comparing results of studies of psychiatric disorders conducted in the United States (e.g., using DSM-III) with studies in other countries (e.g., using World Health Organization criteria). Encourage statewide use of selected maladaptive behavior scales and determine equivalency of item-responses for comparison across states and agencies using different instruments. Recognize the importance of and differences between formal psychiatric diagnosis and maladaptive behavior data.

5. *Bridge the "data gap" between mental health and mental retardation agencies.* Encourage interagency collaboration with regard to data bases on individuals served by mental retardation and/or mental health agencies. Develop uniform reporting standards for information of interest to both agencies. Establish methods of identifying individuals who appear in more than one system.

# Section II: Developmental Aspects of Prevention
# Introduction

ALFRED A. BAUMEISTER

The charge to the authors in this second section is to address research initiatives and prevention strategies from a developmental perspective. The contributors in this section focus on major causes of intellectual disabilities and how these overlap with problems of social, affective, and personality development.

The major causes of mental retardation and other developmental disabilities include (1) genetic disorders, (2) obstetrical and perinatal problems related to prematurity and low birthweight, (3) teratogens and environmental toxins, (4) the myelodysplasias, particularly with reference to nutrition, (5) infectious diseases, and (6) the "new morbidity" stemming from a combination of environmental and biological causes. The intent here is to span the continuum of causation prior to birth and the first few years thereafter. The approach is essentially eclectic in order to synthesize knowledge in these areas and to identify their relevance to both mental illness and mental retardation.

Guiding our presentations and recommendations are the following considerations:

1. Behavioral deviations or disturbances that we associate with mental retardation and mental health problems usually arise and are observed as the developmental process unfolds. There are, of course, abrupt exceptions, but this general principle ought to be reflected in our theory and in our practice. Moreover, ontogenetic aspects of development must become more salient relative to theory construction and intervention programming.
2. Differential diagnosis is often problematic at any point. But one may conclude that especially during the period of early development diagnosis of either condition is particularly difficult, to say nothing of differential diagnosis. There is, in fact, question as to whether differential diagnosis, at an early age, is always helpful or clinically useful. Is it even meaningful to dichotomize artificially the individual into these obviously related forms of adaption? Indeed, fundamental questions can and have been raised about reliability and validity of differential diagnosis, especially among children. There are few diagnostic categories that are valid across the full range of development. This point reflects a major controversy that has divided professional opinion for some time and is reflected in other chapters throughout this book.

3. Developmental determinants and correlates of mental retardation and mental health disorders are typically multivariate and complex involving biological, behavioral, and social phenomena concurrently. If both sets of conditions—that is, impairments in intellectual and affective behavior—are present, we might be advised that the most useful approach is not to try to separate these but rather to understand how this constellation of conditions arose for this particular child.

4. As scant as the data bases are for either type of behavioral disorder separately, in combination we have only the roughest estimates as to incidence and prevalence among children. But there is evidence suggesting that psychiatric disturbances are significantly higher among retarded than among nonretarded people (see Section I). Again, this is a point on which we will find enormous variations in opinion. We can be even less certain about the direction of causality; that is, do psychiatric problems cause retarded behavior or vice versa?

5. A study was recently completed that involved an extensive state-by-state comparative study of mental retardation classification systems (Lowitzer, Utley, & Baumeister, in press). The investigators were astonished by the enormous variability that they found. It is their view that this variability is due, in good measure, to a lack of common and valid data bases concerning mental retardation. Classification, in both fields, is driven less by scientific and professional considerations than by political and financial ones. One of our findings is directly relevant to the issues that have brought this book about. Of the 51 respondents, 48 reported that they were having great difficulty in serving their "dually diagnosed" populations. Aside from the professional and scientific concerns, a major problem was administrative; that is, which state agency would have the primary responsibility? The fact is that no one really seemed to want the responsibility.

This section focuses on some of these issues, including such basic considerations as classification, causation, research priorities, early prevention, and intervention. The authors examine the problem broadly in terms of its behavioral and biological etiologies and manifestations. Some general recommendations along with some that are more specific arise from these considerations.

## Reference

Lowitzer, A.C., Utley, C.A., & Baumeister, A.A. (in press). AAMD's 1983 *Classification in mental retardation* as utilized by state mental retardation developmental disabilities agencies. *Mental Retardation*.

# 6
# The New Morbidity: Implications for Prevention

ALFRED A. BAUMEISTER

A review of the research and clinical literature reveals an abiding and enduring concern with the connection between personality and affective disorders, on the one hand, and mental retardation, on the other. There is, in fact, a larger literature on this subject than one might expect, given certain longstanding administrative and institutional difficulties in organizing and maintaining a systematic basis of research support on this "dual" problem.

It is generally accepted that disorders of psychopathology are much more frequently observed among persons identified as mentally retarded than among nonretarded persons (e.g., Richardson, 1980; Robinson & Robinson, 1976). Both clinical experience and more formal research studies reveal this connection, although dispute still continues over its extent and nature. Kopp (1983) has listed a large number of distinctly biological risk factors for mental retardation that are also associated with emotional problems. There is more serious disagreement over such issues as direction of causality, etiology, symptomatology, and modes of treatment.

Technically, we have made a great deal of scientific and clinical progress, particularly in understanding underlying genetic, epigenetic, and neurological processes. Certainly a new generation of neuroleptics has made a great difference with respect to the treatment of mental disturbances, both psychotic and neurotic. In addition, highly significant advances have been recorded in various forms of behavior therapy, much of which is directed toward treatment of affective problem behavior among mentally retarded children.

But in many important respects our understanding of the basic conceptual, scientific, and intervention issues surrounding this connection has not been greatly clarified. For instance, a critical analysis of research on retarded people who exhibit other types of behavior disorder, such as severe self-injury, obsessive stereotypy, and aggression, leads to the conclusion that the pace of progress to understanding and ultimately effective intervention with and prevention of these disorders has been excruciatingly slow.

One of the most salient aspects of the existing professional literature on this general subject is enormous diversity, mostly in the form of opinion expressed with respect to such fundamental issues as incidence and prevalence, basic and directional causation, and choice of methods of prevention and intervention. Why is it that the same arguments keep resurfacing, and why has scientific and technical progress toward resolving some basic uncertainties been so slow? Also, why has public policy not advanced more rapidly on these fronts?

Contributing to conceptual, scientific, and programmatic confusion are the following factors:

1. Dominant systems of definition and classification that are more directly driven by political, social, and economic considerations than by scientific or professional constraints.
2. Failure to appreciate conceptually, programmatically, and experimentally the enormous inter-individual and intraindividual variability embedded in this constellation of behavior outcomes (Baumeister, 1968).
3. Unwillingness of policymakers and professionals to apply what is known scientifically and technically to both primary prevention and intervention. Indeed, many important decisions regarding prevention initiatives are essentially political, not empirical, a fact that will become all the more salient as new, important, and socially sensitive policy decisions are forthcoming (Baumeister, 1981).
4. Unwillingness to support the research necessary to resolve some of the basic scientific uncertainties. The joint report completed in 1977 by a group of ad hoc consultants to NICHD and NIMH recommended a large number of research priorities that are, in the main, every bit as relevant today as then (Tarjan et al., 1977). Yet these recommendations were never systematically addressed, at least publicly, as a joint planning effort of NIMH and NICHD. A great deal of needed research fell squarely between this bureaucratic crack.
5. Choice of explanatory models that are rooted in concepts whose validity is open to serious question. Diagnostic and screening procedures are not generally based on understanding of the developmental processes as these unfold and elaborate. Understanding of behavior disturbances, both of an affective and intellectual nature, must be couched in the ontogenetic processes that drive and guide individual development among children. It is inconceivable that valid theory and intervention can ever be fashioned without central consideration of these most fundamental developmental issues.

## Prevention

Greater attention should be directed toward some broader aspects of prevention, focusing mainly on subgroups at particular risk. Although the President's Committee on Mental Retardation in a number of earlier reports, has emphasized the need for national prevention programs, in the main, prevention research has not received priority status.

Over the past few decades, children's mortality and morbidity from serious infectious disease have decreased significantly. At the same time an increasing amount of attention has been directed at behavioral, social, and school-related problems – problems that must be considered as health risks in that they produce poor adjustment, physical illness, handicaps, violence, and developmental disabilities. This is what has been termed the "new morbidity" (Haggerty, Roghmann, & Pless, 1975).

Consider the distribution of psychiatric disorders by type and age. The most current and complete data available, obtained from the Department of Health and Human Services, reveal distinct age differences and trends relative to the various mental disorders observed among children. Moreover, the numbers of children diagnosed as sufficiently impaired to be qualified for inpatient services is considerable. Data for 1980, the most recent year for which complete information was available, are presented in Figure 6.1.

Although prevalence estimates are not very precise, on the basis of several recent studies we may conclude that the new morbidity affects a sizable group of children (Butler, Starfield, & Stenmark, 1984). These studies all show that prevalence is strongly linked to socioeconomic status (SES), family status, and other social variables. Data recently obtained from the National Center for Health Statistics show a clear relationship between health status and SES variables. Race and income data are presented in Figure 6.2. Although absolute numbers are greater among white than among black children, the percent figures reveal a marked disproportion of health problems among black children. On the other hand, both in absolute and relative terms, morbidity is much greater among children from poor families. We should be concerned not only with apparently

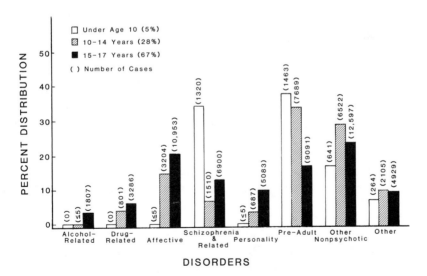

FIGURE 6.1. Percent distribution and number of cases under 18 years of age, to selected inpatient psychiatric services, by age and selected primary diagnoses – United States, 1980. Percentages from *Mental Health Statistical Note No. 175.* U.S. Department of Health and Human Services, April 1986.

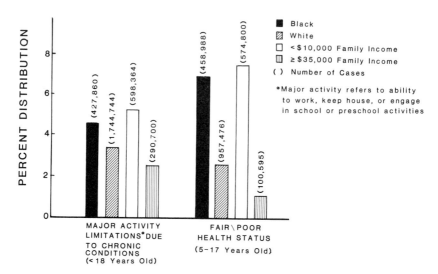

FIGURE 6.2. Percent distribution of persons under 18 years of age with limitation in major activity, owing to chronic conditions, and respondent-assessed health status according to sociodemographic characteristics – United States, 1983. National Center for Health Statistics, 1983. *Vital and Health Statistics*, Series 10, No. 154.

increasing prevalence of the new morbidity but also with implications for the profound social and economic trends currently confronting our society.

There are also a number of scientific lessons contained in these data. One is that classification systems must be revised and elaborated to take into account variability in both cause and effect. Indeed, current evidence now supports the contention that factors initiating a particular behavior problem are not always the same as those factors that maintain the problem. Another is that when considering the developmental aspects of both mental retardation and mental health problems, with a view toward prevention and intervention, the heavily favored linear and additive causation models are not entirely adequate bases on which to fashion meaningful and effective prevention policy.

Perhaps the time has arrived to accept the premise that mental retardation and problems of emotional adjustment should be characterized in absolute and relative terms. By absolute, one is referring to behavior disabilities that would clearly handicap a child in practically any social context. Prenatal factors are a significant cause of severe and profound developmental disability (Moser, 1985) of an absolute nature. For the most part, these reflect distinctly biomedical components, although these too are highly varied both in kind and in effect.

It should be pointed out as well that risk for biological handicaps is not spread evenly across the various socioeconomic or ethnic groups; but, in fact, the risk of biological disorder is linked to the social variables. Relative handicaps, on the other hand, are more context specific in that disability may be behaviorally evident in one environment but not in another. The latter group of affected individuals is larger by far and includes most of those people with mild mental retardation. There are different causal factors in mild and severe retardation and emotional reactivity, a conclusion for which there is now considerable support in the research literature.

It is the mild forms that require us to think in terms of how development in different environments defines intellectual and social competence. This is a consideration that also leads to the conclusion that an adequate system of classification and intervention will require the development of useful and reliable taxonomies of environments. We cannot continue to ignore or discount the fact that relative problems of adjustment must be defined in terms of specific social and environmental demands and constraints that are situationally defined. This is an approach to diagnosis that has not received a great deal of attention in research on early development (Landesman-Dwyer & Butterfield, 1983).

We ought to focus more attention and resources on prevention measures that are contextually relevant. It seems almost axiomatic to assert that prevention of problems is a far superior strategy than that of treating them. Yet, as one reviews the literature, traces funding patterns, and examines efforts state by state, the conclusion is inevitable that concern for primary prevention is not as important as is direct care and, to some extent, intervention.

An example of a condition, essentially preventable, that can cause both intellectual and emotional behavioral disabilities across a wide continuum is fetal alcohol related birth defects. This disease represents the most clearly defined maternal behavior associated with brain maldevelopment.

Baumeister and Hamlett (1986) recently completed a national mail and telephone survey of all the states to determine what is being done to prevent these effects. They also conducted a review of the epidemiology of the disease, particularly with respect to associated demographic factors.

The Centers for Disease Control estimate birth prevalence of fetal alcohol syndrome (FAS) in the range of 1 to 2 per 1,000 live births in the United States. This rate is generally consistent with the data that Baumeister and Hamlett obtained directly from other sources. Alcohol abuse during pregnancy, along with Down's syndrome and spina bifida, is one of the most common causes of mental retardation. Of these three, FAS is clearly the most preventable, at least in behavioral terms, and should be the joint concern of NIMH and NICHD. Four thousand babies, disproportionately represented within minority groups, will be born this year with FAS.

A number of interesting findings emerged from this study. The most general conclusion is that, on a national basis, the effort to prevent FAS and other alcohol-related birth and behavior problems is not encouraging. Indeed, most official state reactions to alcohol consumption are essentially punitive rather than health oriented.

More generally speaking, risk factors do not operate independently but seem most often to interact in such a way as to produce a range of causality, both in absolute and relative terms. Psychosocial and biological risks may be multiplicative in their effects and outcomes, rather than additive.

## Socioeconomic Variables and Outcome

One of the most consistent relationships in the literature is that between socioeconomic status and behavioral adaption. The correlations between these two general factors range from .40 to .60 in every modern industrial society. Incidence rates of mental retardation and mental illness appear to be five and six times greater, respectively, in the lowest as compared with the highest SES level. Are these simply fortuitous correlations or do they have implications for development of more effective and valid models of understanding?

Why is socioeconomic status associated with mental retardation and emotional disturbance? What is the direction of causality? What are the implications for prevention? These are important questions, ones that have been addressed before. Yet their resolution is anything but clear. One fact emerges from an analysis of the relevant literature, much of it of fairly recent origin. Environment, including family background, plays a more significant role than biomedical factors in determining developmental outcome, even among neonates with medical problems (Freeman, 1985). The studies before us show that, except for severe handicaps at birth, dysfunctions—as defined by the new morbidity—are more strongly predicted by family variables and SES. Prevention strategies will have to be based on environmental considerations.

The relatively high risk of mental retardation and psychiatric disorder in lower SES groups is best characterized by a transactional process in which certain children are psychologically and biologically vulnerable to environmental and social variations that predispose them to school, economic, and social failure—the "new morbidity." Many of these conclusions were reached in the widely cited book published by Birch and Gussow (1970), although then there was much more conjecture than data. A number of publications appearing within the past two or three years have added increasingly precise information to the argument.

The environments in which economically deprived children develop are less conducive to good physical, social, and behavioral development than the environments of children not disadvantaged. These differences are deep rooted, fundamental, enduring, and intergenerational—a fact that has not received sufficient attention and respect. As a group, mothers of such children are not so well nourished, they are smaller, and they received less nurturing care as children themselves. When they have their own children, they are younger (frequently teenagers) and they have children more frequently. When she is pregnant, the general health of a woman at the low SES range will be poorer than that of a woman who is better off, and her fetus will be exposed to greater risk of infection, intoxication, and trauma. Prenatal and general health care are less accessible to her, a condition that appears to be growing even more serious owing to recent cutbacks in health care programs. Today, she is far less apt to be married than her richer sister and thus more vulnerable to a number of threats to good child-rearing practices. When they are born, babies of such mothers are, on the average, smaller for gestational age, more likely to be premature, die more readily and more suddenly, are sicker in infancy, suffer a higher rate of accidents, and run a greater risk of neglect than children born into better circumstances. Their mortality is excessively high at birth and beyond. Their illnesses are more frequent, more persistent, and more severe. Their development is a function of maternal health, age, income level, education, habits, and social milieu. During the school years, nutrition may be inadequate, the children miss school more frequently, housing is frequently substandard, and family income is low. These children present a higher rate of learning problems, behavior disturbances, allergies, and speech difficulties (Birch & Gussow, 1970; Freeman, 1985; Laosa, 1984).

Disadvantage, whether economic, educational, or biological, occurs through time, each generation passing on to the next the unfortunate and cumulative consequences of its own experience, as in a circle with no clear beginning and no clear end. Neither the much rehearsed cultural-deficit nor the venerable genetic-inheritance theory is adequate to explain the development of different forms of social competence, economic inequality, and biological vulnerability. There are more sophisticated, albeit complex, developmental models that could form the basis for policy-oriented prevention of some psychopathology (Laosa, 1979).

A number of other indicators ought to be taken into account. Collectively, they also lead to the conclusion that living conditions are causally associated with disability. For example, in 1983, there were over 67 million children in the United States. Of these, 18% were below the poverty line. Among the poverty group, 8.5% had some sort of functional disability. The corresponding figure for the more affluent children was 4%. Of those with disability, only 7% of the non-poverty children were uninsured by private or public sources. For the disabled children in the poverty group, 20% were uninsured (Butler et al., 1984). That difference has a direct effect on both prevention and intervention. Current data state that poverty is again on the increase and that those most affected are the children—particularly minority children.

Miller, in the July 1985 issue of *Scientific American*, presents a very sobering review of some current developments and concludes that recent government cuts have contributed significantly to the change of trend in infant mortality rate. The National Academy of Science in 1985 reported overwhelming evidence that early prenatal care reduces incidence of low birthweight and associated medical and behavior disorders. They also report that social risks, including being unmarried, of an unfavorable age, or poorly educated, are more important than medical risks. The Kauai study, now a classic but still relevant, provides clear evidence of a 10-year growth-related interaction between perinatal factors and the environment into which the child is born (Werner, Brennan, & French, 1971). Boldman and Reed (1977) studied low birthweight in 39 countries and concluded that the major risk factors include rural living, low per capita income, lack of medical services, and low newspaper circulation, among others. Much of this literature has been summarized in a recent book entitled *Prenatal and Perinatal Factors Associated with Brain Disorders*, a major work sponsored by NICHD (Freeman,

1985). Another recent publication, *Black and White Children in America*, presents data showing clear racial differences in these trends.

Low birthweight is associated with mental retardation, cerebral palsy, epilepsy, sensory defects, learning problems, and school failure. Of course, this correlation may be the product of a host of intervening and moderating biological and psychological variables. But, in any case, over the past decade or longer, literature has been accumulated that points to the connection between birth variables and subsequent development as modulated by social factors. This literature begins to tell part of the story: Women who live in adverse economic and social environments are at high risk of giving birth to smaller babies, with associated risks of developmental disability, adjustment problems, and other forms of morbidity.

One recent set of studies is of particular interest because an effort was made to control for genetic confounds by examining twins. Wilson (1983, 1985) has recently presented data concerning risk and resilience in early development among samples of monozygotic and dizygotic twins. In these studies, risk was defined as SGA (small for gestational age) and low birthweight. The low birthweight twins exhibited substantially lower IQs. But there was an interaction in which the upper SES twins recovered completely by the sixth year. The conclusion is drawn that parental education and SES are powerfully related to six-year IQ scores among at-risk infants. Although these data take us into controversial country, public policy will inevitably have to develop along these lines, if for no other reason than abortion is an option and costs of intervention and care are high and growing.

Increased attention needs to be directed at understanding more precisely the epidemiology of the new morbidity, especially the behavioral and social aspects. A new generation of research will have to be aimed at increasing effectiveness of public health initiatives, especially those involving social components. Intervention research needs to be carried out on a systematic and longitudinal basis on a scale sufficient to enlarge our understanding of behavioral correlates. Finally, we need to develop a superior classification system that includes different types of concurrent problems and their interactions coded in terms of quality of adjustments, rather than diseases.

Social, cultural, and economic factors extend widely and deeply into so many important facets of life, including those that concern adaptation. It is clear that environmental elements are the main factors associated with relative and, to a lesser extent, with absolute retardation. Purely technological advances will not be sufficient in themselves to reduce risks associated with the new morbidity.

Our research and programs need to be directed more clearly and meaningfully at real-life problems of human development. Researchers and professionals obviously share this responsibility—but so do federal agencies responsible for research on behavior disability. There is an institutional responsibility to fulfill the public trust, at the very least, by insisting on relevance. For too long we have skirted the most fundamental issues. The problem demands a response consistent with its complexity and significance. When the human and economic costs of emotional and intellectual handicaps are measured against investments in research, prevention, and treatment, it is clear that the response has not been commensurate with the need.

## References

Baumeister, A.A. (1968). Behavioral inadequacy and efficiency of performance. *American Journal of Mental Deficiency, 73*, 477–483.

Baumeister, A.A. (1981). Mental retardation policy and research: The unfulfilled promise. *American Journal of Mental Deficiency, 85*, 449–456.

Baumeister, A.A., & Hamlett, C.L. (1986). A national survey of state-sponsored programs to prevent fetal alcohol syndrome. *Mental Retardation, 24*, 169–173.

Birch, H.G., & Gussow, J.D. (1970). *Disadvantaged children: Health, nutrition and school failure.* New York: Harcourt Brace Jovanovich.

Boldman, R., & Reed, D.M. (1977). Worldwide variations in birth weight. In D.M. Reed & F.J. Stanley (Eds.), *The epidemiology of prematurity.* Baltimore, MD: Urban and Schwartzenberg.

Butler, J.A., Starfield, B., & Stenmark, S. (1984). Child health policy. In H.W. Stevenson & A.E. Siegel (Eds.), *Child development and social policy.* Chicago, IL: University of Chicago Press.

Freeman, J.M. (Ed.). (1985). *Prenatal and perinatal factors associated with brain disorders.* Washington, DC: U.S. Department of Health and Human Services.

Haggerty, R.J., Roghmann, K.J., & Pless, I.B. (Eds). (1975). *Child health and the community.* New York: Wiley.

Kopp, C. (1983). Risk factors in development. In P.H. Mussen (Ed.), *Handbook of child psychology* (4th ed.). New York: Wiley.

Landesman-Dwyer, S., & Butterfield, E.C. (1983). Mental retardation: Developmental issues in cognitive and social adaptation. In M. Lewis (Ed.), *Origins of intelligence: Infancy and early childhood* (2nd ed.). New York: Plenum Press.

Laosa, L.M. (1979). Social competence in children: Toward a developmental, socioculturally realistic paradigm. In M.W. Lent & J.E. Rolf (Eds.), *Primary prevention of psychopathology,* Vol. 3: *Social competence in children.* Hanover: University Press of New England.

Laosa, L.M. (1984). Social policies toward children of diverse ethnic, racial, and language groups in the United States. In H.W. Stevenson & A.E. Siegel (Eds.), *Child development research and social policy.* Chicago, IL: University of Chicago Press.

Miller, C.A. (1985). Infant mortality in the U.S. *Scientific American, 253*(1), 31–37.

Moser, H.W. (1985). Biologic factors of development. In J.M. Freeman (Ed.), *Prenatal and perinatal factors associated with brain disorders.* Washington, DC: U.S. Department of Health and Human Services.

National Center for Health Statistics. (June, 1986). Current estimates from the National Health Interview Survey, United States, 1983. *Vital and Health Statistics*, Series 10, No. 154, DHHS Pub. No. (PHS) 86-1582 (Public Health Service). Washington, DC: U.S. Government Printing Office.

Richardson, S.A. (1980). Growing up as a mentally subnormal young person: A follow-up study. In S.A. Mednick & A.E. Baert (Eds.), *An empirical basis for primary prevention: Prospective longitudinal research in Europe.* Oxford: Oxford University Press.

Robinson, N.H., & Robinson, H.B. (1976). *The mentally retarded child* (2nd ed.). New York: McGraw-Hill.

Tarjan, G., Dornbusch, S.M., Fenichel, G., Graham, F., Richmond, J., & Zigler, E. (1977). *Federal research activity in mental retardation: A review with recommendations for the future.* A report to the Directors of NICHD and NIMH. Washington, DC: U.S. Department of Health, Education and Welfare.

Werner, E.E., Brennan, J.M., & French, F.E. (1971). *The children of Kauai: A longitudinal study from the perinatal period to age ten.* Honolulu, HI: University of Hawaii Press.

Wilson, R.S. (1983). The Louisville twin study: Developmental synchronies in behavior. *Child Development, 54*, 298–316.

Wilson, R.S. (1985). Risk and resilience in early mental development. *Developmental Psychology, 21*, 795–805.

# 7
# Psychiatry, Neuroscience, and the Double Disabilities

JOSEPH T. COYLE

## Introduction

Historically, there has been a notable lack of psychiatric involvement in the evaluation and management of individuals with a developmental disability. Certain factors may account for this deficiency. Psychoanalytic theory, which until recently has played a dominant role in diagnosis and treatment in psychiatry, was generally inapplicable to the types of behavioral problems and psychiatric symptoms that affect the developmentally disabled. Furthermore, the inappropriate institutionalization of developmentally disabled and mentally retarded in state psychiatric facilities has caused justifiable reaction of advocates for the mentally retarded against the stigmatizing effects of such placement and the inappropriate forms of treatment that may have resulted from it.

In the absence of meaningful psychiatric input to the management of the developmentally disabled, psychological and behavioral interventions that use operant conditioning paradigms have gained ascendence in the practical management of their behavioral problems. The seeming advantage of this treatment strategy is that it does not require a mechanistic understanding of the causes of deviant behavior but exploits operant principles to reinforce positive behaviors and extinguish negative behaviors. Nevertheless, this strength must be counterbalanced by the fact that the operant approach is primarily symptom oriented and does not address the developmental level, social understanding, and differing brain etiologies for the behaviors. For example, self-injurious behavior likely has different neuronal causes in the childhood disorders such as Lesch-Nyhan syndrome and pervasive development disorder (PDD).

## Psychiatry and Neuroscience

The last two decades have witnessed an increasing focus in psychiatry on brain mechanisms responsible for deviant behavior in disorders classically considered within the realm of psychiatry, such as the affective disorders and schizophrenia, as well as those disorders with prominent behavioral symptoms, which lie at the interface between psychiatry and neurology, such as Huntington's disease and Alzheimer's disease. The impetus for this shift in focus came from developments both at the preclinical and the clinical levels. The growing appreciation that clinically effective psychotropic medications exert their therapeutic effects by altering the biochemical processes in brain that mediate synaptic neurotransmission has prompted an increasing emphasis on research into the anatomy, physiology, and biochemistry of brain neurotransmitter systems. As a result of the burgeoning research in this area, the number of identified neurotransmitters in the brain has increased 10-fold over the last decade, and a new area of brain research that focuses on neurotransmitter receptors has emerged.

At the clinical level, a shift in focus to a phenomenological categorization of psychiatric disorders, which takes an agnostic stance about psychodynamic causes, has resulted in a cleaner delineation of psychiatric syndromes that appear to be etiologically more homogeneous. This has allowed for more rigorous analysis of the genetic and epigenetic factors that may contribute to the cause of psychiatric disorders such as a schizophrenia, affective disorders, and Tourette's syndrome, to mention a few. Presently, investigators are beginning to exploit molecular genetic approaches such as restriction fragment length polymorphisms (RFLP), which has been used with success in Huntington's disease, to identify genetic loci that are associated with familial transmission of certain psychiatric disorders.

The growth of neuroscientific and molecular biological thinking in psychiatry has not eroded the important foundation in psychological, psychotherapeutic, and behavioral treatment approaches. Nevertheless, there is increasing emphasis on developing objective criteria for the efficacy of behavioral and psychotherapeutic treatment modalities so that they are evaluated by the same rigorous standards required for somatic therapies. In addition, there is increasing appreciation of the interaction between psychological stressors and physiological vulnerabilities. For example, the studies of Falloon (1985) have underlined the impact of the emotional environment in the family on the efficacy of neuroleptic treatment to control the symptoms of schizophrenia.

A salutory development with regard to understanding the pathophysiological basis of behavioral disorders in the developmental disabilities is the increasing attention placed on defining neurotransmitter systems that may be dysfunctional in these disorders and the development of suitable animal models for determining the impact of these abnormalities on brain function and behavior. Our increasing appreciation of the complex processes involved in brain development and the issues of selective neuronal vulnerability should disabuse clinicians and fundamental investigators of assumptions about "nonspecific" damage to brain that cause behavioral and psychiatric symptoms in the developmentally disabled and mentally retarded.

## Alzheimer's Disease: A Precedent

A major impetus for scrutinizing these assumptions about the "nonspecificity" of brain damage comes from the advances made at the other end of the age spectrum with regard to senile dementia. Until approximately a decade ago, the deterioration of cognitive functions that occurred in approximately 5% of individuals over the age of 65 was thought to be a normal consequence of the aging process. However, the demonstration that the brains in a majority of affected individuals exhibited the same neuropathology as those suffering from presenile dementia of the Alzheimer's type gave credence to the hypothesis that senile dementia was in fact a disease process. Nevertheless, it was widely held that the progressive dilapidation of higher cognitive functions, characteristic of senile dementia of the Alzheimer's type (SDAT), reflected a nonspecific, progressive, and global deterioration of cerebral cortical neurons, leading to the pessimistic proposal that it be considered "brain failure."

The application of postmortem analysis of synaptic neurochemical markers to the brains of individuals who had died with SDAT has demonstrated that certain sets of cortical projecting neurons, such as the basal forebrain cholinergic neurons and the locus ceruleus noradrenergic neurons, are profoundly affected whereas many types of local circuit neurons within the cerebral cortex remain largely spared by the process (Coyle, Price, & DeLong, 1983). Furthermore, the neuropathological stigmata diagnostic of Alzheimer's dementia— the neuritic plaques and neurofibrillary tangles—have recently been demonstrated to affect those neurotransmitter systems deficient in the SDAT. Parallel studies at the preclinical level have provided increasing information about the organization, function, and behavioral role played by the neurotransmitter systems that appear to be selectively vulnerable in SDAT. These findings have led to the development of pharmacological strategies to correct the cholinergic deficits in SDAT and to alleviate the cognitive impairments (Mohs et al., 1985).

## Down's Syndrome

The research on SDAT has had direct impact on the most common form of chromosomally based mental retardation—Down's syndrome which is due to trisomy of chromosome 21. Neuropathological studies have demonstrated that virtually all individuals with Down's syndrome develop the neuropathology of Alzheimer's disease by their fourth decade (Wisniewski, Wisniewski, & Wen, 1985). Furthermore, postmortem synaptic neurochemical studies have revealed the selective vulnerability of the cortically projecting cholinergic and nonadrenergic projections that are similarly affected in SDAT (Yates et al., 1983). Thus, the seeds of selective neuronal vulnerability in Down's syndrome appear to be determined by aneuploidy of genes encoded on chromosome 21.

In spite of these observations, remarkably little is known about the pathophysiological basis of mental retardation, the nearly inevitable phenotypic expression in Down's syndrome (Coyle, Oster-Granite, & Gearhart, 1986). Postmortem neuropathological studies have revealed a reduction in cortical mass, selective depletion of cortical inner neurons, and other more subtle structural abnormalities of the brain. However, the developmental basis for these defects and their implications for brain function and ultimately for behavior remain poorly understood and difficult to decipher from human postmortem studies.

Fortunately, some of these questions may be resolved through studies on a mouse model for Down's syndrome – the Trisomy 16 mouse. Such mice are generated by mating mice with stable Robertsonian translocation of chromosome 16 to normal acrocentric mice. Approximately 20% of the conceptuses of this mating exhibit translocation trisomy of chromosome 16 (TS-16). Gene mapping studies have demonstrated that several of the genes located on human chromosome 21 are found on chromosome 16 in the mouse (Reeves, Gearhart, & Littlefield, 1986). Furthermore, these mice exhibit phenotypic characteristics reminiscent of those observed in Down's syndrome, such as a high incidence of cardiac cushion defects, hematological disorders, and craniofacial dysplasia.

Preliminary studies to understand the neurobiology of the TS-16 mouse have revealed selective failures in the fetal development of brain noradrenergic and cholinergic neuronal systems, whereas the markers for the GABAergic neurons appear to be generally within the range of littermate euploid controls (Singer, Tiemeyer, Hedreen, Gearhart, & Coyle, 1984). Furthermore, histological analyses of the fetal TS-16 telencephalon reveal an increased ratio of the thickness of the ventricular germinal zone to the thickness of the entire cortex, which suggests a delay in cortical neuronal differentiation. This finding is consistent with and provides a neuroembryological basis for the reported hypocellularity of the Down's cerebral cortex. Thus, the TS-16 model offers an opportunity for rigorously testing hypothesized mechanisms involved in the genetic processes including altered cell cycle time owing to the aneuploid condition, alterations in cellular characteristics owing to deviant expression of genes encoded on chromosome 16, or abnormalities in placental function.

Since the TS-16 mouse fetus rarely survives to birth, which is equivalent to the mid-second trimester in the human in terms of brain development, critical aspects of brain maturation and aging are not feasible for study in the TS-16 mouse per se. Nevertheless, it is possible to "rescue" the TS-16 neurons to characterize later aspects of synaptogenesis, synaptic maintenance, and plasticity. This can and has been accomplished through various strategies, including the creation of chimeras from euploid and TS-16 conceptuses, culture of TS-16 fetal neurons, or transplantation of fetal TS-16 brain regions into adult euploid mice.

## Cortical Hypoplasia

A variety of insults, including infection, anoxia, malnutrition, and perhaps toxin exposure, can lead to failure of the normal formation of the cerebral cortex during the first trimester of human development and are invariably associated with mental retardation. While such damage could be considered of fairly nonspecific nature, closer scrutiny of fetally induced disruption of the cerebral cortical development has revealed selective alterations in transmitter-specific pathways in response to such damage. A better understanding of these altered synaptic relationships as a consequence of fetal cortical damage might shed light on the pathophysiology of behavioral and cognitive dysfunction associated with them in humans.

To explore this issue in experimental animals, we have exploited the effects of an alkylating agent, methylazoxymethanol acetate (MAM), with a very brief half-life, which kills mitotically active cells (Johnston, Grzanna, & Coyle, 1979). By administering the MAM to pregnant rat dams at the time when the neurons that would form the various layers of the cerebral cortex (days 13 to 18 of gestation) are actively dividing in the fetal brain, relatively specific deletions of fetal cortical neurons could be accomplished. The MAM-treated offspring exhibit rather selective cortical hypoplasia. Synaptic neurochemical analyses have revealed marked alterations in the relationships between cortical intrinsic and afferent systems, especially those derived from the aminergic reticular core, in the hypoplastic cerebral cortex. The concentration of GABAergic neurons in the hypoplastic cortex appeared to be within the range of normal, whereas there was a marked enrichment in the presynaptic markers for noradrenergic, serotonergic, and cholinergic terminals derived from the reticular core. Interestingly, the developmental appearance of the abnormal synaptic relationships varied among the different neurotransmitter systems examined. Further analysis revealed that the cortical afferent projections from the reticular core appeared to develop a quantitatively normal terminal arbor that is compressed within the reduced cortical volume resulting in a functional relative hyperinnervation. Thus, the impact of the lesion must be viewed not only in terms of which neurons are deleted but also which neurons remain and how this affects their synaptic circuitry. Behavioral analysis of these fetally lesioned rats further reveals hyperactivity, impulsivity, impairments in learning, and persistence of immature behaviors (Moran, Sanberg, Antuono, & Coyle, 1986).

## Metabolic and Storage Disorders

Storage disorders can be considered a relatively nonspecific cause of disruption of brain neuronal integrity caused by the accumulation of lipids or glycosides as a result of enzymatic defects in their metabolism. Nevertheless, it must be remembered that these accumulated precursors or products often serve a vital role in the structure and function of neurons and in the processes that mediate chemical neurotransmission. While storage disorders typically result in rather global and early deterioration of motor and cognitive functions, in certain circumstances these heritable disorders can be associated with rather specific psychiatric symptoms such as the occurrence of schizophreniclike symptoms in some patients with metachromatic leucodystrophy (Manowitz, Kling, & Koher, 1978). Such symptomatic manifestations of storage disorders raise the question whether certain brain neuronal systems may be more vulnerable than others.

In support of more specific interactions of storage disorders with processes involved in synaptic neurotransmission, we have demonstrated rather selective disruption of processes involved in specific neurotransmitter function in the brains of cats suffering from GM-1 gangliosidosis, a storage disorder that appears to be identical to its human counterpart. Analysis of several presynaptic components of specific neurotransmitter systems in the cat model at terminal stages of GM-1 gangliosidosis revealed selective impairments in certain parameters (Singer, Coyle, Weaver, Kawamura, & Baker, 1982). Although the levels of the neurotransmitters, glutamate, GABA, and norepinephrine and the specific activity of the biosynthetic enzymes for acetylcholine, GABA, and catecholines were not altered in several brain regions, the specific activities of the high-affinity uptake processes for glutamate, GABA, and norepinephrine, a major route of synaptic inactivation, were markedly decreased. As the GM-1 ganglioside is enriched in synaptic membranes, it would appear that the elevated levels of GM-1 ganglioside may have altered the membrane characteristics, thereby impairing this inactivation mechanism. While the relationship between this defect in neurotransmitter inactivation and progressive symptoms in GM-1 gangliosidosis is unclear, these findings do point to the fact that a storage disorder can have differential effects on processes regulating synaptic neurotransmission.

A number of heritable metabolic defects affect the urea cycle and result in the development of hyperammonemia in affected individuals. In spite of dietary and pharmacological interventions that can control the hyperammonemia in affected individuals, a frequent behavioral complication of the disorder is persistent food refusal. Considerable evidence has implicated serotonin in appetite suppression. In recent studies, rats have been rendered hyperammonemic by chronic infusion of urease, an enzyme that converts urea to ammonia. Hyperammonia caused a significant elevation in serotonin turnover in brain. These preclinical findings have been substantiated in one case of persistent food refusal in a patient suffering from ornithine transcarbamoylase deficiency. This patient was found to have elevated CSF levels of 5-hydroxy-indole-acetic acid (HIAA), the metabolite of serotonin; and, in addition, she exhibited reduced pain sensitivity and abnormalities in rapid eye movement sleep patterns consistent with increased serotonergic activity in brain (Hyman et al., 1986). Dietary manipulation to reduce the availability of tryptophane for serotonin synthesis in brain resulted in marked improvement in feeding and normalization of sleep patterns. Although multiple factors impact feeding behavior, this example demonstrates that manipulation of one of the factors, which appears to be impaired by the metabolic disorder, can positively influence the aberrant behavior.

## Conclusion

Over the last decade, a remarkable growth in understanding of the synaptic and molecular mechanisms involved in brain function has occurred. In particular, the high degree of complexity and specificity of neuronal communication at the synaptic level has been uncovered. Whether the list of neurotransmitters and neuromodulators will continue to expand at the present rate remains unknown. Nevertheless, the application of synaptic neurochemical and immunocytochemical techniques has revealed the chemically encoded wiring of the brain that was unable to be perceived with more classic neuroanatomic approaches. The application of these techniques to studies of postmortem brain material obtained from individuals dying with neurogenerative disorders and, to a more limited extent, developmental disorders has revealed a surprising level of specificity of neuronal vulnerability of certain neurotransmitter systems. Thus, a relatively selective degeneration of reticular core noradrenergic and cholinergic projections that has been described in SDAT also affects Down's syndrome individuals in midlife. Preclinical studies have revealed a relative enhancement of the density of terminal innervation of these two systems in congenitally induced cortical hypoplasia. Additional studies have disclosed the impact of storage disorders and metabolic disorders on selective components of the biochemical processes involved in chemical neurotransmission in brain. Thus, it would appear that disorders that have generally been thought to have rather nonspecific effects on brain structure and function, once examined, are found to have rather selective effects on specific neurotransmitter systems.

It is evident that further efforts need to be made in characterizing the synaptic neurochemical processes in a variety of hereditary and congenital developmental disorders. The limited studies carried out thus far, for example, with Lesch-Nyhan syndrome, provide intriguing hints to metabolically determined dysfunction of the nigrostriatal neurotransmitter system that may provide insight into the dystonic symptoms of this disorder and possibly the self-injurious behavior associated with the disorder. Nevertheless, much more needs to be known about specific syndromes such as Tourette's syndrome, fragile X syndrome, Down's syndrome, and a host of other identified metabolic and storage disorders.

As there is reasonable basis for the belief that neurotransmitters are the ultimate arbiters of information processing in the brain, delineation of neurotransmitter abnormalities in the various developmental disabilities and further elucidation of their physiological and behavioral implications in animal models should lead to a better understanding of the pathophysiological basis of the various behavioral and psychiatric symptoms that may complicate many of these disorders. Such information should provide the foundation for a more rational approach toward the pharmacological, metabolic, and behavioral intervention to alleviate these symptoms. The brains of the developmentally disabled should no longer be considered "black boxes" in which the primary means of symptom management is controlling the contingencies to affect the output. The physiological processes that are likely to be uniquely disrupted in specific disorders should no longer be ignored. For example, the multiple neurotransmitter systems that have been shown to affect sensory processing, pain sensation, and reinforcement point to the several sites at which epigenetic as well as genetically induced developmental disabilities could produce self-injurious behavior. We must move beyond an agnostic consideration of the contingencies that control these behaviors to appreciate the disorder-specific neurobiological mechanisms that are responsible for these behaviors. It seems reasonable that more specific interventions would be more successful and free the patient of behavioral constraints that may be irrelevant.

# Recommendations

Several recommendations are offered that might help correct the current deficiencies in the diagnosis and treatment of behavioral disorders of the developmentally disabled.

First, there must be an increasing emphasis on the delineation of behavioral disorders associated with distinct diagnostic entities. Ignoring the brain pathologies that are likely specific for different structural and metabolic disorders will prevent advances in understanding the causes of their behavioral symptoms. To assist in this endeavor, brain banks need to be established that will allow for the application of current synaptic neurochemical and immunocytochemical methods that have successfully been exploited in clarifying the pathophysiology of Huntington's disease, Parkinson's disease, and Alzheimer's disease. These postmortem studies should be complemented by clinical studies exploiting structural and functional imaging techniques such as positron emission tomography, nuclear magnetic resonance imaging, and BEAM.

Second, support for fundamental neurobiological research relevant to the developmental disorders needs to be augmented. The powerful tools of synaptic neurochemistry, developmental neurobiology, molecular neurobiology, and brain imaging must be implemented to clarify the fundamental processes involved in the causes and symptomatic manifestations of developmental disabilities.

Third, training programs that support the training of child and adult psychiatrists in the behavioral complications of developmental disabilities and their impact on families need to be supported. Preferably, these training programs should be located at large teaching/research centers for developmental disabilities.

Finally, multidisciplinary approaches to the diagnosis and management of the behavioral disorders of the developmentally disabled need to be encouraged. This necessitates a sophisticated biopsychosocial conceptual approach that recognizes the potential contributory role of brain dysfunction in the behavioral disorders.

# References

Hyman, S.L., Coyle, J.T., Parke, J.C., Porter, C., Thomas, G.H., Jankel, W., & Batshaw, M.L. (1986). Anorexia and altered serotonin metabolism in a patient with argininosuccinic aciduria. *Journal of Pediatrics*, 108:705–709.

Coyle, J.T., Price, D.L., & DeLong, M.R. (1983). Alzheimer's disease: A disorder of cortical cholinergic innervation. *Science, 219*, 1184–1190.

Coyle, J.T., Oster-Granite, M.L., & Gearhart, J.D. (1986). The neurobiologic consequences of Down syndrome. *Brain Research Bulletin, 16*, 773–787.

Falloon, I.R.H. (1985). *Family management of schizophrenia.* Baltimore, MD: Johns Hopkins University Press.

Johnston, M.W., Grzanna, R., & Coyle, J.T. (1979). Methylazoxymethanol treatment of fetal rats results in abnormally dense noradrenergic innervation of neocortex. *Science, 203*, 369–371.

Manowitz, P., Kling, A., & Koher, H. (1978). Clinical course of adult metachromatic leukodystrophy presenting as schizophrenia. *Journal of Nervous and Mental Disorders, 166,* 500–509.

Mohs, R.C., Davis, B.M., Johns, C.A., Mathe, A.A., Greenwald, B.S., Horvath, T.B., & Davis, K.L. (1985). Oral physostigmine treatment of patients with Alzheimer's disease. *American Journal of Psychiatry, 142,* 28–33.

Moran, T.H., Sanberg, P.R., Antuono, P.G., & Coyle, J.T. (1986). Methylazoxymethanol acetate cortical hypoplasia alters the pattern of stimulation-induced behavior in neonatal rats. *Developmental Brain Research, 27,* 235–242.

Reeves, R.H., Gearhart, J.D., & Littlefield, J.W. (1986). Genetic basis for a mouse model of Down Syndrome. *Brain Research Bulletin, 16,* 803–814.

Singer, H.S., Coyle, J.T., Weaver, D.L., Kawamura, N., & Baker, H.J. (1982). Neurotransmitter chemistry in feline $GM_1$ gangliosidosis: A model for human ganglioside storage disease. *Annals of Neurology, 12,* 37–41.

Singer, H.S., Tiemeyer, M., Hedreen, J.C., Gearhart, J., & Coyle, J.T. (1984). Morphologic and neurochemical studies of embryonic brain development in murine Trisomy 16. *Developmental Brain Research, 15,* 155–166.

Wisniewski, K.E., Wisniewski, H.M., & Wen, G.Y. (1985). Occurrence of neuropathologic changes and dementia of Alzheimer's disease in Down's syndrome. *Annals of Neurology, 17,* 278–282.

Yates, C.M., Simpson, J., Gordon, A., Maloney, A.F.J., Allison, Y., Ritchie, I.M., & Urghuhart, A. (1983). Catecholamine and cholinergic enzymes in presenile and senile Alzheimer's like disease and Down's syndrome. *Brain Research, 280,* 119–126.

# 8
# Attentional and Neurochemical Components of Mental Retardation: New Methods for an Old Problem

Robert D. Hunt and Donald J. Cohen

## Attention Deficit Disorder with Hyperactivity

Specific cognitive impairments occur within a wide spectrum of overall intelligence. The attentional components that comprise an important dimension of learning deficits include the capacity for both selective and sustained attention. About 3% of American children are estimated to have attention deficit disorder that is often associated with motoric hyperactivity (ADDH), impulsivity, aggression, and conduct disorder. This disorder was previously termed "minimal brain dysfunction," suggesting an organic etiology, and "hyperactivity," which described the most prominent symptom. DSM-III has emphasized the attentional component of this disorder, its onset before age seven, and its persistence. Increasing research and follow-up studies indicate that the impulsivity, distractability, and restlessness may continue into adulthood. Children with this disorder frequently wear out their parents' patience, their teachers' tolerance, and their peers' cooperativeness. They are predisposed to oppositional behavior, defiance of authority, and conduct disorder. ADDH may be a substrate for juvenile delinquency and later adult criminality.

Both genetic and environmental/familial influences contribute to the incidence, clinical pattern, and outcome of this disorder. Genetic studies, using the adoption and twin comparisons, suggest an inherited substrate for this disorder. Parents of affected children have an increased incidence of learning disabilities, depression, hysteria, and alcoholism. This genetic component suggests that the symptoms of some of these children may be mediated by an underlying neurochemical substrate.

Treatment of attention disorder with hyperactivity requires multiple forms of intervention that include special education, behavioral modification, focused psychotherapy, and medication. Selective attentional disruption impairs the learning and function of many individuals with milder forms of mental retardation. Approximately 10% of children with mental retardation also have hyperkinetic symptoms. Inadvertently, our scientific taxonomy has been biased against the study and treatment of selected attentional impairments in the retarded. Attention deficit disorder with hyperactivity is currently defined as a cognitive and behavioral disturbance of children of normal intelligence—and most studies are performed in this population. Regrettably, this limitation has diminished our understanding of the nature of attentional disturbances in precisely those individuals in whom it is most prominent. This exclusion has also impeded studies of the most effective treatment of inattention and hyperactivity within the retarded. To proceed scientifically, we must assess attentional competence in relation to a child's developmental quotient that reflects mental age and extend cognitive and biological evaluation into the developmentally delayed.

## Information Processing

Recent developments in the assessment of information processing suggest that different processes may disrupt attention along temporal and conceptual continua. These cognitive processes include stimulus scanning, selective attention, signal–noise discrimination, vigilance, retrieval from short- and long-term memory, and associative processes that link current and past experiences. An attentional disturbance may be specific to the type of stimulus, the intensity and similarity of distractors, and perhaps the specific psychiatric disorder of the subject. Schizophrenics exhibit difficulty in scanning processes and discrimination of relevant versus irrelevant stimuli. Children with attention disorder are impaired in their ability to sustain attention and to inhibit response to irrelevant stimuli. Using more sophisticated methods, investigators are studying information processing in order to define where in the cognitive sequence specific deficits may occur.

The identification of differential mechanisms of attentional disturbances are now becoming available for studies of the retarded. Assessment of the cognitive competencies of the retarded often reveals a wide range of abilities within an individual. These areas of relative strength or weakness may parallel identifiable regions or circuits of adequate or impaired brain functioning. Conversely, individuals with a specific genetic, metabolic, or anatomic basis for developmental delay may reveal focal or functionally limited cognitive deficits. Study of the interaction between specific cognitive activities and the functioning of the central nervous system may delineate regional or metabolic components of brain functioning. Similarly, behavioral problems—especially aggressive behavior—are often associated with attentional disturbance in the retarded as well as in normally intelligent children. Brain mechanisms that regulate arousal, aggression, and attention appear closely related neurochemically and anatomically. Thus, studies that link distinguishable patterns of cognitive and behavioral disturbance with measures of brain structure and neurochemistry may provide a key to the enigma of brain–behavior interactions. An integrated social, cognitive, and neurochemical assessment may lead to more precise pharmacological treatment of the aggressive, retarded child. Ultimately, this may diminish reliance on neuroleptic medication whose potential for cognitive blunting and late-onset movements is increasingly being recognized.

New methods of cognitive assessment are being applied in the study of the underlying intellectual disturbance of attention deficit disorder. Earlier studies focused primarily on overall measures of intelligence, reaction time, and continuous performance tasks (CPT), such as Kagan's Matching Familiar Figures Task, which assesses cognitive impulsivity, identification of Embedded Figures, which estimates field–ground discrimination, and the Stropp Color Naming Task, which indexes the extent of being stimulus bound.

New cognitive measures that are becoming available for computerized presentation are being developed, in part, by investigators at UCLA and UC–Irvine. These include the use of a Degraded (blurred) Stimulus in CPT, which assesses selective attention and perceptual discrimination as well as vigilance. The Span of Apprehension Task distinguishes parallel versus serial strategies of visual screening. A Memory Scanning Task identifies channel capacity, the effects of spatial organization, and the impact of similar or dissimilar distractions on immediate memory. A Paired Associate Learning Task measures the ability to learn specific, new relationships in varying modalities and assesses the shift from short- to long-term memory. Word Recall Tasks that control for word meaning (category), frequency, imagery, and sequence can be used to assess strategies of encoding and decoding from semantic or episodic memory by measuring free and cued recall and sequential memory of events. These new developments in cognitive assessment can define more precisely where in information processing a specific deficit may lie. These assessments may be linked to increasingly precise neurochemical challenges that may define abnormalities in production, release, or response of a neurotransmitter or peptide system.

## Psychopharmacological Treatment

Developmentally delayed children with attentional disturbances require even more intensive social and educational intervention than that needed for the usual hyperactive child. Greater differentiation of subtypes of attentional and cognitive deficits may assist in planning educational interventions and in more precise selection of pharmacological treatments. The retarded often have special problems in the management of their hyperactivity, inattention, impulsivity, and aggression. More careful systematic studies are needed to define the effectiveness of stimulant medications in the treatment of retarded hyperactive children.

Our recent studies of a new therapeutic agent for attention deficit disorder, clonidine, suggest that it may be an effective alternative to stimulants such as Ritalin in the management of some of the behavioral difficulties of these children. Clonidine decreases their excessive activity and appears to have fewer side effects. The clinical boundaries of the usefulness of clonidine have not yet been established. In low doses, clonidine specifically reduces the activity of the noradrenalin system. Clonidine treatment produced a significant decrease of symptoms as rated on behavioral rating scales (performed weekly by parents and teachers and monthly by clinicians) at 1 and 2 months of active treatment (Figure

8.1). After discontinuing clonidine, patients quickly reverted to pretreatment behavior. About 70% of the children that we have treated improved on clonidine. These findings require further validation in this disorder, but the strategy of treating with a medication that has a very specific mechanism of action may be useful in seeking neurochemical correlates of specific patterns of behavioral disturbances in the retarded.

Federal funding can facilitate an improved understanding of the link between cognitive and neurochemical components of brain functioning. Funding should target methods that aid in understanding the basic mechanisms of these disorders with sufficient clarity to guide treatment and the development of new therapeutic agents. Several scientific methods currently are being developed at major research medical centers which hold promise for identification of disturbances in brain functioning within the retarded. These methods include measures of the response to neurochemical challenge agents, evaluation of receptor binding, brain imaging, and selective psychopharmacology.

## Neurochemical Challenge Studies

Neurochemical challenge studies provide an indirect measure of central brain neurochemistry and receptor responsivity in children and adults with psychiatric disorders. The technique involves the use of a chemical probe that selectively activates or inhibits a specific neurotransmitter system. The brain is organized into very specialized regions or systems that are activated by neurotransmitters. These systems are interconnected in highly specific and well-integrated ways. For example, the limbic system is involved in modulating anxiety, affect, and attentional functioning. The reticular activating system affects arousal and sleep–wake cycles. The synapses that link neurons are interconnected by neurotransmitters that are released from presynaptic vessels and act on receptors located at both pre- and postsynaptic sites. The challenge study involves the administration of a medication that acts at a single well-defined site, which increases or diminishes the activity of a particular neurotransmitter system at a known site. Clonidine is a noradrenergic (NE) agonist that acts primarily presynaptically to reduce NE release; it is also a powerful activator of growth hormone.

We selected this medication because the noradrenalin system may be involved in the symptoms of children with attention disorder. The NE system is important in the regulation of the sleep–wake cycle, vigilance, and in arousal in response to a novel stimulus. This challenge method offers advantages over measuring steady-state levels of a neurochemical in the blood or urine. A single measure of neurochemical is difficult to interpret. An elevated level may reflect increased production or decreased feedback inhibition. The challenge study method assesses the behavioral and chemical responses to a controlled stimulation or inhibition of a neurochemical system.

Prior to participating in this protocol, a child and his family view a movie of other children going through this procedure. After carefully obtaining informed consent, a child is admitted into the hospital. We collect an overnight urine specimen to analyze for baseline catecholamines. The next morning an IV is inserted; at 9 a.m. he receives a single dose of the challenge medication. Blood is drawn at baseline and every half hour for 4 hours. Samples are assayed for metabolites related to neurotransmitter functioning, or the noradrenergic system (norepinephrine and its metabolite MHPG), and related systems (dopamine, HVA, and serotonin, 5HIAA), and also peptides (GH, prolactin, and cortisol). Cardiovascular monitoring of blood pressure and pulse is performed every 10 minutes. Behavior ratings are performed by the adolescent, the nurses, and physician to monitor activity, mood, anxiety, and discomfort. Neuromaturational tasks of visual coordination are administered. The procedure is tolerated well.

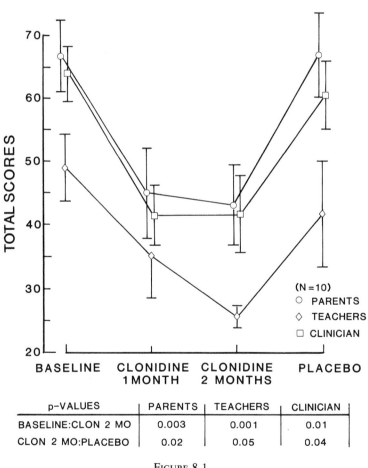

| p–VALUES | PARENTS | TEACHERS | CLINICIAN |
|---|---|---|---|
| BASELINE:CLON 2 MO | 0.003 | 0.001 | 0.01 |
| CLON 2 MO:PLACEBO | 0.02 | 0.05 | 0.04 |

FIGURE 8.1.

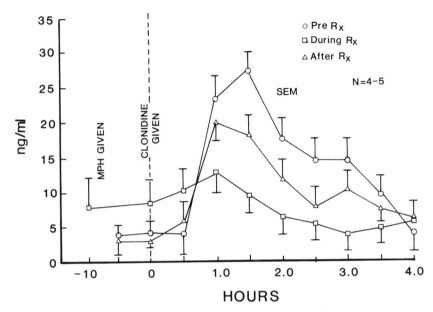

Methylphenidate (MPH) 0.5 mg/kg given orally at 8a.m. to
"During Treatment" Group.

Clonidine 3-4 ug/kg given orally at 9a.m. to all children.

FIGURE 8.2. Plasma growth hormone response to a single dose of clonidine stimulation in children with ADDH. Methylphenidate (MPH) 0.5 mg/kg was given orally at 8 a.m. to the "during treatment" group. Clonidine 3-4 µg/kg was given orally at 9 a.m. to all children.

In our initial study, we found an increase in growth hormone release following the clonidine challenge. Ten ADDH children, before treatment (as you can see in Figure 8.2), had increased level of growth hormone release compared to the response children with Tourette's syndrome and failure to thrive. After chronic treatment with methylphenidate, the GH release was decreased to normal levels. One day following discontinuation of methylphenidate, peak GH levels began to return to normal.

These data illustrate the strategy of measuring the neurochemical response to a very specific challenge agent and determining if this response is altered in children with different diagnoses. This approach could be applied to children with varying subtypes of mental retardation. We are currently developing another challenge method using a medication, yohimbine, that has the opposite effects on the noradrenergic system producing a release of NE and an increase of MHPG. These methods of assessing neurochemical response have not yet been applied to understanding mental retardation.

## Receptor Binding

Another method of assessing neurobiological functioning uses a technique adapted from immunology of assaying the antibodies that block the responsivity of specific types of neurochemical receptors in the brain. An autoimmune response may occur at an early stage of development, producing permanent injury to a specific neurotransmitter system. These methods are currently being applied to the study of autism where an autoimmune insult may have occurred during the early development of the serotonergic system. Other measures of peripheral receptor number and binding may provide an indirect index of brain receptor activity. Techniques such as genetic and amino-acid screening may also lead to identification of deficits treatable by natural or synthetic replacements.

## Brain Imaging

Brain imaging techniques such as the magnetic resonance imaging (MRI) produce remarkably clear pictures of brain structures and tissues without requiring radiation. New techniques are being developed that reflect brain metabolic state and may discriminate regional changes in brain activity. Recently, this technique has identified diffuse, "cottonball-shaped" lesions in the brains of some patients with dementia.

Positron emission tomography (or PET scanning) has even greater potential for defining brain functioning. Specific chemical systems can be labeled with low-dose radiation whose selective regional activity can then be visualized. This technique is promising because of its neurochemical specificity. It can also be used during specific cognitive tasks to reflect brain functioning during a known activity. This method provides an opportunity to link the performance of a cognitive task to the functioning of a neurochemical system and to localize these actions sequentially during brain functioning. Investigators may monitor the local physiological response to a simple burst of light or sound. More sophisticated measures may include the response to complex tasks requiring selective attention, or the differential response to rapid presentation of blurred stimuli, mental arithmetic, problem solving, or memory retrieval tasks. These imaging techniques, which are expensive, have not yet been applied to well-defined groups of retarded individuals.

## Pharmacological Agents

Psychopharmacological agents are being developed whose neurochemical effects are much more precise and whose action in the brain is anatomically more localized. From among this enlarged array of medication, psychopharmacologists can select agents based on their chemical action, thereby producing precisely targeted treatments. The chemical and clinical responses to this new generation of better-characterized agents may inform us conversely about the mechanisms underlying the deficits that they correct. Sophisticated measures of blood level of medications and of their neurochemical effects may be correlated with cognitive and behavioral responses. These agents may provide more precise alternative treatments of some behavioral and possibly intellectual problems of the retarded.

## Summary

In summary, scientific developments now allow more precise measures of cognitive functioning, brain morphology, and neurochemical activity. Collectively, these new methods may differentiate specific mechanisms for various brain deficits. Concurrent use of cognitive, pharmacological, and imaging methods can tell us what is going on, where it is happening, and which neurotransmitters in the brain are doing it. Increasingly, the relationship between brain structure, neurochemistry, and functioning can be interwoven. These methods may define selective causes of mental retardation that may benefit from early identification and more precise treatment. These techniques require further federal investment in basic research to define the parameters of normal response and the effects of development or ontogeny on these systems. Scientists and government should join in ensuring their application to the devastating problems of the mentally retarded.

# 9
# Prevention and Early Treatment of Behavior Disorders of Children and Youth with Retardation and Autism

Travis Thompson

In science as in human affairs more generally, we seem more at home scurrying about undoing the consequences of our own folly than preventing problems in the first place. In the case of developmental disorders, this proclivity is especially evident. That a national initiative to prevent behavioral and emotional disorders among children with retardation and related developmental disorders is long overdue is abundantly clear. However, in planning prevention strategies, it is important that we begin by considering what it is we are trying to prevent or treat.

## Distinguishing Among Types of Behavioral and Emotional Problems

Behavior disorders can be distinguished based on their causal origins and their adaptive features. Of the major forms of psychiatric illness, schizophrenia and major affective disorders appear to be of genetic origin, and, absent evidence to the contrary, there is no reason to believe these disorders are disjunctive for mental retardation. As these disorders evolve ontogenetically, each individual adapts to his or her idiosyncratic history of environmental experiences and demands (cf. Weiner, 1981), depending on the nature of their disorder, other dispositional traits, and features of the specific environment in which they carry themselves (Meehl, 1962).

The manner of expression of these disorders is undoubtedly shaped by the afflicted person's history and current circumstances. However, it seem improbable that environmental interventions alone are likely to prevent or cure these disorders. While environmental interventions may have a place in the prevention and early treatment armamentarium for dealing with such disorders, it would be overly optimistic to assume such treatments will *cure* schizophrenia, mania, or certain types of depressive disorders any more than trying to reinforce differentially the distribution of different types of red blood cells is likely to cure sickle cell anemia.

The special education, habilitation, and behavior analysis literatures reveal that most behavior problems of people with mental retardation, including many with identifiable brain damage, reflect an interaction of impaired cognitive–intellectual functioning with their experience and current circumstances. These problems include those characteristic of personality disorder, adjustment reaction, anxiety, and minor depressive disorders. Typical presenting problems such as aggression, hyperkinesis, social withdrawal, and noncompliance are often secondary to failure to learn to cope socially, vocationally, or academically. The vast majority of behavioral problems of people with mental retardation *are in and of themselves the disorder* and are not symptoms of anything else. Such behavior problems are often responsive to treatment by changing relevant environmental variables, unlike those associated with schizophrenia or major affective disorders. In fact, most behavioral disorders of children with retardation can be prevented or cured by arranging experiences and rearranging current environments to permit them to cope more effectively with their surroundings (Frankel & Forness, 1985; Gardner, 1974; Thompson & Grabowski, 1972, 1977). The term "cure" is used advisedly, for much as an antibiotic may cure an infection, the same infection may flare up again if the conditions giving rise to it are encountered in the future. Similarly, a behavior disorder may be cured, but if the adverse environmental conditions giving rise to it are encountered again, it is likely that a similar problem will arise once again. For most retarded children, prevention and early intervention are synonymous with effective training of parents and early education teaching personnel (Baer, Peterson & Sherman, 1967; Hall et al., 1972; Jewett & Clark, 1979; Kozloff, 1973; Wahler & Fox, 1980; Wilcox & Thompson, 1980).

The fact that psychiatric problems are from 4 to 10 times more common among retarded than nonretarded people is cause for pause (Koller, Richardson, Katz, & McLaren, 1982, 1983; Richardson, 1980; Rutter, Graham, & Yule, 1970; Rutter, Tizard, & Whitmore, 1970). Baumeister and MacLean (1979) reviewed the link between brain damage and retardation, noting that in most individuals with IQs below 50, there is diagnosable brain disease. That a relation exists between brain damage and behavior disorders seems clear. Among the population of children with retardation and autism is a substantial number of children who develop behavior disorders that are minimally and only transiently responsive to environmental intervention. Presenting problems include stereotyped movements, self-injury, unprovoked rage reactions, severe property destruction, and extreme noncompliance. A third family of disorders, which, if not unique to mentally retarded and related developmentally disabled populations, is seen most often in such groups. These disorders involve neuropathological conditions caused by genetic, chromosomal, and pre- or perinatal insults. Kopp (1983) noted in her extensive literature review of risk factors that 17 genetic or chromosomal disorders, 4 common prenatal infections, 3 forms of prenatal chemical exposure, 3 perinatal problems, and 4 forms of postnatal insults cause retardation to various degrees that is commonly associated with behavioral and emotional problems. Collectively, these disorders account for a substantial number of cases of mental retardation and often include people whose emotional and behavioral problems are among the least treatable using current methods. As in the case of schizophrenia, these people exhibit behavioral deviations directly caused by their neuropathology (e.g., explosive rage reactions), but other aspects of their abnormal behavior may be indirect products of their disorder (e.g., noncompliance).

Stereotypes and self-injury are illustrative. These two pervasive problems are common symptomatic behavior classes associated with several types of disorders and appear to result from both direct biochemical causes as well as indirect responses of the person to the environment. Self-injury may come about through several different mechanisms (Baumeister, 1978; Carr, 1977; Schroeder, Schroeder, Rojahn, & Mulick, 1980; Wieseler, Hanson, Chamberlain, & Thompson, 1985): (1) Lesch-Nyhan self-mutilation is provoked by a biochemical state brought about by a genetically induced metabolic error; (2) self-injury may also, inadvertently, be positively reinforced by parents and staff who attempt to stop a child from hurting himself or herself; (3) other self-injury may be negatively reinforced by caregivers who accidentally teach retarded children to hurt themselves by promptly terminating all demands as soon as the child begins to injure himself or herself; and (4) in some cases self-injury is apparently endorphin reinforced by release of endogenous opiate agonist (and its occupation of the Mu opiate receptor) contingent on self-inflicted injury (Bernstein, Hughes, Mitchell, & Thompson, 1985; Sandman et al., 1983). In any given case, the *initial cause* may gradually shift so a different mechanism *maintains* the self-injury from that which originally gave rise to it. Thus, self-injury may arise as a by-product of a perceptual homeostatic mechanism (Berkson, 1983) or a defect in communication development (LaVigne & Donnellan, 1986), but once full-blown, it may gradually change into self-abuse maintained by reinforcing effects of pain-elicited endorphin release. This distinction has important implications for differentiating prevention efforts from treatment, since it may be necessary to use very different approaches at the two points in time.

## Priorities in Prevention and Treatment

In many instances, the single most effective way to prevent emotional behavior disorders among people with retardation is to prevent prenatal neuropathology. Consider, for example, the fact that one of 750 live births exhibits fetal alcohol syndrome (FAS), and in some high risk populations that figure is as high as one in 100 (Hanson, Streissguth, & Smith, 1978; May, Hymbaugh, Aase, & Samet, 1983). By treating the conditions giving rise to FAS, the associated emotional and behavior problems commonly associated with FAS could be avoided. It follows that any effort to prevent or intervene early in life must begin with a clear picture of what it is one is trying to prevent or treat. Though this may seem obvious, there is considerable disagreement about priorities. Since there are several subtypes of behavioral and mental health problems with very different etiologies and current regulating conditions, one would not expect the same prevention or early treatment methods to be especially effective with them all.

The majority of people remaining in large segregated residential facilities and those who repeatedly fail in smaller community programs do so because of extremely violent behavior, severe self-injury, or bizarre, repetitive behaviors that are unacceptable in most community settings. These people have often received a wide array of treatments that did not significantly improve their condition. In truth, we know very little about effective treatments for some people having such behavior disorders. In many cases, failure to provide effective treatment can be life threatening or may mean a life in restraints or chronic administration of high daily dosages of neuroleptic drugs (with the associated risk of tardive dyskinesia) as the only alternatives. It seems increasingly clear that many of the current untreatable problems will be found to have specific biological etiologies and regulating conditions that can either be prevented or treated neurochemically. In short, it would seem prudent to invest our limited research resources in developing prevention and treatment approaches for those behavior disorders that are the most severe and for which few if any effective treatments already exist.

## Lack of Federal Leadership

Though the need for research in behavior disorders of the mentally retarded and other developmentally disabled people has been recognized for many years (Tarjan, et al., 1977), regrettably, neither of our lead federal agencies (the National Institute on Mental Health and the National Institute for Child Health and Human Development) has demonstrated commitment to these issues. While a good deal of excellent basic biomedical and behavioral research is currently being sponsored by NICHD concerning underlying mechanisms in development, it is often unclear whether such work, even if it were totally successful, would have any relevance to the issues at hand. The question is not whether such research should be funded at all, but whether, after 20 years of such efforts, it is time that more than a fraction of 1% of our federal health research dollars is invested in the urgent needs of our mentally retarded citizens with behavior disorders and other mental health problems, and a relatively smaller portion of the federal research budget should be invested in basic science areas concerned with normal development, which have already been well funded for the past two decades. Government scientific programs that fail to address the urgent needs of the people they are intended to serve, especially when those needs are central to the mandated missions of those agencies, make themselves vulnerable targets for legitimate public and congressional scrutiny.

## Recommendations

1. It is recommended that the NIMH, NINCDS, ADD, NIHR, and NICHD jointly fund a 10-year national research initiative in behavioral and emotional disorders of persons with mental retardation, to be coordinated and administered by NICHD.

2. A first step in such a program should involve establishing four regional centers for applied and related basic research, research training, and dissemination of research findings – focusing on problems of mental health and behavioral disorders of mentally retarded people with related developmental disorders. In preparing RFPs for these centers, the foregoing issues should be made central features. Such centers should clearly demonstrate a biobehavioral approach to behavior disorders of people with retardation and autism, which should include such disciplines and specialty areas as biological psychiatry, clinical psychology, neuropharmacology, applied and experimental behavior analysis, behavior genetics, behavioral pharmacology, special education, and policy research.

3. It is also recommended that these agencies issue jointly and/or separately RFAs with overall agency research budgets allocated in proportion to the beds occupied nationally by mentally retarded autistic and other developmentally disabled individuals (as a proportion of total beds occupied by persons with other disorders plus those occupied by persons with retardation and related developmental disorders). Such RFAs should provide for individual research grants, program project grants, interdisciplinary training grants, and career development awards.

4. Existing research review committees of ADAMHA, the DRF, and NICHD do not possess the expertise to evaluate research and/or training proposals in this area. To facilitate proper review of grant applications in this complex and unique area, it is recommended that a specialized Initial Review Group (IRG) be established under the joint administrative auspices of NICHD, NIMH, NIHR, and NINCDS and coordinated by the associate directors of the cooperating agencies. Membership on such an IRG should be based specifically on experience and expertise in mental retardation and research directly relevant to the prevention and treatment of behavioral disorders of the mentally retarded.

5. Programmatic separation of retarded from autistic and other related developmentally disordered children and youth should be discontinued. To fail to do so would perpetuate a facetious practice that may be useful for bookkeeping purposes but makes little sense either therapeutically or for prevention.

6. Such a national program should be applied in that both short- and long-term objectives are to develop preventative methods and treatments for mentally retarded and other developmentally disabled children, adolescents, and young adults with severe behavior disorders. While research on related normative behavioral, cognitive developmental, or basic neurobiological questions may be of interest, such activities ought not distract from the urgent work of such specialized research centers.

7. It is recommended that significant focus of the activities of such centers should be on effective dissemination of research knowledge. While publication of pamphlets, conducting one- and two-day parent and teacher workshops, and in-school advertising campaigns may be better than doing nothing,

there is little evidence that such procedures have a significant impact on preventing retardation and associated behavior disorders. On the other hand, a good deal is known about prevention and early intervention of some developmental problems, problems that are frequently associated with behavior disorders. For example, compliance with prenatal dietary health care and maternal chemical use regimens can prevent retardation and the associated behavior disorders. Use of automobile restraint devices can reduce one of the most common causes of infantile brain damage. Behavior problems secondary to communication disorders can be reduced by using appropriate home and preschool educational and language intervention methods. Though improved treatments would be welcome in such instances, the *real* problems are in devising methods of implementing known effective procedures on a societally meaningful scale. Policy research designed to develop methods of implementing effective procedures should be among our highest priorities.

## Conclusion

In his history of society's care of the mentally retarded, Leo Kanner quoted Martin Luther's recommendation that, "If I were the Prince, I should take this child to the Moldau River which flows near Dessau and drown him." While we no longer drown our mentally retarded brothers and sisters, the changes in care and treatment of our mentally retarded citizens have not been commensurate with other changes in our society since Martin Luther's day. Major improvements have taken place in education and residential services since the 1960s, but as a society we have failed to make a serious commitment to developing effective treatments for the most grievous problems of our retarded children and youth. Most shamefully, we have done very little to prevent them. It is time we did so.

## References

Baer, D.M., Peterson, R.F., & Sherman, J.A. (1967). The development of imitation by reinforcing behavioral similarity to a model. *Journal of the Experimental Analysis of Behavior, 10*, 405–416.

Baumeister, A.A. (1978). Origins and control of stereotyped movements. In C.E. Meyers (Ed.), *Quality of life in severely and profoundly retarded people: Research foundations for improvement*. Washington, DC: American Association on Mental Deficiency.

Baumeister, A.A., & MacLean, W.E. (1979). Brain damage and mental retardation. In N.R. Ellis (Ed.), *Handbook of mental deficiency* (2nd ed.). Hillsdale, NJ: Lawrence Erlbaum Associates.

Berkson, G. (1983). Repetitive stereotyped behaviors. *American Journal of Mental Deficiency, 88*, 239–246.

Bernstein, G., Hughes, J., Mitchell, J., & Thompson,T. (1985, November). *Treatment of self-injurious behavior with opiate antagonists*. Presented at the annual meeting of the American Academy of Child Psychiatry, Houston, TX.

Carr, E.G. (1977). The motivation of self-injurious behavior. *Psychological Bulletin, 84*, 800–816.

Frankel, F., & Forness, S.R. (1985). Educational and clinical behavioral approaches to the child and adolescent with dual disabilities. In M. Sigman (Ed.), *Children with emotional disorders and developmental disabilities: Assessment and treatment.* Orlando, FL: Grune & Stratton.

Gardner, W.I. (1974). *Children with learning and behavior problems.* Boston, MA: Allyn & Bacon.

Hall, R.V., Axelrod, S., Tyler, L., Grief, E., Jones, F.C., & Robertson, R. (1972). Modification of behavior problems in the home with a parent as observer and experimenter. *Journal of Applied Behavior Analysis, 5*, 53–64.

Hanson, J.W., Streissguth, A.P., & Smith, D.W. (1978). The effects of moderate alcohol consumption during pregnancy on fetal growth and morphogenesis. *Journal of Pediatrics, 92*, 457–460.

Jewett, J., & Clark, H.B. (1979). Teaching preschoolers to use appropriate dinnertime conversation: An analysis from school to home. *Behavior Therapy, 10*, 589–605.

Koller, H., Richardson, S.A., Katz, M., & McLaren, J. (1982). Behavior disturbance in childhood and early adult years in populations who were and were not mentally retarded. *Journal of Preventive Psychiatry, 1*, 453–468.

Koller, H., Richardson, S.A., Katz, M., & McLaren, J. (1983). Behavior disturbance since childhood among a 5-year birth cohort of all mentally retarded young adults in a city. *American Journal of Mental Deficiency, 87*, 386–395.

Kopp, C. (1983). Risk factors in development. In P.H. Mussen (Ed.), *Handbook of child psychology* (4th ed., Vol. 2). New York: Wiley.

Kozloff, M.A. (1973). *Reaching the autistic child: A parent training program.* Champaign, IL: Research Press.

LaVigne, G.W., & Donnellan, A.M (1986). *Alternatives to punishment: Solving behavior problems with non-aversive strategies.* New York: Irvington Publishers.

May, P.A., Hymbaugh, K.J., Aase, J.M., & Samet, J.M. (1983). Epidemiology of fetal alcohol syndrome among American Indians of the Southwest. *Social Biology, 30*, 374–387.

Meehl, P.E. (1962). Schizotaxia, schizotype and schizophrenia. *American Psychologist, 17*, 827–838.

Richardson, S.A. (1980). Growing up as a mentally subnormal young person: A follow-up study. In S.A. Mednick & A.E. Baert (Eds.), *An empirical basis for primary prevention: Prospective longitudinal research in Europe.* Oxford: Oxford University Press.

Rutter, M., Graham, P., & Yule, W. (1970). *Neuropsychiatric study in childhood.* London: Spastics International Medical Publications and Heinemann.

Rutter, M., Tizard, J., & Whitmore, K. (Eds.). (1970). *Education, health and behavior.* London: Longmans.

Sandman, C., Datta, P., Barron, J., Hoehler, F.K., Williams, C., & Swanson, J.M. (1983). Naloxone attenuates self-abusive behavior in developmentally disabled clients. *Applied Research in Mental Retardation, 4*, 5–11.

Schroeder, S.R., Schroeder, C.S., Rojahn, J., & Mulick, J.A. (1980). Self-injurious behavior: An analysis of behavior management techniques. In J.L. Matson & J.R. McCartney (Eds.), *Handbook of behavior modification with the mentally retarded.* New York: Plenum Press.

Tarjan, G., Dornbusch, S.M., Fenichel, G., Graham, F., Richmond, J., & Zigler, E. (1977). *Federal research activity in mental retardation: A review with recommendations for the future.* A Report to the Directors of NICHD and NIMH of the Department of Health, Education and Welfare. Washington, DC: U.S. Government Printing Office.

Thompson, T., & Grabowski, J.G. (1972). *Behavior modification of the mentally retarded.* New York: Oxford University Press.

Thompson, T., & Grabowski, J.G. (1977). *Behavior modification of the mentally retarded* (rev. ed.). New York: Oxford University Press.

Wahler, R.G., & Fox, J.J. (1980). Solitary toy play and time out: A family treatment package for children with aggressive and oppositional behavior. *Journal of Applied Behavior Analysis, 13*, 23–29.

Weiner, H. (1981). Contributions of reinforcement schedule histories to our understanding of drug effects in human subjects. In T. Thompson & C.E. Johanson (Eds.), *Behavioral pharmacology of human drug dependence.* NIDA Research Monograph 37. Washington, DC: U.S. Government Printing Office.

Wieseler, N.A., Hanson, R.H., Chamberlain, T.P., & Thompson, T. (1985). Functional taxonomy of stereotypic and self-injurious behavior. *Mental Retardation, 23*, 230–234.

Wilcox, B., & Thompson, A. (Eds.). (1980). *Critical issues in educating autistic children and youth.* Washington, DC: U.S. Department of Education, Office of Special Education.

# Conclusion

ALFRED A. BAUMEISTER

The preceding chapters have indicated that prevention and early intervention have to be viewed from a biobehavioral, developmental perspective that must be approached in a multidisciplinary fashion. In this regard, the authors of this development/prevention section offer several general recommendations. Specific recommendations are also included within the individual contributions of authors.

1. The current research and training resources allocated to NICHD, NIMH, NINCDS, and NIHR should be reallocated and redistributed according to the number of residential beds and educational placements in the United States for mentally retarded children and adults.
2. Four regional centers for research, research training, and dissemination should be mandated to address issues related to the developmental aspects of mental retardation and mental health. These would be selected from among those Mental Retardation Research Center applicants who will be under competitive review within the next two years.
3. NIMH should establish a special Initial Review Group with expertise in mental retardation and behavior disorders. NIMH is urged to set aside research and program funds specifically for this population, in an amount proportional to the number of beds and educational placements in the United States for mentally retarded children and adults.
4. Better forms of accountability need to be developed with respect to research, service, and training in this area. Federal funds to the states should be tied to this mechanism of accountability by providers. These include both residential services and education programs. Special consideration should be given to states that develop *effective* as contrasted with cosmetic programs.
5. Much more policy-oriented research needs to be conducted, especially concerning dissemination and technology transfer mechanisms.
6. Finally, we urge the concerned agencies to adopt the specific recommendations for research contained in the 1977 report entitled "Federal Research Activity in Mental Retardation: A Review with Recommendations for the Future."

# Section III: Clinical Research and Training Introduction

FRANK J. MENOLASCINO

In this section, we have a quartet of contributions made by four internationally known psychiatrists who have each spent more than a quarter of a century working with persons with mental retardation and concomitant mental illness.

In Chapter 10, Dr. Menalascino provides an overview of the key diagnostic and treatment issues involved in providing direct services to the dually diagnosed population. He uses the framework of the DSM-III classification system of mental disorders to review the diagnosis and treatment of persons with mental retardation who concurrently exhibit syndromes of mental illness. Disorders such as schizophrenia, organic brain syndromes, adjustment disorders, personality disorders, affective disorders, psychosexual disorders, and anxiety disorders are reviewed, including clinical data from his ongoing studies at the University of Nebraska—one of the largest data base systems concerning the dually diagnosed in our country.

In Chapter 11, Dr. Szymanski distills his personal experiences via the interdisciplinary team approach to the mentally retarded/mentally ill that he has developed at the Boston Children's Hospital. This chapter presents essential guidelines for constructing and operating a modern evaluation program and underscores the limitations of the various diagnostic tools and techniques. He also provides his reflections on the strengths and weaknesses of using the DSM-III system for differential diagnostic considerations in persons with mental retardation. He points out that our knowledge and skills in these complex areas are still in the early stages and offers specific recommendations for future directions. Practitioners will find his concerns and reflections extremely helpful in initiating new programs or further developing their current services for mentally retarded/mentally ill citizens.

Colleagues who are discouraged about ever having the necessary financial resources to develop a large interdisciplinary treatment program, particularly within a larger health care setting, will note that Dr. Evangelista provides a very pragmatic and "do-able" model on how to serve this dually diagnosed population. She provides us some unique insight into some of the major problems faced by this group of complex individuals and notes that if these problems are not addressed directly, they will preclude successful treatment and placement.

Practitioners who provide direct individualized treatment to the dually diagnosed population (e.g., psychiatrists, psychologists, and psychiatric social workers) will find Dr. Loomis' chapter on the challenges of the psychiatric examination in this population to be extremely helpful. Very few professionals have had the breadth and length of clinical experience as Dr. Loomis in providing individualized psychiatric evaluations and resultant treatment prescriptions. He provides multiple helpful tips on how to enhance our success with these complex patients. For example, a professional cannot expect to conduct a psychiatric interview simply by "scaling down" to their mental age or otherwise minimally modifying the process for persons with mental retardation. Instead, the developmentally oriented interview, replete with attention to delayed language considerations, with the focus on concrete (versus abstract) requests for interactions, and the modified interview techniques from child psychiatry are all necessary. The reader will find this chapter carries this one-to-one interactional focus directly into useful components and approaches to individualized treatment programs.

In essence, the four authors in this section provide a unique contribution to this book via their own wealth of clinical experiences, insights, and reflections— based on successes and failures during their more than 100 years of combined clinical experiences as practitioners and researchers in the topical area of mental illness in the mentally retarded.

# 10
# Mental Illness in the Mentally Retarded: Diagnostic and Treatment Issues

FRANK J. MENOLASCINO

## Introduction

The coexistence of mental retardation and mental illness in the same individual presents unique challenges to mental health professionals both in terms of diagnosis and treatment. The mentally retarded/mentally ill comprise a complex group of persons whose needs are often poorly identified and who are often referred from agency to agency in fruitless efforts to obtain help. These challenges are heightened by the recent national deinstitutionalization movement, which has focused on integrating mentally retarded children and adults into the mainstreams of family and community life. As the more complex individuals with mental retardation are served in community-based programs, mental health professionals have increasingly been confronted with the challenge of meeting their needs within the confluences of family and community life.

This chapter focuses on the diagnostic and treatment challenges presented by the mentally retarded/mentally ill as well as an analysis of what the appropriate care and treatment of this population can bring to the field of psychiatry in general. The diagnostic challenges are immense because the patient often cannot verbally express himself or herself and at times the behavioral symptomatology is atypical owing to the mental retardation. Treatment challenges also are immense because of a number of intrinsic and extrinsic factors such as the nature and degree of mental retardation itself and society's response to persons considered to be "deviant."

## Diagnostic Dimensions

The diagnosis of mental illness in mentally retarded persons requires the sensitive application of general diagnostic procedures. Owing to the coexisting mental retardation, the clinician must rely more on the signs (observed behaviors) and less on the symptoms (verbally reported distress or dysfunction) that characterize the various psychiatric disorders, especially in those individuals with more severe degrees of mental retardation. There are a number of recent studies that show that the mentally retarded fall prey to the same types of mental illness that befall people with normal intellectual abilities (Craft, 1959; Donoghue, Abbas, & Gal, 1979; Duncan, 1935; Hunsicker, 1938; Innes, Kidd, & Ross, 1968; Matson & Barrett, 1982; Menolascino, 1965, 1983, 1986; Menolascino Ruedrich, Golden, & Wilson, 1985; Mercer, 1968; Payne, 1968; Reid, 1972; Reis, 1985; Reiss, Levitan, & McNally, 1982; Rosenoff, Handy, Plesset, 1935; Ruedrich & Menolascino, 1984; Shellhaas & Nihira, 1969; Sovner & Hurley, 1983; Weaver, 1946; Williams, 1972).

In our most recent work with this population of mentally retarded/mentally ill individuals, we noted 543 instances of this dual diagnosis. This study was conducted at the Nebraska Psychiatric Institute and reviews the mentally retarded persons admitted for acute psychiatric care from July 1, 1979 through June 30, 1985. In this six-year study, the entire range of psychiatric diagnoses was found in the mentally retarded (Table 10.1). The highest frequency was schizophrenia, 25%; followed by organic brain disorders, 19%; adjustment disorders, 19%; personality disorders, 13%; affective disorders, 8%; psychosexual disorders, 6%; anxiety disorders, 4%; and other mental disorders, 6%. These 543 cases were evaluated by an interdisciplinary team using diagnostic criteria based on the American Psychiatric Association's (1980) DSM-III. The sample ranged in ages from 3 to 76 years. Males and females were found in approximately equal numbers. All levels of mental retardation were found.

## Schizophrenia

Schizophrenia remains the most frequently reported type of major mental illness in mentally retarded individuals. In this study, 138 patients (25%) displayed indices of both mental retardation (since very early in life) and schizophrenia (the onset of the latter having been noted usually during late adolescence). Striking examples of schizophrenic symptoms included bizarre behavior, persistent withdrawal, echolalic speech, and affective unavailability in mentally retarded persons who had clearly regressed from higher levels of social adaptive functioning. These individuals displayed very clear developmental indices of propfschizophrenia (i.e., schizophrenia that was engrafted on distinct earlier indices of mental retardation).

## Organic Brain Syndrome

The diagnosis of organic brain disorder with an *allied behavioral* or *psychotic* disorder was diagnosed in approximately 19% of the total sample. Mentally retarded persons diagnosed as having an organic brain disorder with psychotic reactions presented a different clinical picture than schizophrenia because (1) the underlying organic brain disorder and symptoms were prominent, (2) their out-of-contact behaviors were not the type commonly seen in schizophrenia, and

TABLE 10.1. A review of mentally retarded/mentally ill patients at NPI (unduplicated count) for the period from July 1, 1979 through June 30, 1985.

| Psychiatric diagnosis | Ages (yr) | | | | | | | | Total |
|---|---|---|---|---|---|---|---|---|---|
| | 1-5 | 6-10 | 11-15 | 16-20 | 21-25 | 26-30 | 31-35 | 36+ | |
| **Schizophrenic disorders** | | | | | | | | | |
| Catatonic type | | | 1 | 4 | 2 | 1 | | 2 | 10 |
| Paranoid type | | | | 8 | 5 | 3 | 4 | 10 | 30 |
| Undifferentiated type | | | | 15 | 8 | 10 | 5 | 15 | 53 |
| Residual type | | | | | 4 | 13 | 13 | 15 | 45 |
| | | | | | | | | | 138 |
| **Organic brain disorders** | | | | | | | | | |
| Behavioral reaction | | 4 | 11 | 7 | 13 | 6 | 8 | 6 | 55 |
| Psychotic reaction | 1 | 1 | 2 | 2 | 10 | 14 | 8 | 5 | 43 |
| Presenile dementia | | | | | | | | 7 | 7 |
| | | | | | | | | | 105 |
| **Adjustment disorders** | | | | | | | | | |
| Childhood and adolescent | 5 | 4 | 10 | 25 | | | | | 44 |
| Disturbance of conduct | | 3 | 5 | 10 | | | | | 18 |
| Adulthood | | | | | 15 | 12 | 9 | 5 | 41 |
| | | | | | | | | | 103 |
| **Personality disorders** | | | | | | | | | |
| Schizoid | | | | 2 | 4 | | | | 6 |
| Paranoid | | | | | | 2 | 1 | | 3 |
| Narcissistic | | | | | | 2 | 4 | 1 | 7 |
| Avoidant | | | | 1 | 2 | 1 | 1 | 2 | 7 |
| Passive aggressive | | | | 5 | 4 | 2 | 5 | 6 | 22 |
| Antisocial | | | | 1 | 8 | 7 | 2 | 5 | 23 |
| | | | | | | | | | 68 |
| **Affective disorders** | | | | | | | | | |
| Unipolar manic disorder | | | | 4 | 2 | 1 | | | 7 |
| Bipolar affective | | | | | 2 | | | 3 | 5 |
| Major depression, recurrent | | | 5 | 4 | 4 | 9 | 5 | 5 | 32 |
| Cyclothymic disorder | | | | | 1 | | | | 1 |
| | | | | | | | | | 45 |
| **Psychosexual disorders** | | | | | | | | | |
| Fetishism | | | | 1 | | | | | 1 |
| Transvestism | | | | 2 | 1 | | | 1 | 4 |
| Zoophilia | | | 1 | | | | | | 1 |
| Pedophilia | | | 1 | 1 | 4 | 2 | 1 | 3 | 12 |
| Exhibitionism | | | 1 | 1 | 2 | 1 | | 1 | 6 |
| Ego-dystonic homosexuality | | | 1 | 1 | | | | | 2 |
| Disorder not elsewhere classified | | | | 3 | 2 | 1 | 1 | 1 | 8 |
| | | | | | | | | | 34 |

TABLE 10.1. *(Continued)*.

| Psychiatric diagnosis | Ages (yr) | | | | | | | | |
|---|---|---|---|---|---|---|---|---|---|
| | 1-5 | 6-10 | 11-15 | 16-20 | 21-25 | 26-30 | 31-35 | 36+ | Total |
| Anxiety disorders | | | | | | | | | |
| Generalized anxiety | | | | 2 | 1 | 2 | 2 | 2 | 9 |
| Posttraumatic stress | | | | 2 | 2 | 1 | 2 | 3 | 10 |
| Obsessive compulsive | | | | | | | | 1 | 1 |
| | | | | | | | | | 20 |
| Other mental disorders | | | | | | | | | |
| Pervasive developmental | 2 | 5 | 7 | 2 | | | | | 16 |
| Anorexia nervosa | | | 3 | 2 | 1 | | | | 6 |
| Oppositional | | | 2 | | | | | | 2 |
| Substance use | | | | | 3 | | 1 | 2 | 6 |
| | | | | | | | | | 30 |
| N = 543 | | | | | | | | Total | 543 |

(3) their personality structures did not show progressive involvement of multiple segments of personality functioning.

## Adjustment Disorders

Although the category of adjustment disorders is perhaps overused in the assessment of nonretarded individuals, it tends to be employed infrequently in the mentally retarded/mentally ill population. In this study, 19% of the cases involved adjustment disorders. In our experience, adjustment disorders are most frequently caused by inappropriate social–adaptive expectations or unexpected changes in externally imposed life patterns. The presence of mental retardation can make it difficult for the person to process and cope with personal and familial changes; for example, changes in teachers or the separation of parents. Persons with these disorders respond rapidly to interpersonal and environmental support, combined with individual psychotherapy and family counseling to realign the parents' or the residential/educational personnel's unrealistic expectations or goals.

## Personality Disorders

Personality disorders (13%) occurred in mentally retarded individuals whose abnormal behaviors were based primarily on extrinsic factors and had no distinct etiological relationship to the symptom of mental retardation. The presence of personality disorders in 13% of the sample suggests that these disorders are not an infrequent psychiatric handicap for mentally retarded citizens. Those with mild mental retardation are most susceptible to this disorder. They possess the cognitive ability to almost fit into society yet cannot quite integrate themselves without early intervention and support.

## Affective Disorders

These disorders (i.e., bipolar affective disorders and unipolar depressive reactions) were noted in approximately 8% of this sample. They represent difficult diagnostic challenges because of the "masked" depressive features so often noted in the retarded. Furthermore, the frequently noted delayed language development in the retarded produces a major diagnostic roadblock to eliciting vegetative and allied somatic indices of depression. The dexamethasone test is a very helpful biological marker in this diagnostic area. Interestingly, once the diagnostic parameters of these affective disorders are clarified, these individuals responded very well to standard antidepressive treatment regimes.

## Psychosexual Disorders

Although there is little literature available on the topic, 6% of our sample had psychosexual disorders, with the largest grouping being pedophilia. It is difficult to assess the nature of this disorder. In general, the mentally retarded in this study appeared to have neither greater nor lesser sex drives than any other persons. Yet years of institutionalization and societal segregation left some with deviant sexual responses. Institutionalized retarded persons often are subjected to little privacy and stimulation. Public nudity and open masturbation become a way of life. Most have never received guidance in sex education or the development of personal relationships. Many lead isolated and lonely lives.

## Anxiety Disorders

Reviews of anxiety disorders in the retarded have suggested that their frequency is quite low. These reports have prompted speculation as to whether the complexity of anxiety disorder is beyond the adaptive limits of the more severely retarded. These studies tend to attribute anxiety phenomena in the retarded to factors associated with atypical developmental patterns in conjunction with major indices of disturbed family functioning. Our sample included 20 mentally retarded individuals (4%) with anxiety disorders. These disorders were clearly linked to exogenous factors such as chronic frustration, unrealistic family expectations, and persistent interpersonal deprivation.

## Other Mental Disorders

The remaining diagnoses (6%) included such disorders as anorexia nervosa, oppositional disorders, substance abuse, and pervasive developmental disorders. The clinician needs to be prepared to discover any of the psychiatric disorders found in the normal population.

## Other Sample Characteristics

All levels of mental retardation were seen in our study group. Of the 543 persons studied, approximately 25% were mildly retarded, 55% moderately retarded, and 20% severely/profoundly retarded. Each level presents special challenges in diagnosis and treatment. The severely retarded are characterized by a high frequency of central nervous system impairments and multiple handicaps, especially sensor deficits and seizure disorders. This population has a high vulnerability to psychiatric disorders. Moderately retarded persons are vulnerable to problems in personality development because of their slower rates of development and concrete approaches to problem solving. The mildly retarded are quite similar to their nonretarded peers.

A major focus in the "at-risk" status of retarded individuals for concurrent mental illness centers around developmental problems in communication. For example, most of the low to moderate and severely retarded persons in this study had significant language and communication dysfunctions. Because of their limited ability to process information (both qualitatively and quantitatively), personality disorganization could occur rapidly, and they subsequently reacted with a variety of primitive behaviors. These behaviors in the severely retarded are atypical forms of communication; that is, nonverbal ways of responding to the apparently confusing and perplexing interpersonal world around them. Accordingly, it is crucial to take into account the impact of delayed communication levels in assessing the needs of the mentally retarded/mentally ill.

Another important factor is the frequency and type(s) of allied medical disorders found in this population. More than 34% were found to have one or more major medical disorders (such as epilepsy, cerebral palsy, diabetes mellitus, and hypothyroidism). The most frequent allied medical disorder was seizure disorders, which affected more than 21% of this sample. These major medical disorders exacerbate the already complex coexistence of mental retardation and mental illness (e.g., instances of postseizure confusion may often further impair their interpersonal and intrapersonal transactions) and thus further complicate diagnostic and treatment challenges.

## Treatment Dimensions

The psychiatric treatment of the mentally retarded/mentally ill provides profound insight into the very foundations of psychiatry. The mentally retarded/

mentally ill can give us deep insight into the basic human needs of all persons and the clinician's values and posture toward those in need. The eloquent simplicity of the mentally retarded person's emotional life should remind the clinician of the interdependence of all persons. Their often silent cries for help should remind the clinician of the depth of their need for emotional support—support that all persons need. These reminders can and should lead the clinician to seek bonding and interdependence for all persons.

The clinician's posture toward the patient shapes the use of all treatment modalities, much like Itard's posture toward Victor, the Wild Boy of Aveyron, led him to treat Victor in a very loving manner and to seek ways to integrate him into community life—a posture that led Itard to teach bonding to Victor. Lane (1976) reports in his treatise on the Wild Boy that Victor initially was a "disgustingly dirty child affected with spasmodic movements, and often convulsions, who swayed back and forth ceaselessly like certain animals in a zoo, who bit and scratched those who opposed him, who showed no affection for those who took care of him; and who was, in short, indifferent to everything and attentive to nothing." Yet, five years later Itard described Victor in a dramatically different manner. "As the ever-increasing number of his desires made his contacts with us and our attentions to him more and more frequent, his underlying heart at last opened to unequivocal feelings of gratitude and affection." He was soon able to demonstrate to his caregiver "a radiant facial, expression" as an "affectionate son who, of his own free will, comes and throws himself in the arms of the one who has given him life."

Like Itard's work, the psychiatric care and treatment of mentally retarded/mentally ill individuals has as its goal the teaching of bonding so that the individual can remain in, or reenter, the confluence of family and community life. The treatment process needs to focus on and respectfully deal with persistent aggression, self-injury, withdrawal, and self-stimulating behaviors. It needs to provide a mechanism to develop an active psychiatric treatment structure through which the clinician can create multiple opportunities to teach the value of human presence and reward in spite of the mental retardation and mental illness.

This underlying treatment goal embodies a professional posture that weds affection and tolerance with the objective of teaching bonding between the caregiver and the patient. At the start, the mentally ill/mentally retarded person will often display behaviors that clearly indicate that they do not want anything to do with the clinician: for example, screaming, biting, kicking, scratching, and avoiding. At this initial point, the clinician superimposes his or her treatment posture on the disturbed person with the aim of teaching the value of human presence and reward. Regardless of the psychiatric diagnosis or level of retardation, the underlying goal is to teach bonding, to form that affectionate relationship that existed between Victor and his caregiver, Madame Guerin, the heroine of Itard's work with Victor. It was she who, over the years, cared for him and who bonded with him. It was into her arms that he threw himself—as a son into his mother's arms. As important and essential as Itard's pedagogy was, it was Madame Guerin who treated him "kindly and who gave into his tastes and inclinations with all the patience of a mother and the intelligence of an enlightened teacher."

## Treatment Approach

The mentally retarded/mentally ill are often the last to be served, the least likely to be served, and the most subject to abuse. Many are left abandoned in custodial care settings—much like Victor was left in Aveyron—to fend for themselves and frightened by those around them. It is necessary to translate a humanizing and liberating posture into reality. In the initial treatment sessions, the clinician needs to focus on teaching equitable interactions to the person in spite of often intense maladaptive behaviors through a process of constant redirection toward appropriate behaviors. These complex mentally retarded persons will tend to "win" most of the initial interpersonal transactions via obstinacy, refusal to sit, screaming, or striking self or the caregiver. The caregiver must understand this stage of rebellion against "outside" interference and energetically continue to attempt to engage the person in a series of concrete and specific developmental activities. The caregiver must focus on the teaching of interactional equity while at the same time tolerating the initial barrage of heightened maladaptive behaviors. The caregiver must not view violence, self-injury, or withdrawal as willfully destructive or aggressive acts, but rather as the person's basic protective mechanism for coping with a world that has, prior to active treatment intervention, presented itself to him or her as quite meaningless and even absurd. This initial interactive relationship can best be achieved through a constant and sincere display of warmth, tolerance, and uncritical acceptance, constantly and patiently redirecting the person toward participatory behaviors. The role of any treatment modality, whether psychotherapy or psychoactive drugs, must be to establish bonded relationships.

The following three case studies reflect our recommended treatment process for helping the mentally retarded/mentally ill person enter the threshold of bonding. The first two case studies focus on specific, developmentally oriented treatment processes. In the third case study, the delicate balance between the use of psychoactive medications and developmental teaching to gain interactional equity and eventually bonding with the mentally retarded/mentally ill person is demonstrated.

### Case 1

Case 1 was a 26-year-old man who had been institutionalized since he was 14 years old. He was admitted to the Nebraska Psychiatric Institute with chief complaints of continuous pica (ingesting potentially dangerous objects or materials) and markedly aggressive behavior toward others in his immediate environment. He had a diagnosis of severe mental retardation and chronic undifferentiated schizophrenia. He had a spit fistula and a gastrostomy. These surgical interventions had been performed (prior to admission to our hospital) because he had swallowed several objects that lodged in his esophagus and had caused erosion of his esophagus and allied serious infections. He had no speech nor any other manner of expressive language. His self-care skills were minimal. He was able to follow one-step instructions, although he often required physical prompting. He was brought to our program in restraints. We did not use punishment or aversive stimulation— contrary to previously reported uses of such negative procedures in similar clinical cases. Our intent was to focus on teaching him humanizing, participatory behaviors and thereby decrease his maladaptive behaviors.

We evolved a developmental program for him that included (1) a full-day program on and off the living unit in order to create opportunities to teach reward, (2) allowing him to remove himself momentarily from tasks at any time, (3) redirecting him back to tasks or interactions with nonverbal cues and rewarding him with praise for his participation, (4) one-to-one staffing during the first 10 days of his treatment program, and (5) environmental and stimulus control so as to prevent the pica as much as possible (see Figure 10.1).

*Specific Comments.* Case 1 began to demonstrate equitable interactions by the 26th session. His pica significantly decreased and he began to respond favorably to demands placed on him.

The first major presenting problem in redirecting Case 1 from his high-frequency pica behavior was to set up a treatment environment in which his severe pica could be prevented while a bond was being established. Such environmental control consisted of two measures: (1) a seating arrangement that made it difficult (but not impossible) for him to grab available objects and (2) control of all teaching materials.

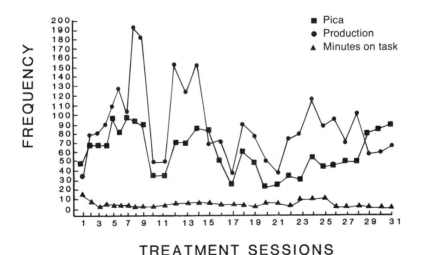

TREATMENT SESSIONS

FIGURE 10.1.

The second major problem that he presented was the lack of any means of expressive communication. He could not speak nor could he indicate his needs through signs or gestures. Indeed, he presented a very blunted affect. This problem was difficult because an important preventive technique is to discern precursor behaviors in order to avoid behavior problems. It was necessary to identify quickly more subtle signs—the only one being brief stares toward the object that he wanted to ingest.

The third presenting problem was to extend his on-task time from initially less than a minute to over 30 minutes without a break. The primary techniques used to extend his attention to tasks and interactions were (1) the use of errorless teaching techniques; that is, he was presented tasks to complete in such a way as to increase the probability that he would respond correctly and thereby earn verbal and tactile praise; and (2) giving him hands-on physical praise at the completion of each task or interaction.

## Case 2

Case 2 was a 14-year-old adolescent boy diagnosed as severely mentally retarded with Cornelia de Lange's syndrome. He resided with his natural family until 10 years of age, at which time he was placed in a community-based group home. He had been attending a school for multiply handicapped children. He was admitted to the Nebraska Psychiatric Institute program because of severe self-abusive behaviors, primarily continuously picking at his neck and failing to attend to tasks. He had minimal self-care skills. He had no spoken language. He was able to make a few gestural signs such as "eat" and "drink." Again, we used no punishment or any other negative techniques (see Figure 10.2).

*Specific Comments.* The first presenting problem was that he would refuse to sit and perform a task. In the first session, he roamed the room for 40 minutes, ignoring verbal and gestural cues to sit. Over the course of this first 40 minutes, his wandering and inappropriate attention-seeking behavior were ignored and he was periodically redirected to a task. Through this process of ignoring and redirecting, he quickly learned that he would only be rewarded for participating with his caregiver on a task.

The second challenge, once he sat at the table, was to focus his attention on the task at hand, while he picked at his neck at a high frequency. He also encumbered the treatment process by aggressively insisting on keeping a towel wrapped around his neck and various objects in his hands. Group home staff had encouraged this as a substitute for his neck-picking. As he sat in the first and forthcoming sessions, these objects were gradually removed from his possession.

The third presenting problem was to redirect him from his neck-picking to the task. The following was done: He was instructed to "sit . . . (and) put his hands on the table." He was then given the sign "to put" and given verbal and tactile praise for correct matching. Incorrect responses were ignored and he was redirected. This physical assistance was faded out by the 10th session. This entire treatment

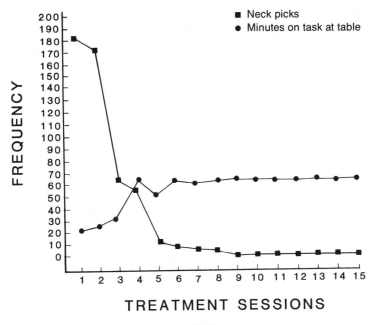

FIGURE 10.2.

process focused on gaining interactional equity with tolerance and warmth. This was attained as indicated in the increase of his on-task behavior and the elimination of his neck-picking. It should be emphasized that initially the task and daily structure serve as vehicles to ignore, redirect, and teach reward.

## Psychoactive Medications

Another important dimension to the treatment of mentally retarded/mentally ill persons is the use of psychoactive medications as a tool to assist in leading the person to instructional control. A delicate balance must be struck between the use of psychoactive medications and ongoing behavioral intervention. While excellent reviews of the clinical use of psychopharmacological agents in mentally ill/mentally retarded persons are available, there are relatively few objective studies that stress the balance between the use of psychoactive medications and developmental programming. The balance that we examine has little to do with an "either–or" posture toward the exclusive use of either psychoactive medication or behavioral management approaches—always maintaining the goal of assisting the person to move toward meaningful human engagement.

The three basic rationales for using psychoactive medications are (1) to aid persons who display marked motoric overactivity, (2) to aid persons who display marked motor underactivity, and (3) to aid persons whose overall behavior is slowly (or rapidly) escalating into "out-of-contact" behaviors (e.g., psychosis).

In a balanced treatment regime (i.e., combined use of psychoactive medications and behavioral programs), the following basic processes typically occur:

1. *Initiation phase.* There is noted the gradual effect of the psychoactive medication's dampening of the excessive amounts of inappropriate behaviors to the point where programming efforts can "take hold." This initial dampening effect of the psychoactive medication must be monitored closely and sensitively in order to avoid sedative effects; behavioral availability is the goal, not disorganization or depression of cognitive processes.
2. *Catching-on phase.* As the initial dampening effect of the psychoactive medication joins forces with the intensive developmental programming (i.e., energetic one-to-one efforts to gain instructional control), the acquisition of appropriate behaviors and skills begins to accelerate, multiplying by their own power, and the inappropriate behaviors begin to decelerate, usually in inverse proportion to the accelerating rate of appropriate learning acquisitions.
3. *Reduction phase.* Once the second phase begins to stabilize, it is time to focus on the slow reduction and/or elimination of the dosage levels of psychoactive medications used in the previous two phases. Concomitantly, intensive developmental programming must continue and extend further into extrinsic interpersonal transactions (i.e., interactional equity), which can permit the recently acquired behavioral improvement to both stabilize and begin to generalize across other interpersonal environments.

## Case 3

In this case study, we examine the balance between the use of psychoactive medications and developmental programming. Case 3 was a 26-year-old man who had resided in a community-based group home and attended a sheltered workshop for the last eight years. Prior to this, he had been institutionalized for eight years. He had been diagnosed as severely mentally retarded with organic brain syndrome with psychotic reactions. Behaviorally speaking, upon admission to the Nebraska Psychiatric Institute's program, he displayed the following behaviors: persistent screaming, pacing, biting, hitting, and scratching (see Figure 10.3).

*Specific Comments.* By the 12th treatment session, his highly aggressive behaviors dramatically decreased through intensive developmental programming and the balanced use of psychoactive medications.

The first presenting problem was to reduce his highly uncontrollable behaviors to a more manageable level through the use of psychoactive medications. Indeed, prior to taking data on Case 3, he ran after staff for over 2 hours, refusing to sit for even a moment. He was placed on a regime of Navane (15 mg BID), which brought his behaviors to a manageable level between the first and second treatment sessions. This was later reduced to 5 mg BID and then increased back to

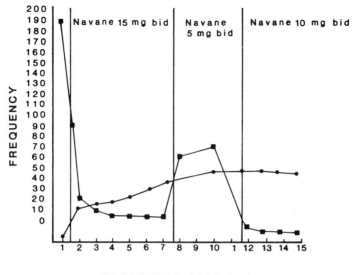

TREATMENT SESSIONS

■ Hits, bites, pinches, scratches

● Minutes on task per hour session

FIGURE 10.3.

10 mg BID because his behaviors significantly worsened during the seventh to tenth treatment sessions.

Another challenge, as treatment took hold, was to eliminate his last remaining undesirable behavior—jumping out of his seat about once every 5 minutes. The solution to this problem was twofold. First, it was necessary to sense when he was about to jump up. This became fairly predictable for he would go off-task momentarily and begin to say, "water," or "coffee," or "potty" repeatedly. When these precursor behaviors occurred, he was more intensely rewarded for any participatory behaviors.

The next presenting problem was to attempt to gradually reduce the Navane. In his case, this reduction almost immediately brought about a dramatic increase in his maladaptive behaviors and his unavailability to continued treatment. Therefore, his treatment team decided to return to a higher dosage and give the developmental intervention process more time to "catch on."

If there are problems in the initiation or catching-on phases— as in the third case study—three questions should be asked relative to the psychoactive medication management: (1) Is it the correct medication? (2) Is it the right dosage: too little, too much, or possible negative side effects? (3) Is the correct administration schedule of the medication being used? These questions clearly underscore the need for constant and rapid feedback between all the cooperating professionals and other caregivers.

The balance between the use of psychoactive medications and developmental/behavioral programming is delicate. Just as behavioral techniques are gradually faded in and out, the use of psychoactive medications should be faded in the same way. The primary purpose of the medication should be to help the person arrive at a state of interactional equity. It is clearly an adjunctive treatment component of any balanced treatment approach.

## Conclusion

We have presented our experiences with diagnostic and treatment techniques in serving the mentally retarded/mentally ill. These factors involve a redefinition of the clinician's posture toward this population as well as the gentle application of modern treatment technology. We have emphasized that no technology is of use without a redefinition of our posture toward this population – a posture that leads these complex handicapped persons to the threshold of treatment and meaningful human engagement. The primary treatment tools at our disposal are the principles of applied behavioral analysis and, where appropriate, the balanced use of psychoactive medications.

The mentally retarded/mentally ill can become significantly engaged in developmental programming that sequentially moves them toward meaningful integration into the educational, vocational, and residential sets of experiences that can embellish their lives in the community.

The challenge is to question our posture toward all persons with special needs and to translate our diagnostic and treatment approaches into actions that result in bonding and interdependence. The mentally retarded/mentally ill can teach us that the goal of treatment is not to eliminate disruptive or destructive behaviors, but rather to teach new sets of humanizing behaviors that focus on our solidarity with all persons, leads us to open ourselves up to bonding, and gives up deep insight into the elemental human need for mutual love.

## References

American Psychiatric Association. (1980). *Diagnostic and statistical manual of mental disorders*, Vol. III (DSM-III). Washington, DC: Author.

Craft, M. (1959). Mental disorder in the defective: A psychiatric survey among inpatients. *American Journal of Mental Deficiency, 63*, 829–834.

Donoghue, E.C., Abbas, K.A., & Gal, E. (1979). The medical assessment of mentally retarded children in hospitals. *British Journal of Psychiatry, 117*, 531–532.

Duncan, A.G. (1935). Mental deficiency and manic depressive insanity. *Journal of Mental Science, 82*, 635–641.

Hunsicker, H.H. (1938). Symptomatology of psychosis with mental deficiency. *Proceedings of the 62nd Annual American Association on Mental Deficiency, 43*, 51–56.

Innes, G., Kidd, C., & Ross, H.S. (1968). Mental subnormality in northeast Scotland. *British Journal of Psychiatry, 114*, 35–41.

Lane, H. (1976). *The wild boy of Aveyron*. Cambridge, MA: Harvard Press.

Matson, J.L., & Barrett, R.P. (1982). Affective disorders. In J.L. Matson & R.P. Barrett (Eds.), *Psychopathology in the mentally retarded* (pp. 121–146). New York: Grune & Stratton.

Menolascino, F. (1965). Emotional disturbance and mental retardation. *American Journal of Mental Deficiency, 70*, 248–256.

Menolascino, F.J. (1983). Overview. In F.J. Menolascino & B.M. McCann (Eds.), *Mental health and mental retardation: Bridging the gap* (pp. 3–64). Baltimore, MD: University Park Press.

Menolascino, F.J. (1986, May). *Differential diagnosis: Clinical research challenges in the mentally ill/mentally retarded*. Paper presented at the 26th annual meeting of the New Clinical Drug Evaluation Unit (NCDEU), Key Biscayne, FL.

Menolascino, F.J., Ruedrich, S.L., Golden, C.J., & Wilson, J.E. (1985). Diagnosis and pharmacotherapy of schizophrenia in the retarded. *Psychopharmacology Bulletin, 21*, 316–322.

Mercer, M. (1968). Why mentally retarded persons come to a mental hospital. *Mental Retardation, 6*, 8–10.

Payne, R. (1968). The psychiatric subnormal. *Journal of Mental Subnormality, 14*, 25–34.

Reid, A.H. (1972). Psychoses in adult mental defectives: I. Manic–depressive psychoses. *British Journal of Psychiatry, 120*, 205–212.

Reis, R.K. (1985). DSM-III implications of the diagnoses of catatonia and bipolar disorder. *American Journal of Psychiatry, 142*, 1471–1474.

Reiss, S., Levitan, G., & McNally, R. (1982). Emotionally disturbed mentally retarded people: An underserved population. *American Psychologist, 37*(4), 361–367.

Rosenoff, A.J., Handy, L.M., & Plesset, I.R. (1935). The etiology of manic–depressive syndromes with specific references to their occurrences in twins. *American Journal of Psychiatry, 91*, 725–762.

Ruedrich, S.R., & Menolascino, F.J. (1984). Dual diagnosis of mental retardation and mental illness: An overview. In F.J. Menolascino & J.A. Stark (Eds.), *Handbook of mental illness in the mentally retarded* (pp. 45–81). New York: Plenum Press.

Shellhaas, M.D., & Nihira, K. (1969). Factor analysis of reasons retardates are referred to an institution. *American Journal of Mental Deficiency, 74*, 171–179.

Sovner, R., & Hurley, A.H. (1983). Do the mentally retarded suffer from affective illness? *Archives of General Psychiatry, 140*, 1539–1540.

Weaver, T.R. (1946). The incidence of maladjustment among mental defectives in a military environment. *American Journal of Mental Deficiency, 51*, 238–346.

Williams, C.E. (1972). A study of the patients in a group of mental subnormal hospitals. *British Journal of Mental Subnormality, 17*, 29–41.

# 11
# Integrative Approach to Diagnosis of Mental Disorders in Retarded Persons

Ludwik S. Szymanski

## Introduction

The fact that retarded persons exhibit mental disorders even more frequently than nonretarded ones has been well documented in the literature reviewed by Dr. Russell in Chapter 3. As pointed out by him, as well as by other writers (Szymanski, 1980), one of the major obstacles to progress in the field of mental health of persons with mental retardation has been the lack of clear and universally accepted diagnostic terminology of mental disorders.

The term "psychiatric diagnosis" is usually equated with the "diagnostic label," which is actually only an abbreviated general code, useful in grouping disorders for administrative or research purposes. For clinical purposes, a more elaborate and expanded diagnostic formulation is needed that describes the individual's problems, strengths, environment, and so on. Establishing such an expanded diagnosis is probably the most important phase of mental health care since it is a prerequisite to treatment intervention tailored to the particular individual's needs, rather than a mere diagnostic label. In multiaxial classification systems such as DSM-III (American Psychiatric Association, 1980), this information may be coded on different axes, which provide a more detailed and individualized description of the patient.

This chapter focuses on the manner in which a diagnosis of mental disorders in persons with mental retardation might be made and an adaptation of the conventional diagnostic criteria to the problems posed by this population.

## The Diagnostic Process

The following description is based on the clinical practice of the staff at the Developmental Evaluation Clinic at the Children's Hospital, Boston. Many mental health facilities serving retarded clients do not have all the services that are available at this interdisciplinary teaching clinic where most of the clients need to be seen by multiple disciplines. Still, the principles of integrating interdisciplinary information into a comprehensive diagnostic formulation are applicable in different settings serving various degrees of handicapping conditions. The diagnostic process can be divided into the preevaluation and evaluation stages.

## Preevaluation stage

Retarded persons (similarly to children) are rarely self-referred and the referral is usually initiated by a caregiver following a change in the person's behavior. Typically, the behavior becomes disruptive; less frequently, a client who does not disturb others will be referred, such as a withdrawn and depressed person (Szymanski & Biederman, 1984). Caregiver attitude and tolerance are important as well. Sometimes, there is no change in the client's behavior, and the referral is precipitated by a change in caregiver's tolerance of a preexisting behavior. Not infrequently, the referral is an expression of a caregiver's anger, for example, because of a reduction in staffing or a physician's decision to reduce the client's dose of a neuroleptic medication.

## The Evaluation Stage

### REVIEW OF THE HISTORY

Obtaining an accurate history might be a problem with retarded clients, especially in institutions, because of poorly maintained records. The caregivers may know only about the client's behavior during their shift, providing only such history that supports their "agendas" [both manifest and latent (Szymanski, 1977)], such as having the patient put on medication. Not infrequently, we found that a client referred because of "aggression" and "attention getting" had a history of schizophrenia and multiple hospitalizations. Therefore, reviewing all records and interviewing all caregivers, including direct-care staff, are essential (Bailey, Thiele, Ware, & Helsel-De Wert, 1985).

The history providing description of symptoms should be longitudinal, correlated with other concurrent events such as environmental stresses, medical illnesses and procedures, and the administration of psychotropic medications. Graphic visualization of the data may be particularly helpful. This might help to resolve, for example, a question of whether there is a cyclicity in the client's clinical presentation.

### COMPREHENSIVE EVALUATION

A psychiatric diagnostic evaluation of a retarded person has to be comprehensive (Menolascino & Bernstein, 1970). This might range from critical assessment of past evaluations by other disciplines to a full interdisciplinary assessment. For this reason, the diagnosticians should be the most trained professionals available, such as child psychiatrists (even if the retarded patient is an adult), since training in the three crucial areas—biological, psychosocial, and developmental—is essential.

PATIENT EXAMINATION

Clinical diagnostic techniques with retarded persons have been described extensively (Menolascino & Bernstein, 1970; Philips, 1966; Szymanski, 1977, 1980) and therefore are mentioned only briefly. Both observation and active patient interview, verbal and nonverbal, are essential. Directiveness and limit setting, without leading questions to which retarded persons are particularly susceptible (Sigelman, Budd, Spanhel, & Schoenrock, 1981), are necessary, as is "tuning-in" to the patient's communication level. Surprisingly many clinicians, especially those with psychodynamic background, do not expect that one can talk to a retarded person and neglect this part of the assessment (Szymanski, 1980).

ASSESSMENT

This stage includes both analysis and synthesis of the collected data. The symptomatic behaviors are assessed in light of the patient's cognitive level, social experience, life experience, and circumstances. For instance, is a stereotypic behavior site specific, is it related to certain antecedents and/or staff reactions? Abnormal behaviors should not be dismissed as an expected part of one's retardation or explained as an inevitable result of "organicity" inherent in mental retardation (Philips, 1966). This misconception has also been described as a diagnostic "overshadowing," a tendency to ignore psychopathology if the patient is known to be retarded (Reiss, Levitan, & Szyszko, 1982).

DIAGNOSTIC FORMULATION

At this stage, the diagnostician might be ready to make a formal diagnosis. This should also include a description of the patient's strengths, weaknesses, environmental liabilities, and supports.

INTERVENTION PLAN

This is obviously the reason for the diagnostic referral in the first place. To be effective, the recommendations have to be comprehensive, take into account all the client's needs, and be well integrated with recommendations of other disciplines. At this point, the clinician's broad training (as described earlier) proves its importance. On the other hand, narrowly specialized clinicians tend to focus primarily on their area of expertise, such as drug treatment.

INFORMING CONFERENCE

The importance of this diagnostic phase is matched only by the frequency with which it is neglected. At this point, the diagnostician's knowledge is shared with the caregivers and the client (whenever possible) in a manner understandable to them. Specific techniques useful at this stage have been described previously (Szymanski, 1980).

FOLLOW-THROUGH

Even if the referral was purely for a consultation, it is the diagnostician's responsibility to follow up on the recommendations, at least in making appropriate referral for recommended services.

## Other Diagnostic Tools and Techniques

Recently, there has been growing interest in the use of structured interview schedules and rating scales. Instruments such as DIS and SADS have been developed (for nonretarded persons), but reports on their reliability as compared with clinical interviews are still contradictory (Anthony et al., 1985; Helzer et al., 1985; Klerman, 1985). Instruments designed specifically for assessment of certain disorders have recently been used with retarded persons. Kazdin, Matson, and Senatore (1983) successfully used the Beck Depression Inventory and the Zung Self-Rating Depression Scale and reported that they significantly correlated with each other and with the clinical diagnosis. Senatore, Matson, and Kazdin (1985) reported on the use of psychopathology assessment instruments developed by them for retarded adults. The correlations between informant and self-report versions were relatively low, but it seemed to be of value in screening individuals for referral for a more comprehensive assessment. Aman, Singh, Stewart, and Field (1985) have developed an Aberrant Behavior Checklist for retarded persons, especially for follow-up on the effects of treatment. Its reliability appears, so far, to be rather limited and it was not suggested as a tool for routine diagnosis.

An approach of promise would be adaptation of empirically derived instruments for behavioral profiling, such as those developed by Achenbach (1980) and Achenbach and Edelbrock (1979), based on clustering behaviors that tend to occur together. This would be particularly useful for research and might lead to closer delineation of clinical syndromes.

The value of projective tests in diagnosis is still debated. Gittelman (1980) reviewed literature on this subject and concluded that there was no evidence that these tests could distinguish reliably between various diagnostic categories or be predictive of outcome.

In summary, these approaches are important since they offer a structured and reproducible way of obtaining comprehensive histories and conducting a clinical interview and can be administered by less trained personnel, which in turn could help more trained professionals to standardize their assessments. At the present stage, they seem to be particularly useful for epidemiological surveys, screening, and follow-up on treatment effects, rather than for making a definitive diagnosis in an individual; especially since clinical judgment has to be made concerning the validity of the history and the need for ancillary examinations, particularly medical ones. Further research is obviously needed.

## Differential Diagnosis – Physical Disorders

Physical disorders may often manifest in behavioral and emotional symptoms. In the classic studies of Hall, Popkin, Devaul, Faillace, and Stickney (1978), in 658 psychiatric outpatients, careful medical evaluation including blood chemistries showed that 9.1% had a medical disorder causative of the psychiatric symptoms, and 77% of these had not been previously recognized. The most frequent disorders were cardiovascular and endocrine. In the second study, 46% of 100 patients in a state hospital were found to have a medical disorder causative of or exacerbating their symptoms (Hall, Gardner, Stickney, LeCann and Popkin, 1980).

These findings may be very relevant to persons with mental retardation who are often multiply handicapped and have associated physical disorders, receive medications with many side effects, and may have difficulty in describing somatic complaints. For these reasons, a careful medical assessment is necessary, even if the presenting symptoms are behavioral/emotional in nature.

## Classification of Mental Disorders

Rutter (1978) and Cantwell (1980) have pointed out that an adequate classification system should (1) be valid, (2) classify disorders and not patients, (3) differentiate between disorders, (4) have a developmental framework, and (5) be practical and useful. The DSM-III, introduced in 1980, to some degree reflected the above principles. Its most important features included the following (Spitzer & Cantwell, 1980):

1. A statement conceptualizing what a mental disorder is.
2. Nonetiological, descriptive approach.
3. Systematic description of each disorder.
4. Diagnostic criteria.
5. Multiaxial classification.

In an early field trial of DSM-III (draft), Cantwell, Russell, Mattison, and Will (1979) found the average agreement of raters with the expected diagnosis was 50%, and the interrater agreement was 54% for Axis I, and it was better for broader, rather than for narrow, categories (Mattison, Cantwell, Russell, & Will, 1979). It was noticed that as opposed to DSM-II, the multiaxial system enabled more frequent recording of both the major psychiatric syndromes and specific developmental disorders (Russell, Cantwell, Mattison, & Will, 1979).

The DSM-III has not been evaluated in a similarly rigorous way with retarded persons, although some authors mentioned that the patients they studied were diagnosed in accordance with DSM-III criteria (Eaton & Menolascino, 1982; Gostason, 1985).

# Specific Disorders

Current knowledge of epidemiology of specific mental disorders in retarded persons are not discussed here since it has been comprehensively reviewed by Dr. Russell in Chapter 3. I shall only echo that it is clear that, as a group, retarded persons exhibit the same mental disorders as nonretarded persons, although sometimes the clinical presentation may be modified by the communication problems the patient might have, environmental factors, and other factors mentioned previously. It is difficult to evaluate the literature on this topic for a number of reasons, such as varied and often idiosyncratic diagnostic criteria for mental retardation and mental disorders used by different researchers and biased, preselected study populations. Even recently, when the DSM-III has been the accepted classification, some reports that start with a sort of modern incantation, a statement that the diagnoses were made by DSM-III criteria actually use idiosyncratic terms that are not part of DSM-III. Therefore, the existing literature should be reviewed critically.

Because of time limitation, I shall review only some of the major psychiatric syndromes in retarded persons, in respect to the diagnosis (with particular emphasis on the use of DSM-III), problems in establishing the diagnosis, and prevalence.

## Mental Retardation

DSM-III criteria are essentially the same as those of the American Association on Mental Deficiency, and the reliability of this diagnosis is generally high (Cantwell et al., 1979; Mattison et al., 1979). The placement of this diagnosis on Axis I has been criticized since DSM-III was introduced. Rutter and Shaffer (1980) pointed out that mental retardation reflected abnormal level, rather than type of functioning, and therefore should be coded on a separate axis (Rutter, Shaffer, & Shepherd, 1975); also grouping two major diagnoses on one axis reduced the possibility that both, if coexisting, would be diagnosed (Cantwell et al., 1979; Russell et al., 1979). Kendell (1980, 1983) suggested coding it on Axis II, which would thus group together lifelong and stable handicaps (Williams, 1985a, 1985b). The last view has also been supported by the Committee on Mental Retardation and Developmental Disabilities of the American Academy of Child Psychiatry. In the revised version of the DSM-III published in 1987, Mental retardation, Pervasive Developmental Disorders, and Specific Developmental Disorders are grouped together as Developmental Disorders, which are coded on Axis II.

The fifth digit codes behavioral symptoms requiring attention or treatment and that are not a part of another disorder. The intention here is to code nonspecific behaviors that can be attributed to mental retardation alone. This seems to reflect, however, the misconception described by Philips (1966), that a maladaptive behavior of a retarded person is a function of the retardation. This fifth digit code seems to be useful only to clinicians inexperienced with retarded patients, who can lump here the symptoms that they do not understand. No behavior is unique to mental retardation, and different individuals may manifest exactly opposite behaviors. If a behavior is of such severity that treatment is required, a specific diagnosis should be sought. For these reasons, our committee recommended abolishing this fifth digit code. It is not used in the DSM-III-R (Revised).

## Pervasive Developmental Disorders (PDD)

In the DSM-III, PDD includes infantile autism, PDD-childhood onset, and "atypical" PDD, differentiated mainly by arbitrary age of onset of 30 months. While the broad PDD category has been relatively easy to diagnose, the subcategories did not seem to reflect clinical reality. The relationship of the PDD to psychotic disorders has been a focus of controversy. Following early ideas, including those of Kanner, infantile autism (IA) has been seen as a form of psychosis. However, later studies are convincing that these are separate disorders, and this seems to be the accepted view at the present (Campbell & Green, 1985). However, some of these individuals might in later life develop a psychotic disorder, and then both diagnoses should be coded. The DSM-III-R (revised) divides PDD into autistic disorder and PDD, not otherwise classified (NOS).

Mental retardation professionals frequently see adults with a typical residual form of IA. However, Eaton and Menolascino (1982) did not find it in their sample of 168 retarded persons 6 to 76 years of age. Gostason (1985) did not diagnose a PDD in his sample of 132 retarded adults. In our own original sample of 237 children, there were 9 cases (5 IA and 4 PDD) among 111 nonretarded and 20 (9 IA and 11 PDD) among 126 retarded children. PDD was diagnosed in 15% of 155 retarded adults.

## Psychotic Disorders

Psychosis has probably been grossly overdiagnosed in retarded persons. Many mental health professionals still have the tendency to diagnose psychosis in retarded individuals on the basis of strange (in their perspectives) behaviors, such as self-stimulation, talking to self, or aggressive outbursts. More recently, following the Rogers decision (on administration of antipsychotics to incompetent persons), diagnosis of psychosis has been seen by some as necessary to justify to the courts the use of these drugs. In the earlier years, the distinction between retardation and schizophrenia was not that clear (Reid, 1972). Kraepelin thought that manneristic movements of some retarded persons were diagnostic of early schizophrenia and proposed the term propfschizophrenie for these cases. Other early writers thought that retarded persons cannot develop genuine schizophrenia, or that psychosis occurring in them is of a special type (Earl, 1934). However, in the years to follow, no evidence was gathered that there is a special form of schizophrenia in retarded persons. Reid (1972) described 12 schizophrenic-retarded patients, and Heaton-Ward (1977), who found 42 such cases, felt that schizophrenia in retarded patients could be diagnosed on the basis of usually accepted criteria; but this diagnosis would be impossible to make in patients unable to communicate sufficiently verbally. In patients who are nonverbal, symptoms such as gross disorganization of behavior and behavioral episodes suggesting hallucinations and deterioration may help to establish the diagnosis, but the residual category of "atypical psychosis" might have to be used. Positive past and family history will support the diagnosis.

Eaton and Menolascino (1982), in 24 of 168 retarded persons aged 60 to 76, noted altered affect, bizarre rituals, and interpersonal distancing, which were judged to be a clear mark of schizophrenia. Gostason (1985) diagnosed schizophrenic and paranoid disorders in 4 of 51 retarded persons. In our sample, psychosis was diagnosed in 17% of mildly/moderately and 30% of severely/profoundly retarded adults. The most frequent subcategory was atypical psychosis followed by schizoaffective, schizophrenia, and paranoid disorder.

Besides the usual problems in the differential diagnosis of psychotic disorders, we noticed several issues particularly relevant to retarded persons. The first one was of a lonely adult, often living at home, tending to isolate himself, talk to himself, and voice unrealistic expectations. On closer questioning and observation, it would become evident that no genuine hallucinations or delusions were present, but the patient had an "imaginary friend," which one might consider developmentally appropriate. The second, reverse problem would occur when the patient was labeled by the staff as an attention getter, but on close assessment, progressive deterioration and disorganization could be found. In a third situation, discussed below, both psychotic and depressive symptoms coexisted, and one could mask the other.

Another problem has been recognized relatively recently. Following the trend of a rational approach to the use of antipsychotics in retarded persons, many who had been on these agents for years (often for no clear reason) have been taken off them. In some, a variety of behavioral symptoms emerged, some resembling psychosis. Chouinard and Steinberg (1984) refer to supersensitivity psychosis in which there is an increase in the number of synapses and postsynaptic neuronal overactivity following "chemical denervation" by the drug. The differential diagnosis from relapse of the original psychosis may be difficult, especially since these symptoms might disappear spontaneously only after a prolonged period. The diagnosis may be suggested by presence of positive symptoms of schizophrenia and emergent dyskinesia.

In summary, the available knowledge indicates that the same psychotic disorders occur in retarded as in nonretarded persons. In both groups, they may result in cognitive impairment to some degree; they may be diagnosed in mildly retarded and verbal persons by the usual criteria but, in the more severely handicapped, mainly on the basis of general and severe behavioral and social disorganization.

## Affective Disorders

In this section, depression is discussed as an illness rather than as a state of mood. Depressive disorders are probably the most underdiagnosed category of mental disorders of retarded persons for reasons such as the misconception that depression (as an illness) does not occur in this population, and also professionals' ignorance of its clinical presentation (Szymanski & Biederman, 1984). Retarded persons with depression may go unnoticed since they may not be usually disturbing to others and their mood could be confused with the passivity "expected" of a retarded person. Gardner (1967), reviewing the early literature, noticed lack of definite data and also contradictory theoretical predictions of high vulnerability of retarded individuals to depression, owing to their experience of rejection, failure, and inconsistent mothering. This was contradictory to beliefs that retarded persons could not develop depression because their low intelligence precluded development of low self-esteem. Later, literature on depression in retarded persons, mainly case reports, was reviewed by Sovner and Hurley (1983). Still, such reports have been infrequent and even recently, Eaton and Menolascino (1982) did not diagnose depressive disorders in their respective samples. Gostason (1985), in his study of a representative sample of retarded persons, diagnosed atypical depression in 1 of 75 mildly, and none among 57 moderately and below, retarded persons.

On the other hand, manic–depressive illness has been described more frequently, starting with the later part of the last century. More recently, Reid (1976), Heaton-Ward (1977), and Rivinus and Harmatz (1979) reported on a series of retarded patients with diagnosis of manic–depressive illness. Gostason (1985) diagnosed cyclothymic disorder in two of his cases.

In our clinic, depressive disorders were diagnosed in 14% of mildly/moderately and 6% of severely/profoundly retarded children (including dysthymic disorder and adjustment disorders in which depressive mood predominated). Among adults, this diagnosis was made in 13%, including major depression and dysthymic disorder, as well as manic–depressive and cyclothymic disorders.

The DSM-III criteria can be used for diagnosis of affective disorders in retarded persons, but one has to bear in mind that the clinical presentation may be altered somewhat and depends on patient's communication skills, particularly verbal–conceptual. In mildly retarded ones, verbalizations of dysphoric mood, low self-image, "feeling sick," and so on are common, while in less verbal ones, the diagnosis will be based more on behavioral and vegetative symptoms. Pre-existing aggressive, self-stimulatory, and self-abusive behaviors might be intensified. In both cases, sad appearance, as well as family history, will support the diagnosis. The Dexamethasone Suppression Test (DST) might be used, although the earlier enthusiasm about it has diminished as the frequency of false positive results has been recognized. In some cases, there might be need to resort to a therapeutic trial with antidepressants.

In differential diagnosis of affective disorders in retarded persons, there are four major considerations:

1. *Dementia*, particularly in adults with Down's syndrome in whom Alzheimer's disease has been described as occurring more frequently than in the general population. Certain similarities between persons with Down's syndrome and Alzheimer's patients have been described (see also Coyle, Chapter 7). Included here are biochemical features (decreased activity of cholinergic enzymes such as choline acetyltransferase and acetylcholine esterase) and similarity in dermatoglyphics (Cutler, Heston, Davies, Haxby, & Schapiro, 1985). However, while the neocortical plaques and neurofibrillary tangles consistent with Alzheimer's disease have been found in up to 100% of these adults over 40 years of age (Malamud, 1964), they are not necessarily accompanied by a clinical dementia. Ropper and Williams (1980) found these neuropathological changes in the brains of all 20 patients over 30, with Down's syndrome, whom they studied, but clinical dementia was reported in only 3 of them. Similar conclusions were reached by Cutler et al. (1985) on the basis of literature review and their own experience. They state that although some memory impairment and other cognitive changes are found in older persons with DS, they are usually not evident before the mid-forties. Precipitous diagnosis of dementia in these patients may be disastrous since the caregivers may accept an attitude of therapeutic nihilism and abandon a patient who might actually have a treatable depression.

2. *Reaction to major environmental stress*, similar to one seen in geriatric patients precipitously relocated ("relocation syndrome"), may lead to symptoms such as weight loss, withdrawal, confusion, and disorientation (Cochran, Sran & Varano, 1977). Some of these patients might also be genuinely depressed.

3. We encountered an interesting situation in some profoundly retarded individuals. Following a loss of a direct-care staff who had cared for them for many years, symptoms such as interpersonal withdrawal, hypomotility, irritability, and loss of weight appeared. For practical purposes, these cases were very similar to *Reactive Attachment Disorder of Infancy*, although the DSM-III requires onset in the first eight months of life (changed in DSM-III-R to five years).

4. *Medical disorders*, such as hypothyroidism, especially in persons with DS and side effects of medications.

## Organic Disorders

"Organicity" has been one of the most misused and overdiagnosed terms in the mental retardation field, mostly as the result of psychiatrists' obsession with classifying mental disorders into organic and nonorganic, their misconception that all disordered behaviors of retarded persons are due to brain damage, and the inadequacies of previous classification systems. The DSM-III acknowledges that labeling a disorder as nonorganic does not imply that it is independent of brain processes since all psychological processes depend on brain function. It removes the misleading and overgeneralizing DSM-II subdivision into "psychotic", "nonpsychotic", reversible, and irreversible disorders (Lipowski, 1980). It requires that clinical presence of the brain syndrome be recognized and that specific organic factors judged etiologically related to the organic mental state be demonstrated rather than implied (except in certain and clear circumstances). Two gross categories were recognized in the DSM-III. *Organic brain syndromes*, without reference to etiology were subdivided into: (1) delirium and dementia, (2) amnestic syndrome and organic hallucinosis, (3) organic delusional and affective syndromes, (4) intoxication and withdrawal, and (5) atypical or mixed organic brain syndrome. The term *organic mental disorder* was used if etiology was known (e.g., multi-infarct dementia). In the DSM-III-R organic mental disorders are divided into: demetias arising in the senium and presenium; psychoactive substance-induced organic mental disorders; and organic mental disorders associated with Axis III physical disorders or conditions whose etiology is unknown. The fact that retardation, perhaps with an additional neurological disorder such as epilepsy, exists and that the person has abnormal behavior does not warrant "organic" designation unless, for example, temporal or other association could be documented and suggests etiological connection of the latter with the former. Such association may be implied when a behavioral syndrome is present that is well known to be specifically associated with a particular brain dysfunction, such as personality change of "frontal lobe syndrome" or in temporal lobe epilepsy (Bear, 1979; Bear, Freeman, & Greenberg, 1984) such as obsessive religiosity, hypergraphia, hypo- or hypersexuality, or "stickiness" of mental functioning. In the literature, however, this designation has been used liberally and idiosyncratically. Reported prevalence of these disorders has varied greatly. Menolascino (1970), surveying 95 persons with Down's syndrome, diagnosed chronic brain syndrome with behavioral reaction in 17 who exhibited behaviors such as hyperactivity, impulsiveness, and short attention span. An additional four, who manifested periods of uncontrollability and withdrawal, were given diagnoses of OBS with psychotic reaction. Eaton and Menolascino (1982) diagnosed organic brain syndrome with behavioral reaction in 18.4% and with psychotic reaction in 11.4% of their sample. These patients had findings and/or histories of neurological, etiologically significant factors and symptoms such as inappropriate acting out, impulsivity, and frequent tantrums. These psychotic patients differed from schizophrenic ones in that they did not have hallucinations and did not show "progressive involvement of multiple segments of functioning." Gostason (1985) diagnosed atypical OBS in 27 of 57 moderately/severely retarded and in 2 of 75 mildly retarded. He used evidence of symptoms such as perseveration, lassitude, indecision, and agitation to justify the diagnosis (although it did not conform to DSM-III criteria). In our clinic, using strict DSM-III interpretation, we diagnosed an organic disorder in approximately 4% of retarded patients.

In summary, a better definition of organic disorders (or better adherence to DSM-III intention) is needed, as well as a better assessment of retarded patients for the presence of organic structural and physiological factors, including iatrogenic ones, which do not merely coexist but can be proved to cause psychopathology. This could enable specific treatment in some cases. To that end, as described earlier, the diagnostic assessment should be comprehensive and biobehavioral. On the other hand, precipitous diagnosis of organicity, based on nonspecific symptoms, should be avoided since it often leads to therapeutic nihilism (Lipowski, 1980).

## Effects of Diagnostic Labeling

The purpose of diagnostic labeling (the formal diagnosis) is obviously to capitalize on its positive effects—such as improving communication between professionals, providing specific treatments if available, and obtaining epidemiological data important for administrative and research purposes. However, responsible professionals must keep in mind the negative effects and try to minimize them. So far, little is known about effects of combined diagnoses of mental retardation and mental disorder on others' attitudes toward the labeled individual. However, we know about the many negative effects of each diagnostic label separately. These are based chiefly on ignorance, and the use of the diagnosis to classify and stereotype people rather than disorders. We do know that mentally retarded and mentally ill people are often feared, rejected, and met with stereotypic (usually negative and lowered) expectations, as well as excluded from services and segregated. While such segregation might offer temporary shelter, as well as the raison d'etre for a new provider industry, it is contrary to the principles of normalization and mainstreaming and against the individual's long-term interests. Classifying a person in such general terms as "mentally retarded," "mentally ill," "emotionally disturbed," "dually diagnosed," or "behaviorally disturbed," lumps together a mildly depressed person, a floridly psychotic, and obsessive–compulsive, but tells us nothing about their problems and needs (Szymanski & Grossman, 1984). Creating special programs to which persons are sent only on the basis of such general diagnosis is not justifiable. Hopefully, we shall develop the means by which administrators can classify clients on the basis of needs and not labels, as is done under Massachusetts special education law (Public Laws Chapter 766) (see also the chapters in Section VII).

# Discussion

Our knowledge of mental disorders in retarded persons is still in an early stage. To advance it, a number of developments are needed.

First, the current classification system (DSM-III) should be improved to be more adaptable to retarded patients. It should be more developmentally oriented; diagnosis of certain disorders (e.g., depression and schizophrenia) should be made possible in nonverbal patients. Criteria for organic disorders should be clarified. Nonspecific behaviors, such as self-abuse and aggression, should be linked with a disorder syndrome or they might be coded in an appropriate "atypical" or otherwise not specified category.

Second, better diagnostic techniques and tools should be developed to assess severely/profoundly retarded and nonverbal persons.

Third, caution should be exercised in inventing new syndromes for retarded persons unless they can be linked with underlying pathology rather than merely with the fact that the person is cognitively impaired.

Fourth, it is the responsibility of the diagnosticians and professionals to do the utmost to prevent misuse of the diagnosis (such as categorizing people rather than disorders) and to ensure its proper use. General terms, lumping together people on the basis of diagnosis, such as the deindividualizing terms "the dually diagnosed," should not be used.

Fifth, there is an acute need for comprehensively and eclectically trained mental health clinicians and researchers to work with retarded patients. Since one deals here with a relatively small, "orphan" patient population, public funding for their training and research will be needed, not very different from support provided in developing "orphan drugs."

# References

Achenbach, T.M. (1980). DSM-III in light of empirical research on the classification of child psychopathology. *Journal of the American Academy of Child Psychiatry, 19*, 395–412.

Achenbach, T.M., & Edelbrock, C.S. (1979). The Child Behavior Profile: II. Boys aged 12–16 and girls aged 6–11 and 12–16. *Journal of Consulting Clinical Psychology, 47*, 223–233.

Aman, M.G., Singh, N.N., Stewart, A.W., & Field, C.J. (1985). The Aberrant Behavior Checklist: A behavior rating scale for the assessment of treatment effects. *American Journal of Mental Deficiency, 89*(5), 485–491.

American Psychiatric Association. (1980). *Diagnostic and statistical manual of mental disorders*, 3rd Edition (DSM-III). Washington, DC: Author.

Anthony, J.C., Folstein, M., Romanoski, A.J., Von Korff, M.R., Nestadt, G.R., Chahal, R., Merchant, A., Brown, C.H., Shapiro, S., Kramer, M., & Gruenberg, E.M. (1985). Comparison of the lay interview schedule and a standardized psychiatric diagnosis. *Archives of General Psychiatry, 42*, 667–675.

Bailey, D.B., Thiele, J.E., Ware, W.B., & Helsel-De Wert, M. (1985). Participation of professionals, paraprofessionals and direct-care staff members in the interdisciplinary team meeting. *American Journal of Mental Deficiency, 89*, 437–440.

Bear, D.M. (1979). Temporal lobe epilepsy—a syndrome of sensory–limbic hyperconnection. *Cortex, 15*, 537–584.

Bear, D.M., Freeman, R., & Greenberg, M. (1984). Behavioral alterations in patients with temporal lobe epilepsy. In D. Blumer (Ed.), *Psychiatric aspects of epilepsy*. Washington, DC: American Psychiatric Press.

Campbell, M., & Green, W.H. (1985). Pervasive developmental disorders of childhood. In H.I. Kaplan & B.J. Sadock (Eds.), *Comprehensive textbook of psychiatry*. Baltimore, MD: Williams & Wilkins.

Cantwell, D.P. (1980). The diagnostic process and diagnostic classification in child psychiatry—DSM-III. *Journal of the American Academy of Child Psychiatry, 19*, 345–355.

Cantwell, D.P., Russell, A.T., Mattison, R., & Will, L. (1979). A comparison of DSM-II and DSM-III in the diagnosis of childhood psychiatric disorders: I. Agreement with expected diagnosis. *Archives of General Psychiatry, 36*, 1208–1213.

Chouinard, G., & Steinberg, S. (1984). New clinical concepts on neuroleptic-induced supersensitivity disorders: Tardive dyskinesia and supersensitivity psychosis. In H.C. Stancer, P.E. Garfinkel, & V.M. Rakoff (Eds.), *Guidelines for the use of psychotropic drugs*. New York: SP Medical and Scientific Books.

Cochran, W.E., Sran, P.K., & Varano, G.A. (1977). The relocation syndrome in mentally retarded individuals. *Mental Retardation, 15*, 10–12.

Cutler, N.R., Heston, L.L., Davies, P., Haxby, J.V., & Schapiro, M.B. (1985). Alzheimer's disease and Down's syndrome: New insights. *Annals of Internal Medicine, 103*, 566–578.

*Diagnostic and statistical manual of mental disorders*, Vol. III (DSM-III). (1980). Washington, DC: American Psychiatric Association.

Eaton, L.F., & Menolascino, F.J. (1982). Psychiatric disorders in mentally retarded: Types, problems and challenges. *American Journal of Psychiatry, 139*, 1297–1303.

Earl, C.J. (1934). The primitive catatonic psychosis of idiocy. *British Journal of Medical Psychology, 14*, 231–253.

Gardner, W.I. (1967). Occurrence of severe depressive reactions in the mentally retarded. *American Journal of Psychiatry, 124*, 142–144.

Gittelman, R. (1980). The role of psychological tests for differential diagnosis in child psychiatry. *Journal of the American Academy of Child Psychiatry, 19*, 413–438.

Gostason, R. (1985). Psychiatric illness among the mentally retarded. A Swedish population study. *Acta Psychiatrica Scandinavica*, Supplement.

Hall, R.C.V., Popkin, M.K., Devaul, R.A., Faillace, L.A., & Stickney, S.K. (1978). Physical illness presenting as psychiatric disease. *Archives of General Psychiatry, 35*, 1315–1320.

Hall, R.C.W., Gardner, E.R., Stickney, S.K., LeCann, A., & Popkin, M.K. (1980). II. Physical illness manifesting as psychiatric disease. *Archives of General Psychiatry, 37*, 989–995.

Heaton-Ward, A. (1977). Psychosis in mental handicap. *British Journal of Psychiatry, 130*, 525–533.

Helzer, J.E., Robins, L.N., McEvoy, L.T., Spitznagel, E.L., Stoltzman, R.K., Farmer, A., & Brockington, I.F. (1985). A comparison of clinical and diagnostic interview schedule diagnoses. *Archives of General Psychiatry, 42*, 657–666.

Kazdin, A.E., Matson, J.L, & Senatore, V. (1983). Assessment of depression in mentally retarded adults. *American Journal of Psychiatry, 140*, 1040–1043.

Kendell, R.E. (1980). DSM-III: A British perspective. *American Journal of Psychiatry, 137*, 1630–1631.

Kendell, R.E. (1983). DSM-III: A major advance in psychiatric nosology. In R.L. Spitzer, J.B.W. Williams, & A.E. Skodol (Eds.), *International perspectives on DSM-III*. Washington, DC: American Psychiatric Press.

Klerman, G.L. (1985). Diagnosis of psychiatric disorders in epidemiologic field studies. *Archives of General Psychiatry, 42*, 723–724.

Lipowski, Z.J. (1980). A new look at organic brain syndromes. *American Journal of Psychiatry, 137*, 674–678.

Malamud, N. (1964). Neuropathology of organic brain syndromes associated with aging. In C.M. Gaitz (Ed.), *Aging and the brain*. New York: Plenum Press.

Mattison, R., Cantwell, D.P., Russell, A.T., & Will, L. (1979). A comparison of DSM-II and DSM-III in the diagnosis of childhood psychiatric disorders: II. Interrater agreement. *Archives of General Psychiatry, 36,* 1217–1222.

Menolascino, F.J. (1969). Emotional disturbances in mentally retarded children. *American Journal of Psychiatry, 126,* 168–179.

Menolascino, F.J. (1970). Down's syndrome: Clinical and psychiatric findings in an institutionalized sample. In F.J. Menolascino (Ed.), *Psychiatric approaches to mental retardation.* New York: Basic Books.

Menolascino, F.J. & Bernstein, N.R. (1970). Psychiatric assessment of the mentally retarded child. In: N.R. Bernstein (Ed.), *Diminished people.* Boston: Little, Brown.

Philips, I. (1966). Children, mental retardation and emotional disorder. In I. Philips (Ed.), *Prevention and treatment of mental retardation.* New York: Basic Books.

Reid, A.H. (1972). Psychosis in adult mental defectives. *British Journal of Psychiatry, 120,* 205–212.

Reid, A.H. (1976). Psychiatric disturbances in the mentally handicapped. *Proceedings of the Royal Society of Medicine, 69,* 509–512.

Reiss, S., Levitan, G.W., & Szyszko, J. (1982). Emotional disturbance and mental retardation: Diagnostic overshadowing. *American Journal of Mental Deficiency, 86,* 567–574.

Rivinus, T.M., & Harmatz, J.S. (1979). Diagnosis and lithium treatment of affective disorder in the retarded: Five case studies. *American Journal of Psychiatry, 136,* 551–554.

Ropper, A.H., & Williams, R.S. (1980). Relationship between plaques, tangles and dementia in Down's syndrome. *Neurology, 30,* 639–644.

Russell, A.T., Cantwell, D.P., Mattison, R., & Will, L. (1979). A comparison of DSM-II and DSM-III in the diagnosis of childhood psychiatric disorders: III: Multiaxial features. *Archives of General Psychiatry, 36,* 1223–1226.

Rutter, M. (1978). Classification. In M. Rutter & L. Hersov (Eds.), *Child psychiatry.* London: Blackwell Scientific Publications.

Rutter, M., & Shaffer, D. (1980). DSM-III: A step forward or back in terms of the classification of child psychiatric disorders? *Journal of the American Academy of Child Psychiatry, 19,* 371–394.

Rutter, M., Shaffer, D., & Shepherd, M. (1975). *A multiaxial classification of child psychiatric disorders.* Geneva: World Health Organization.

Senatore, V., Matson, J.L., & Kazdin, A.E. (1985). An inventory to assess psychopathology of mentally retarded adults. *American Journal of Mental Deficiency, 89,* 459–466.

Sigelman, C.K., Budd, E.C., Spanhel, C.L., & Schoenrock, C.J. (1981). When in doubt say yes: Acquiescence in interviews with mildly retarded persons. *Mental Retardation, 18,* 53–58.

Sovner, R., & Hurley, A. (1983). Do the mentally retarded suffer from affective illness? *Archives of General Psychiatry, 40,* 61–67.

Spitzer, R.L. & Cantwell, D.P. (1980). The DSM-III classification of the psychiatric disorders of infancy, childhood and adolescence. *Journal of the American Academy of Child Psychiatry, 19,* 356–370.

Szymanski, L.S. (1977). Psychiatric diagnostic evaluation of mentally retarded individuals. *Journal of the American Academy of Child Psychiatry, 16,* 67–87.

Symanski, L.S. (1980). Psychiatric diagnosis of retarded persons. In L.S. Szymanski & P.E. Tanguay (Eds.), *Emotional disorders of mentally retarded persons*. Baltimore, MD: University Park Press.

Szymanski, L.S. & Biederman, J. (1984). Depression and anorexia nervosa of persons with Down syndrome. *American Journal of Mental Deficiency, 89*, 246–251.

Szymanski, L., & Grossman, H. (1984). Dual implications of dual diagnosis. *Mental Retardation, 22*(4), 155–156.

Williams, J. (1985a). The multiaxial system of DSM-III: Where did it come from and where should it go? I. Its origins and critiques. *Archives of General Psychiatry, 42*, 175–180.

Williams, J. (1985b). The multiaxial system of DSM-III: Where did it come from and where should it go? II. Empirical studies, innovations and recommendations. *Archives of General Psychiatry, 42*, 181–186.

# 12
# Comprehensive Management of the Mentally Retarded/Mentally Ill Individual

LILIA A. EVANGELISTA

The management of the developmentally disabled population is difficult, and many professionals have devoted time and energy for methods to deal effectively with the individual problems presented by this population. In the person with *both* mental retardation and mental illness, the presenting clinical problems are more magnified and complicated. Therefore, this "dual diagnosis" population, which has been well addressed in other chapters in this section, tends to fall between the cracks since so few professionals want to deal with them, even in the medical field. These dually diagnosed individuals tend to get shuffled between the mental retardation and the mental health facilities, and few professionals claim acceptance for the full responsibility of their management. The purpose of this chapter is to offer the reader a descriptive analysis of both the diagnosis and management of this subpopulation from a developmental perspective. This approach perhaps differs from the other programs managed by psychiatrists and described throughout this book (e.g., Menolascino in Nebraska, Gualtieri in South Carolina, and Szymanski and Sovner in Boston), not to mention the management of programs by psychologists (such as Gardner and Matson), in that it does not take place in a large research-training-service facility. While such isles of excellence are essential, the less fortunate facilities may be tempted to despair with their own limitations. Hopefully, this brief chapter on how to establish an affordable and available team approach will be encouraging to the practitioner.

The more modern management approaches to the mentally retarded/mentally ill population is a comprehensive view that begins at the time an "at-risk" disorder is recognized. An initial comprehensive evaluation of a child suspected of being at high risk for a developmental disability should be initiated. At minimum, this encompasses a psychosocial assessment, a developmental pediatric examination, a psychological evaluation, and a speech and language (with audiological) evaluation when warranted. Upon gathering clinical evidence that an emotional/behavioral problem might exist, a psychiatric assessment is then required. Often, among our mentally retarded/mentally ill population, one has to distinguish whether the behavioral findings are purely psychiatric in nature or a manifestation of a neurological condition such as seizures or neuromuscular disorders.

As clinicians, we are then obligated to rule out all other possible causes of atypical behaviors other than an emotional one. In the event that the behavioral disorder is emotional in nature, the psychiatric clinician involved needs to work in full cooperation with the other medical specialists and team professionals in the management of the mentally retarded/mentally ill individual. The responsibilities of the clinicians do not cease upon diagnosis but, in fact, just begin. Mental retardation/mental illness is a lifetime condition that can improve or modify under treatment. Educational and vocational needs and community involvement, which are totally dependent on early intervention, have to be planned by an interdisciplinary team, as well as enhanced by the pediatric and psychiatric input and, perhaps, leadership.

Our approach involves assessment in our evaluation clinic where the team members discuss the case and usually arrive at a clinical impression/diagnosis with specific recommendations. Thereafter, the findings and recommendations are discussed with the parents—who are fully advised of their rights to agree or disagree and/or to seek a second opinion if they so desire. Most of the time, the parents agree to the findings and recommendations. The parents are a vital part of the child's management. Thus, they should be made an integral component in the planning and treatment implementation process of the mentally retarded/mentally ill individual's destiny.

# Education

## Preschool

Usually, a preschool program is recommended for early treatment/intervention. In this aspect, the school and the clinical team should be communicating as often as necessary in the management of the child. In our experience, the earlier the proper intervention is instituted, the more chances the mentally retarded/mentally ill individual has in ameliorating, controlling, or redirecting their behaviors. This type of intervention makes the individual's behavior more functional and acceptable to society.

Often, there are very few programs that are geared to deal with the mentally retarded/mentally ill population since insufficient numbers of clinicians and preschool teachers—nationwide—are trained to deal with this special population.

## School Age

Children with mental retardation/mental illness benefit greatly from accepting educational systems. The child who has experienced acceptance in a preschool program has a smoother transition to the regular educational system than do other children at risk. Their problems seem to diminish, and the children adjust and perform better than the mentally retarded/mentally ill child who enrolls for the first time at a later age. The younger the mentally retarded/mentally ill child is served by the educational staff, the better his or her chance to be assisted in the improvement of his or her function.

## After 21-Years Program

### Day Treatment/Employment

When the disabled individual turns 21 years of age (in some states like Michigan, it is 25 years of age), he or she is no longer the responsibility of the Board of Education. Mentally retarded/mentally ill individuals need to continue their habilitation training and need to be enrolled in a Day Treatment/Vocational Program depending on their skill and level of work function and disability. If they are not able to obtain such service, many stay home and regress. The client should work at the level at which he or she is capable. Certainly, the new supported work model designed to provide transitional services to this population should be utilized.

### Recreation

All people need social expression and the mentally retarded/mentally ill person needs to have social experiences at whatever level that he or she can participate and enjoy. Recreation programs can bring joy to these individuals and, in our experience, the mentally retarded/mentally ill individuals can participate in dancing, sports activities, trips, and outings that are accepting and supportive of them.

### Respite Program

The care of a disabled person by the parents is a continuous one. It can be tedious, long, enduring, and fatiguing. Caring for such individuals can intensify family tensions and anxieties. The parents and siblings of dually diagnosed clients need to be relieved, even for a short period, of this tension, and the mentally retarded/mentally ill individual benefits as the energies of the family are renewed. The availability of respite programs prolongs the ability of families to care for their own and thereby forestall the specter of institutionalization.

### Residential/Community Living

Living arrangements that provide for various levels of care are necessary based on the level of adjustment and disability of each client. Community living, be it an ICF/MR, group home, or supervised individual apartment living, is a great step toward normalization and to some independence away from the family. The mentally retarded/mentally ill individual responds positively to these types of living arrangements, affording a flexible system for those who regress or advance. Having these individuals in the community also helps in the education of society via the presence of this population and making society aware of its responsibility in accepting and caring for them.

## Management
### General Medical/Dental/Nursing

The mentally retarded/mentally ill individual often has a great need for specialized health care, except they are often unable to express specifically the symptoms and problems that they are experiencing in order to obtain the necessary care. The medical profession must therefore be sensitive in the observation and interpretation of the disabled individual's behavior and to differentiate these behavioral features from basic clinical manifestations of various medical disorders. In our clinical experience, we have observed some mentally retarded/mentally ill individuals who have such high tolerance to pain that, at times, they may have developed medical problems that have gone undetected until a close examination was conducted. Upon regular and close observation of these individuals, the clinicians are able to detect medical problems early and thus prevent some catastrophic sequelae.

### Behavior Management

There have been different methods attempted in dealing with the various behavior disorders. Some are successful and some are not. Thus, it is incumbent on us to try and determine which are the best and most suitable methods to use. It is quite apparent that various methods can be applied to the same individual at different times for different behavioral problems. Therefore, the clinician should not persist in using the same method for all circumstances. Different environments and circumstances require different tactics. Flexibility is important.

## Types of Treatment Interventions
### Psychotropic Medications

The general impression of the resolution of a behavior disorder is through the use of medication. Some professionals, especially in the educational system, believe that medication is the best answer complemented by a neurological exam with an EEG analysis. We, the clinicians in this field, know that it is not that simple. Different behavior/psychiatric disorders respond to specific psychotropic medication or a combination of medications. Some mentally retarded/mentally ill individuals become drowsy so that, although the medication has subdued their behavioral disorder, they become nonfunctional. Therefore, the dosage and type of psychotropic medication should be monitored on a regular basis. Blood levels and other appropriate laboratory tests should be regularly obtained to determine the therapeutic level(s) of the medication and see if potential side effects are developing. Long-term use of some medications can produce serious side effects (e.g., tardive dyskinesia). A balanced treatment approach is necessary and must focus on maintaining the lowest dose of medication possible and complement it with behavior/developmental interventions.

## Behavior/Developmental Interventions

In our experience, some, if not the majority, of MR/MI clients function better and can be managed solely via behavioral intervention. Their ability to reach their optimum level of functioning in such areas as socialization, vocational and academic areas, and adaptive behavior, can more readily be achieved if the type of behavioral intervention utilized is appropriate, effective, and timely. Some behavior interventions are short term and others are long term, depending on the circumstances of application and the consistency and constancy of the applications. A few of the behavior/developmental interventions are bonding and tension reduction.

*Bonding.* Bonding is a very important initial method to develop with a mentally retarded/mentally ill client. Once this is established, management and response of the client becomes more positive. (See McGee, Chapter 18, for a more lengthy explanation.)

*Tension Reduction.* Some of the methods utilized to reduce tension are swimming and physical exercises. Our experience shows that clients with behavior disorders benefit from the above activities. The reduction of tension allows the individual to respond more smoothly to his surroundings, relate more appropriately to other clients and staff, and perform different task-oriented activities that eventually lead to constructive and long-term functional achievement and, at the same time, diminution, if not control, of the behavior disorder.

# Recommendations

1. Incorporation of courses and/or practical training on the developmentally disabled/mentally retarded/mentally ill in the curriculum of the various college programs especially in medicine, nursing, dentistry, psychology, and education.
2. Education of the public, including legislators, of accurate facts about the disabled population, especially of the mentally retarded/mentally ill.
3. Formulation of reconcilable rules and regulations regarding the developmentally disabled/mentally retarded/mentally ill by the federal, state, and local agencies. Accountability is a *must* in program monitoring, but it should be at a reasonable level without sacrificing direct care. At this time, professionals and providers are overburdened by paperwork under the guise of accountability. The current rules often do not account for the origin and continuation of aberration. Instead, they blame aspects of an aberration on the persons or agency working with the clients having the aberration.

4. Better and clearer delineation between the mental health and the mental retardation/developmental disabilities agencies on their respective responsibility in the care and welfare of the mentally retarded/mentally ill individual.
5. More supportive services and follow-up of deinstitutionalized mentally retarded/mentally ill individuals.
6. Establishment of specialized programs for the mentally retarded/mentally ill individuals with the full cooperation of the government agencies and expedition of the approval process. These government agencies should work hand-in-hand with the professionals/service providers to provide effective programs.
7. All persons, including the developmentally handicapped, are entitled to sexual expression. However, those developmentally handicapped persons that are noncompetent to make decisions regarding self-care, safety, and handling of funds are not capable of making a decision independent of a caretaker. The decision by such a person to have sex becomes the responsibility of the caretaker and the consequences of the act are related to the competency and care that the caretaker exerts. A noncompetent, developmentally disabled person therefore does not have the right to consent to a sexual act without the expressed permission of the caretaker. However, some severely handicapped have relative levels of autonomy. In the context of that autonomy, sexual expression does not occur without the knowledge of the caretaker. The caretaker must provide pregnancy guidance and control, prophylaxes, and disease control to offset any loopholes in their care.

# 13
# Psychiatric Examination of Mentally Retarded Persons: General Problems and Challenges

EARL A. LOOMIS, JR.

Problems of assessment in this field are so numerous, complicated, and individualized that it renders their use in treatment as unduly cumbersome at this time. Professionals in this field of endeavor quickly realize that the psychiatric examination by itself is not adequate to address the necessary multiple parameters of the symptom of mental retardation and thus the process becomes very complex when a dual diagnosis of mental retardation and mental illness are *both* present. I am specifically referring to the psychiatric portion of presumably *multiphasic* assessment capabilities. Failing the latter, the psychiatrist is often challenged to provide answers that tax his or her knowledge, skills, and wisdom. Nevertheless, he or she is often challenged with just such a demand for service and recommendations.

The purpose of this chapter, which concludes this section on diagnostic issues, is to share with the reader the challenge and importance of the psychiatric examination as well as its implications for treatment. With a paucity of research studies in this area, the hypotheses postulated in this chapter are based on empirical research from my clinical practice. This chapter is designed to provide a practical guide to the clinician in the quest for a differential diagnosis toward a treatment program.

My own professional approach to psychiatric evaluation is, first of all, to place myself into the context of my patient and his setting and problems. If I cannot visualize something of his world through his eyes and something of his self-presentation through the eyes of his peers, parents, significant others, and surroundings—I feel already at a disadvantage. This is, unfortunately, how many of us feel in the settings within which we must exercise responsibility and sometimes authority well beyond that which we might choose.

Having used what means we do have—records, informants, our prior experience with our professional informants, and our queries about the occasion for the current referral or consultation—we go to meet the patient. We are naturally interested in how he is introduced to us, how he responds to the introduction, and how separation from the person bringing or accompanying or introducing him transpires. Herein, we closely note the presenting evidences of chronological age, mental age, dependence on the accompanying caregiver, and the presence of superficial signs of bonding, bonding failure, or pathological symbiotic bonding.

Other phenomena that we can see, hear, or smell in the diagnostic setting/transactions are already impinging on the examiner and lead to questions and concerns: the patient's appearance, posture, gait, gestures, grooming, movements, and responses to the presence of the examiner engage our interest. A most important observational dimension for me is the importance of the extent to which the subject can (or does) indicate capacity for bonding, connectedness with another person, and capacity to declare his state of fear, curiosity, distress, discomfort, dysfunction, or concern. Can this patient recognize me as part of a new (or familiar) interpersonal transaction? Does the patient disclose expectations, curiosity, help-seeking behavior? Or am I apparently ignored, misidentified, or actively rejected? My assignment and activities so far may be reasonably difficult with a verbal patient. What about the situation with a nonverbal patient? Here I come face-to-face with one of the major challenges in examining retarded persons. One cannot assume, as one might with neurotic and even some psychotic patients who are of average intelligence, that "a misunderstanding is often deliberate." Indeed, one must take responsibility for the misunderstandings and make every possible attempt to avoid their entering as deceptively misleading data. An example of the latter occurs every time I examine a certain female patient in her forties. Every question she is asked is answered in the affirmative. Is she too hot? Yes. Too cold? Also, yes. Isn't this a contradiction? Yes, it's a contradiction. Enthusiastic compliance in verbal response is not only one form of automatic obedience in this lady, but also one that has misled many who have accepted her initial self-declarations. For she will tell you and/or agree with anything if you ask her in the right fashion. She is a self-leading witness, a prosecutor's dream or nightmare.

A similar misinformation nightmare is the patient who complains of abuse to one examiner, only to deny same when confronted with another examiner. Is this, or is this not, the patient's attempt to divide and conquer his treatment team, or is he telling each person the portion of his truth that they want to hear or can tolerate? Why and how *failure of repression* allows a patient to tell one story to a "neutral" examiner and quite another story to someone closer to his routine existence may remain conjectural. That sort of diagnosis pitfall strains the fabric of our teamwork, our credulity, and our basic trust. One learns to validate these types of diagnostic double-binds-in-the-making.

Though the above-noted concerns and dilemmas may discourage us from trusting the dual diagnosis patient's own verbal productions, the opposite course seems to me of greater danger. Therefore, I tend to credit the statements of the patient as being reflective of *his reality* or at least of one of his realities. To discount the words he gives me not only deprives me of this input but also undermines the mutual trust between patient and doctor without which I work at a still greater disadvantage. Better to risk my own need to be infallible than to undermine my patient's need to be heard and to lose *his* truth in *his* declarations. The diagnostic principle here is that we ignore the testimony of the intellectually impaired at our peril. Only recently this principle has been underscored again in the case of the testimony of sexually abused persons. Such testimony must be heeded. It may not be impeccable, but it points to a truth. The child may not have been the victim of the accused, but the child has most likely, most certainly, been *someone's* victim.

In the years in which our St. Luke's Hospital group puzzled over differential diagnosis of retardation and autism, we were challenged with the problem of interpreting the nonverbal communication of our young patients whom we followed during a longitudinal series of clinical observations between their 13th and 48th months of life. We clearly noted the value of play analysis in the nonspeaking child: their spontaneous behavior around play materials, especially the uses— conventional and unconventional—to which they are put, the presence or absence of thematic material, and the extent to which original and ingenious problem solving accompanies limitations of intelligence or of interpersonal competence and comfort. Here the examiner is declared by the child to be animate or inanimate, human or animal, and all without words. Here ego functions are demonstrated, from motility control to modulation of affective expression and discharge. Here cognitive levels and cognitive impairment, immaturity, or distortion raise their heads. Here coping and defense functions, or their absence, are demonstrated.

Before and beyond play came physical and voice contact. Especially with infants and persons with severe mental retardation, the nonverbal parameters become very important: the capacity to cuddle, to respond to a soothing voice, or to initiate contact or reject it are all messages; reactions to movement through space, to being rocked, swung, upended, twirled, and put through active or passive ranges of motion. These diagnostic techniques constitute replicable measures of the range of nonverbal communications that are present in the dual diagnostic young patient.

Interpersonal competence, familiarity with human rituals of greeting and farewell, imparting information, the ability to signal for help, and promiscuous or indiscriminate intimacy with strangers are other cues to which we must be sensitive. Toleration of distance and/or closeness, confinement or freedom, crowds versus one-on-one settings all tell their tales. The DSM-III diagnostic system (American Psychiatric Association, 1980) only minimally refers to these diagnostic parameters and mostly only in connection with early infantile autism and pervasive developmental disabilities.

Menolascino and McGee (1983) stress that two major hurdles for the examination of the retarded/mentally ill patient are his lack of communicative speech and the distorting or modifying effect of the retardation on the otherwise evident and pathognomonic signs of specific mental disorders. These developmental handicaps bring up the question (Menolascino & Stark, 1984): "How do the same symptoms and signs declare themselves differently (or atypically) in mentally retarded persons?" My approach to this diagnostic challenge is to explore the following three parameters. First, we must be careful to assess our misexpectations.

Second, we must clearly focus on "at least two ages" of each mentally retarded man or woman—their chronological age and their mental age. Third, we must be alert to the extent that their treatment or mistreatment by the nonretarded world has induced secondary symptoms or supplementary symptoms. These secondary symptoms include the consequences of neglect, separation from and loss of family, institutional abuse secondary to interpersonal crowding and associated loss of privacy, enforced loneliness, enforced intimacy or pseudointimacy, sexual exploitations including temptation and denial, constantly changing child-care workers and personnel rosters over the years, and no opportunities to learn bonding, wholesome self-image, and even primitive interpersonal and social survival skills—to list only some of the gravest. Some have been left without coping skills to face abuse, deprivation, atrocities, and hideous and seductive sights and sounds. Some have been imprisoned with criminals and perverts, hospitalized with psychotics of average intelligence, and have been placed in homes that are unwelcome in the communities or in homes ill adapted to growth, development, learning, and loving. Society has denied chances for apprenticeship and useful work; leisure time has not yet been sanctified or dignified, especially for those who do no useful work to "justify their right to leisure" (Kiernan & Stark, 1986).

If, as I claim, the foregoing issues require attention in examining and arriving at a diagnosis and treatment plan or a mentally ill/mentally retarded child or adult, how in the world do you convey such concepts, categories, procedures, and skills to professional trainees so that they can learn about the diagnostic challenges herein? (See also Matson, Chapter 17.) In a way I am thrown back on a parable: A famous scholar and appraiser of jade was sought out by a wealthy man who aspired to become a qualified judge of jade. The jade authority finally consented to accept the apprentice for $10,000 and his promise to follow instructions absolutely and ask no questions during a prolonged training period. The pupil was told to present himself daily and that each day he would be given a piece of jade to hold. He sat for hour after hour, session after session, holding specimen after specimen in his hands. His exasperation mounted and he was finally restrainable no longer by the prohibition. The pupil burst out to his teacher, "Not only have you taken my good money, not only have you kept me incommunicado hour after hour holding onto your precious treasures in silence, now you have given me a piece of fake jade!"

Watching examinations through one-way interview screens or on videotapes, serving as coexaminer in repeated situations with similar and different patients, sharing in the development of models and constructs, and taking part in research projects as observers, participant and nonparticipant, judges, and as follow-up evaluators and therapists—all these seem to help impart both the skills and the confidence to undertake these difficult diagnostic tasks.

One may ask: Is this a valid scientific approach to diagnosis—especially differential diagnosis? Not yet! Just as the stethoscope preceded the EKG and the physical examination the laboratory tests, so too the skills of observation, dialogue, and play with mentally ill/mentally retarded young persons may constitute both the route and also a continuing conduit to contact with our patients.

Machines and mechanically imposed procedure may be more scientific, but possibly also less human. Of all people, those with a dual diagnosis can least afford to be depersonified.

Making a virtue out of necessity does not justify delaying further research in favor of purely intuitive approaches. Neither does the absence of fully standardized procedures belie the value of the subjective and intuitive clinical approaches both of which we learn to use to the advantage of these very complex patients.

## Current Psychiatric Diagnostic Issues

### Tradition of the Missing Psychiatrist

As Gualtieri points out in Chapter 15, this current state of affairs refers to psychiatry's past turning away from interest and responsibility for mentally retarded persons. Only a few, mostly child psychiatrists, have shared this concern and have struggled to share newly acquired knowledge of developmental, dynamic, and neuropsychopharmacological approaches with the educators, pediatricians, psychologists, and neurologists who had more or less replaced the abdicated psychiatrists.

### Tradition of Either/or Mental Retardation or Mental Illness

Except for disorders of infancy and childhood, no significant attention seems to have been paid to the presence of mental illness in mentally retarded persons by the DSM-III drafters. Many, if not most, psychiatrists eschew putting a second or third diagnosis into Axis I if there is already a retardation diagnosis present, a point made by Szymanski in Chapter 11. Moreover, numerous research studies and the clinical experience of Dr. Sovner, a psychiatrist, also indicate that there have been no consistent efforts to delineate the difference between the presence of a conjoint psychiatric diagnosis and simply a behavior habit or trait that is unacceptable or annoying (Sovner & Hurley, 1983). These demand clarifications where possible, lest necessary and available specific therapies be denied appropriate application.

### Absence of Adequate Speech in Many Patients

We are forced in such cases to depend more on signs than on symptoms, more on overt behavior than on affective, appetitive, or volitional state. We have to learn how to validate nonverbal communication, perhaps using signing or another substitute for words and/or conventional gestures and signals. The absence of speech does not absolve us from considering the patient's affect and the possible meaning of his symptoms and life goals to himself.

## Absence of an Adequate Clinical History

In many patients, there is a paucity of clinical information provided to the examiner—especially developmental history information. I have often found that patients and families could provide more of this direly needed diagnostic information, even years later. Also, in some cases, amytal interviews (narcoanalysis or narcosynthesis) and/or hypnosis have unlocked the otherwise inaccessible elements of the mildly retarded person's clinical and/or developmental histories.

## Variation in the Appearance of the Syndromes and Disorders in Persons with Mental Retardation

*Simple.* Allowances must be made for the mental age and the constricted or special experiences of the mentally retarded person that may serve as a substrate on which the propf-schizophrenia, propf-mania, or propf-depression is engrafted.

*Complex.* Complexity introduced by institutionalization refers to special exposure to unconventional or bizarre scenes and scenarios: nudity, pedophilia, stereotyped behaviors, and regimentation, to mention only a few possible sources of negative interpersonal modeling, traumatic interaction, or the absence of normal interpersonal bonding and acquisition of mutual interdependence as a source of inner and outer reward, comfort, stimulation, and teaching—the gist of our common humanity (i.e., good mothering and fathering, neighboring, and teaching).

## Tensions and Pressures Between the Mental Health and the Mental Retardation Establishments

The tensions and pressures have major implications for ongoing clinical management, staffing, and treatment. For example, in the state of Georgia it is difficult to get a mentally ill/mentally retarded person admitted anywhere for acute (if emergency) psychiatric treatment. The mental retardation hospital was until 1987 forbidden by statute to accept emergency admissions; the psychiatric hospital declines to accept persons with mental retardation. In case of a grave emergency, especially when accompanied by a court order, persons with mental retardation may be admitted to the general admission wards of the state (regional) mental hospitals. The hospital administration and staff tend to regret and resent this for they are ill-equipped to care for such patients, have no facility or success in transferring them to a mental retardation facility, and tend to find these patients "clogging" their admission ward by long stays (i.e., five to six times the length of stay of those of nonretarded patients). The patients in each group—and their respective families—also resent the intermingling of the two populations, particularly with different age levels.

## Summary

Hopefully, this chapter has provided the reader with both a philosophical mind set and a pragmatic guide to conducting the very important first step, the psychiatric interview, which leads the clinician toward a differential diagnosis and enables a significant treatment intervention, which at this writing is more of an art than a science.

## References

American Psychiatric Association. (1980). *Diagnostic and statistical manual of mental disorders*, 3rd Edition (DSM-III). Washington, DC: Author.

Kiernan, W.E., & Stark, J.A. (1986). *Pathways to employment for adults with developmental disabilities*. Baltimore, MD: Paul H. Brookes Publishing Company.

Menolascino, F.J., & McGee, J.J. (1983). Persons with severe mental retardation and behavioral challenges: From disconnectedness to human engagement. *Journal of Psychiatric Treatment and Evaluation, 5*, 187–193.

Menolascino, F.J., & Stark, J.A. (Eds.). (1984). *Handbook of mental illness in the mentally retarded*. New York: Plenum Press.

Sovner, R., & Hurley, A.D. (1983). Do the mentally retarded suffer from affective illness? *Archives of General Psychiatry, 40*, 61–67.

# Conclusion

FRANK J. MENOLASCINO

The major advantage of having practitioners, who have for so long been intimately involved in the dilemma of services and ongoing research study of the special population reviewed in this book, as contributors is that they have long reflected on the necessary recommendations for meaningful and needed changes, along with policy changes that need to be implemented on a national level, in order to improve our treatment success rate with this challenging population. These practitioners have directly witnessed, during their clinical interactions with these complex retarded citizens, environments wherein they daily work to try to aid them; and thus the listed recommendations below for national changes in services, research, and training areas are grounded in clinical realities.

## Research Recommendations

1. We need to establish a national data bank system using epidemiological analyses to arrive at an accurate prevalence rate of mental illness in the mentally retarded. A corollary of this data bank would be attention to the identification factor of the major risk factors related to mental illness in the mentally retarded and those recurrently noted intrapersonal and interpersonal barriers to successful placement in the community.
2. Research into the nature of mental illness in the mentally retarded must be a major focus of the proposed regional treatment centers and also the currently operational University Affiliated Program(s) network throughout our country (see Section IV).
3. We need to develop easy to administer assessment instruments that can be used by parents and school personnel as well as front-line treatment/management staff in the community, to provide objective data for early intervention and effective treatment efforts for retarded persons who display allied indices of mental illness.
4. Research is direly needed on the dissimilarities in the diagnosis of mental illness and mental retardation with a particular focus on clarifying the

currently nonspecific behavioral symptom descriptors such as "self-injurious behaviors" and "noncompliant behaviors." The singular symptom management approach, to date, has not been very helpful in our understanding or ability to provide professional help. The recasting of these symptom descriptors within the larger scope of mental illness syndromes will permit clearer research approaches.

5. Research must be supported into the new treatment modalities that have placed particular emphasis on developing nonpunishment treatment interventions (i.e., alternatives to aversive treatment techniques). Beyond the pressing need for a wider range of treatment interventions is the humanistic–legal dimension wherein punishment does not fulfill protection and advocacy guidelines.

6. The high frequency of seizure disorders associated with mental illness in the mentally retarded, especially in the more severe levels of mental retardation, needs to be investigated further in order to better control seizures and attempt to alter their often adverse role in heightening the incidence and severity of mental illness in the mentally retarded.

7. Greater financial support for research activities is needed to fund a wide array of research projects via a special study section, which directly focuses on the topic of mental illness in the mentally retarded. This is an area of a major national policy "blindspot" since neither the NIMH nor the NICHHD have addressed the need for *special* attention (i.e., by establishing a special study section in these national research thrusts) to this subpopulation of the mentally retarded. The research focus must be on the diagnostic and treatment issues pertinent to this population, and not a vague offshoot of the national focus on mental illness in the nonretarded, or the overfocus on developmental issues rather than mental illness (i.e., disease) issues.

8. We need to establish a national collaborative research study, using a series of centers across our country (e.g., as in the past NIMH national studies on depression) concerning appropriate guidelines for psychopharmacological interventions in the treatment of mental illness in the mentally retarded. This topical area remains in the shadow of modern treatment approaches to the mentally ill/mentally retarded population. Anecdotal impressions on the efficacy of psychoactive drugs in the retarded must be replaced by large scale national collaborative studies.

9. We need research on balanced treatment approaches which involve the orchestration of psychopharmacological approaches, behavioral techniques, environmental restructuring, self-esteem techniques (etc.) and their selective applications in various settings.

10. A national system for the dissemination of clinical and research information on this special topic must be developed (and extended) so that those who are providing daily contact with this population can quickly assess the rapidly emerging body of knowledge on this topic.

# Training Recommendations

1. We need a national commitment involving the training of direct-care workers and parents in the use of the wide variety and number of successful treatment/management approaches that are currently available.
2. Active incorporation of modern treatment approaches to this population must become an integral part of our interdisciplinary training programs with a specific emphasis on key diagnostic issues and effective treatment/management approaches.
3. We need to develop groups of specialized clinical teams, across our country, who are willing to provide direct ongoing clinical services to this population. This resource can also be used for in-service workshops for psychiatrists, psychologists, social workers, vocational rehabilitation nursing, child-care and cottage-care workers, and other professionals involved in this field as an indirect way of accomplishing this task.
4. We need to foster the development of regionally located educational sites for fellowships, seminars, and institutes devoted to this research topic.
5. Encouragement to establish specific training programs in this area within our 126 medical schools (i.e., in both the basic sciences and the clinical years) must be coupled with increased clinical practicums and residency training programs in this area. Although this challenge has been a difficult task to accomplish to date, it should be noted that the specter of national oversupply of physicians, the greatly increased interest of medical schools in children's programs, and the increasing national focus on preventive approaches hold great promise.

# Policy Recommendations

1. We need a national focus on both quality control and accountability of the current and future treatment programs for this complex population, especially since they have (historically and now) been so prone to abuse or not served at all, with ongoing monitoring by various federal and state agencies.
2. The National Institute of Handicapped Research could serve as the key federal agency involved in the dissemination and transmission of technology and information concerning modern treatment programs and training availability. It could provide direct dissemination of this information via publications and audiovisual materials.
3. The National Institute of Child Health and Human Development, via its direct contractual relationships with the University Affiliated Programs, could serve as the major federal agency with the primary responsibility for research in this dual diagnosis area. Their direct funding involvement with the Mental Retardation Research Centers, which have now reached their first 20 years of

existence, should be used as a base to encourage these centers to redirect their focus into this vital area of unmet national need on behalf of the mentally retarded/mentally ill.

4. The National Institute of Mental Health could provide greater research emphasis on specific research areas such as schizophrenia, affective disorders, and anxiety. Additional research in each area is in desperate need of specific investigation into the apparent differences in the diagnostic categories (e.g., as to the diagnostic assessment of schizophrenia in the severely retarded) and the needed special treatment modalities.

5. The Office of Special Education and Rehabilitation Services, along with the Administration on Developmental Disabilities, will need to continue to play a coordinating role in encouraging the important transition of developmentally disabled individuals into the community wherein their behavioral/emotional disorders should not preclude them from seeking maximal services in the residential and vocational areas.

# Section IV: Clinical Treatment Issues
# Introduction

FRANK J. MENOLASCINO

The readers of the eight chapters contained in this section should find the treatment strategies recommended by these extraordinary authors extremely helpful in their day-to-day service to persons who are mentally retarded and mentally ill. Rarely will you find a more comprehensive analysis of treatment issues with this population. The authors provide us with unique insights into successful treatment approaches because they all have national and international reputations built on years of *direct* clinical experience as well as directing productive research and teaching programs. All have published major texts in their respective areas of expertise as it applies to this population. This section should provide practitioners with both a primary text and handy reference guide in developing skills for themselves or their staff in providing direct-care services.

Few individuals are more eminently qualified to review the use of behavior therapies with persons who are mentally retarded than William Gardner. His texts and chapters on the use of behavioral approaches during the last 20 years are classics (i.e., *Behavior Modification in Mental Retardation*) that have frequently been referenced. In addition, Gardner is a superb writer whose contributions are always thoroughly referenced and comprehensive. In Chapter 14, he provides the reader with a historical understanding of the past, present, and future evolution of behavioral therapy, including excellent visual diagrams of this complex and popular approach. He concludes with guidelines for the application of behavioral techniques that all practitioners should find essential in assisting them in their clinical services.

Thomas Gualtieri is an articulate young psychiatrist who has already made a number of outstanding contributions to this field (i.e., *Psychiatric Treatment Manual*). He has served as an anchor and motivating factor in the provision of quality services to this dually diagnosed population in North Carolina. In Chapter 15, he reviews the problems, obstacles, and solutions to serving this population vis-á-vis the role of neuropsychiatry. He succinctly reviews the historical reasons for psychiatry's lack of interest with mentally retarded persons. Gualtieri also examines a number of issues in neuropsychiatry— from psychopharmacology to neuropsychology—which provide the framework for successful treatment approaches. He follows with a number of recommendations and solutions for the major obstacles postulated, punctuated with some revealing personal experiences that perhaps explain why his views might appear to be radical or excessive. The reader of this chapter should find this personal sharing a moving experience.

One of the most intriguing chapters in this section is written by Richard Kunin, an orthomolecular psychiatrist whose extensive clinical experience in the treatment of persons who are mentally retarded with concomitant behavior disorder is extremely rare. Dr. Kunin introduces the reader to the role and potential contributions of orthomolecular psychiatry. Certainly, nutritional research has significantly increased in the last decade to the point where it is beginning to play a major role in the treatment of various health concerns ranging from cancer and cardiovascular disease to mental health disorders. The role of nutrition in its application to the treatment of various cognitive deficits with persons who are mentally retarded has received considerable attention and debate since Dr. Ruth Harrell's 1981 study on megavitamin therapy, which indicated dramatically improved intellectual functioning in mentally retarded children. Although follow-up studies have not been able to duplicate these findings, it has produced a wealth of information and interest in this field, which Dr. Kunin reviews in Chapter 16. He first presents a model of nutrition and its role in the treatment of disease entities, followed by guidelines in the use of orthomolecular approaches. A case study analysis helps to illustrate these tenets along with an excellent review of tardive dyskinesia—a major irreversible side effect of medication sometimes found in the treatment of this group of individuals.

Few psychologists have achieved as much recognition in this field as Johnny Matson. Noted for his extensive number of publications in this field, including comprehensive textbooks (i.e., the award winning *Handbook of Mental Retardation*), Matson has made numerous contributions, particularly in the areas of depression and the use and development of diagnostic techniques. His extensive clinical experience is obvious in Chapter 17 and he provides the reader with unusual insight into treating children who are dually diagnosed. Matson concludes his chapter with recommendations for further research on how to improve our technology in treating this complex population.

Certainly one of the most talked about, debated, and controversial areas of discussion in recent years is the use of aversive techniques. Three chapters by McGee, Thompson et al., and a follow-up response by McGee provide the reader with healthy debate and review of this entire area. McGee first postulates his nationally acclaimed "gentle teaching" approach with its central goal of bonding, which he describes as being a complete antithesis to punishment and submission (i.e., aversive techniques). McGee carefully describes the major tenets of "gentle teaching", which draws on the behavioral science of applied behavior analysis.

Thompson, Gardner, and Baumeister team up in their discussion on the ethical issues involved in the intervention process of severe behavioral disorders of mentally retarded persons. They call for a more careful systematic analysis and additional research on how durable are the treatment effects and which procedures are most effective with which individuals and under what circumstances.

McGee follows up with a response to this chapter of Thompson, Gardner, and Baumeister via a delineation of the misuses of behavioral technology along with his concerns over inadequate safeguards. Judging by the recent position statements released by the American Association on Mental Retardation, the Association for Persons with Severe Handicaps, and the Association for Retarded Citizens – U.S., Chapters 18 to 20 should be extremely stimulating to the reader who has an interest in this hotly debated area.

The last chapter in this section focuses on the rapidly expanding area of behavioral psychopharmacology. Robert Sovner is extremely well qualified to write an overview of this area. In addition to publishing (as chief editor) the acclaimed *Psychiatric Aspects of Mental Retardation Reviews*, Dr. Sovner has extensive experience as a consulting psychiatrist to numerous facilities throughout the New England region.

Sovner first describes the use and abuses of this field, then describes the correct and critical role that a behavioral psychopharmacologist can and should play. His call for a new subspecialty in this field is a welcome respite, particularly in the treatment of maladaptive behavior. He concludes this important chapter with recommendations on how to monitor adverse drug reactions and strategies on ways to implement drug withdrawal trials.

In summary, practitioners who work with the dually diagnosed population and who need to update their skills should find this entire section one that they can frequently use as a reference in meeting their daily treatment challenges.

# 14
# Behavior Therapies: Past, Present, and Future

WILLIAM I. GARDNER

## Introduction

A range of psychological treatment approaches are available for use with mentally retarded individuals who present mild to profound mental health difficulties (Barrett, 1986; Matson & Barrett, 1982; Menolascino & Stark, 1984; Sigman, 1985). One group of approaches, termed *behavior therapies*, is based on various theories of human learning and related concepts of psychological development and functioning (Bellack & Hersen, 1985; Bellack, Hersen, & Kazdin, 1982).

Behavior therapy techniques are among the most frequently used in attempts to treat the multiple emotional and behavioral difficulties presented by persons with mental retardation. Numerous illustrations are provided in the research and clinical literature of the potential therapeutic efficacy of behavioral approaches with such problems as physical aggression and related conduct disorders, eating disorders, self-injury, stereotypy, pica and coprophagy, psychogenic vomiting and ruminating, attention deficit disorders, fears and phobias, obesity, anxiety disorders, enuresis and encopresis, personality disorders, and various symptoms associated with depression, psychoses, and autism (Gardner & Cole, 1984b; Whitman, Scibak, & Reid, 1983). Some clinical researchers even suggest that, in some instances (e.g., severe self-injury), behavioral procedures may well be, while not ideal, at least the most effective treatment among *currently* available alternatives (Favell, 1982). It is acknowledged, however, that even at best, behavior therapy approaches do not offer ultimate solutions.

In addition to being among the most frequently used therapeutic procedures, the behavior therapies are also the most thoroughly researched of the psychological approaches available to the clinician. In recognizing that "scientific research does not include anecdotal, subjective accounts of intervention and outcome, no matter how authoritative the source" (Favell, 1982, p. 532), the behavioral clinician frequently uses scientific research methods to evaluate the adequacy of the therapy procedures being used. In so doing, effective behavior therapy approaches are supported and less effective ones are discarded. More specifically, behavior therapists, with the tradition of applied behavior analysis, characteristically use the strategy of repeated measures of single individuals, or of small groups of individuals, in evaluating the usefulness of various treatment proce-dures. In preparation for this chapter, some 600 research studies were identified that reported the effects of various behavioral treatment procedures on clinical problems presented by mentally retarded individuals. In contrast, in searching the scientific literature, only a handful of research studies were located that evaluated the effects of other forms of psychological therapies in treatment of the mentally retarded. This does not imply that alternative treatment approaches are not effective. Rather, it is merely being reported that a scientific basis for the efficacy of other approaches is not available in the professional literature.

Thus, contemporary behavior therapy approaches are grounded in conceptual models of human learning and behavior and also enjoy a significant degree of empirical support. The most influential of these models of behavior and related concepts from experimental psychology and experimental psychiatry are depicted in Figure 14.1. Concepts from these models are used to hypothesize about the development of behavioral and emotional pathologies and additionally to derive treatment procedures to modify those variables assumed to be critical in creating and maintaining the psychological difficulties. Although the majority of behavioral treatment research and practice has been based on operant or rein-forcement interpretations of the development, maintenance, occurrence, and alteration of psychological symptoms, the other learning-oriented models of

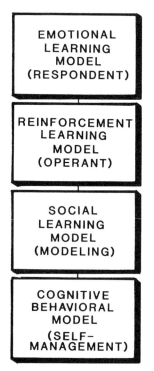

FIGURE 14.1. Models of learning and behavior associated with behavior therapy.

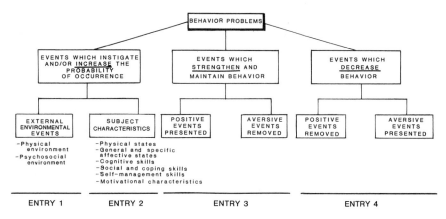

FIGURE 14.2. Multicomponent behavioral assessment and treatment model.

human functioning are exerting an increasing influence on research and clinical activities (Bellack et al., 1982).

## Multicomponent Assessment and Treatment

In recognition of the complexity of the behavioral and emotional difficulties presented by mentally retarded individuals, the behavior therapist uses a multicomponent assessment and treatment model, depicted in Figure 14.2, as a basis for understanding and modifying these mental health difficulties. Behavioral diagnosis is concerned with understanding the multitude of factors currently contributing to the person's difficulties. The objectives of assessment are threefold: (1) to identify the various internal and external conditions under which the problems are likely to occur, (2) to hypothesize about the various functions served by the problem behaviors, and (3) to identify various client-specific personal characteristics that contribute to the person's difficulties. A clinical understanding of these client-specific personal characteristics is essential if *effective* and *durable* therapeutic changes are to occur.

This multicomponent view represents the traditional operant explanations of psychological difficulties as well as more recently developed social skills, anxiety management, and cognitive behavioral and coping skills explanations (Gardner Cole, 1984b). This multicomponent view also interfaces satisfactorily with a medical model in recognizing that physical factors (e.g., brain impairment, chemical imbalance, and neurotransmitter difficulties) may contribute to a major or minor extent to the difficulties presented by any specific client (Sovner & Hurley, 1986). Thus, behavior therapy may be provided in combination with medical treatment to ensure a comprehensive therapeutic program.

Entries 3 and 4 of the model focus on the effects of problem behaviors of various procedures that manipulate contingent consequences. These include both positive and negative reinforcement and punishment procedures. Entry 1 includes a description of external environmental factors (e.g., excessive performance demands) that, when present, instigate or increase the likelihood of problem behaviors.

Entry 2 variables include those internal conditions that, in isolation and when combined with external events, instigate or increase the likelihood of problem behaviors. Examples of these events include *physical states* (e.g., pain, fatigue, and menses), *affective states* (e.g., anger and anxiety), and *cognitive variables* (e.g., covert verbal ruminations of a provoking nature and paranoid ideas). Entry 2 also includes consideration of *skill areas and characteristics* that, owing to their low strength or absence, increase the likelihood of problems. In illustration of these behavioral deficits, an adolescent, when taunted by peers or criticized by adults, may react aggressively because he either does not have alternative interpersonal skills in his repertoire or, if present, the skills to self-manage these are absent or inefficient. A final client characteristic of significance in understanding any difficulties and in selecting effective interventions is the person's *motivational features*. Knowledge of client-specific positive reinforcers (e.g., adult approval, peer acceptance, and having control over others) as well as the variety and relative influence of aversive events that control behavior (e.g., rejection by peers, adult reprimand, and anxiety) are of central importance in behavioral programming.

In summary, some Entry 2 client characteristics such as excessive negative emotional arousal may, *by their presence*, increase the likelihood of occurrence of the difficulties. Other client variables, such as conflict-resolution skills and motivation to please adults or to abide by rules of social behavior, *by their absence or low strength*, render the client more vulnerable to various problems under stress conditions (Gardner & Cole, 1985).

## Behavior Therapy Approaches

Although most behavioral practitioners would agree in principle with the potential value of this multicomponent assessment and treatment approach, clinical practice all too frequently deviates significantly from this model. This is especially evident in treating chronic, excessively occurring behavior symptoms presented by the severely and profoundly developmentally disabled person with multiple psychological difficulties. Treatment approaches designed to suppress these behavioral excesses may be selected in the absence of a suitable clinical assessment of the multiple factors that produce the behavioral symptoms. As has been noted in previous papers, various behavioral procedures, especially those involving aversive consequences, are subject to misuse by the untrained or uninformed clinician. In efforts to be effective and efficient in producing treatment effects, especially in the face of limited resources, the practitioner may be prone to select those behavior therapy procedures that serve to produce rapid suppression of the presenting behavioral symptoms. Such practices create concerns of an

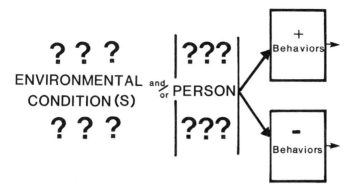

FIGURE 14.3. Clinical assessment process of the skill development therapy approach.

ethical, legal, and long-term treatment effectiveness nature. Except in highly selected instances, such practices *do not* represent adequate behavior therapy practice (see also McGee, Chapter 18).

To place this concern in perspective, it is valuable to recognize that behavior therapy procedures may be grouped into two major categories, the skill development therapy approach and the punishment therapy approach. Concepts associated with each therapy approach give direction to the type and intent of the procedures selected for use by the practitioner.

## Skill Development Therapy Approach

A primary group of behavior therapy procedures is based on the previously described clinical assessment model that seeks to identify potential environmentally based and client-based factors that contribute to the occurrence of the problem behaviors and/or emotions. By focusing on the combination of environmental conditions and person variables that result in prosocial behaviors and minimizing or eliminating those that produce aberrant behaviors, the client is provided with new coping skills to manage future stress. Figure 14.3 depicts this clinical process. Based on client-specific assessment results, various behavior therapy procedures are selected to accomplish one or more of the following:

1. Eliminate the problematic behavior through removal of those consequent events hypothesized to maintain the behavior—an *extinction procedure* (e.g., removing social attention and physical contact when self-abusive behavior is occurring; removing specific sensory stimulation associated with stereotypy).
2. Replace the problematic behaviors with prosocial ones that serve the same or similar function for the individual—a *skill building procedure*. Reinforcement procedures of shaping specific replacement skills and a range of other differential reinforcement procedures, modeling, social skills training, emotional (re)training, token economies, and the like illustrate the behavior change

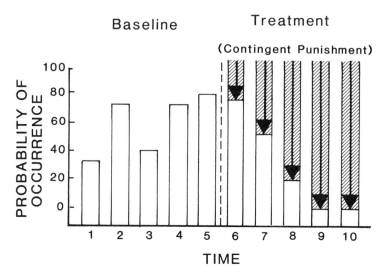

FIGURE 14.4. Punishment therapy approach.

tactics of this approach (e.g., reinforcing adaptive behavior under the conditions that result in anger and aggression).

3. Remove those stimulus conditions that control the behavior—*a stimulus control procedure* (e.g., reduce demands and thus decrease aggression, reduce excessive anxiety or fear and thus reduce isolation).

This multicomponent *skill development* approach represents the more desirable of the two behavior therapy approaches and is favored by the vast majority of behavioral researchers and clinicians. By attending to the *complex* of factors that potentially contribute to a person's mental health difficulties and by focusing on the development of a range of socially appropriate and adaptive coping skills, the potential for long-term maintenance of therapeutic gains is optimized. To accomplish this, a comprehensive behavior therapy program most typically will make use of combinations of the various therapeutic procedures described.

## Punishment Therapy Approach

The second group of therapy procedures, derived from operant-based and related concepts and depicted in Figure 14.4 as the punishment therapy approach, is designed to *inhibit* or *suppress* the occurrence of aberrant behaviors. The procedures are based on experimental data that demonstrate a relationship between behavior-contingent aversive consequences and behavior suppression or deceleration. As illustrated in Figure 14.4, after reliable measurement is obtained of the rate of occurrence of the target symptom (e.g., pica, aggression, self-injurious behavior, and stereotypy), the contingent aversive consequences are presented following occurrence of the symptom. Over a number of treatment sessions, if treatment is successful, the behavior followed by the aversive consequences is effectively suppressed; this suppression is maintained, at least temporarily, by the potential of such aversive consequences being repeated in the future.

One subset of punishment procedures involves the presentation of aversive conditions contingent on the occurrence of aberrant behaviors (e.g., an aversive consequence is presented immediately following aggression, pica, self-injurious, destructive, or other harmful actions). Such aversive consequences are selected on the basis of the severity of the problem behavior as defined by its intensity, potential harmfulness to self or others, and/or the extent to which it interferes with the person's availability to other therapeutic or habilitative program approaches. Aversive consequences have ranged from quite intrusive events, such as aversive electrical stimulation, aromatic ammonia, and physical restraint, to such less intrusive but nonetheless aversive conditions as water mist sprayed in the person's face, lemon juice squirted in the person's mouth, overcorrection, and facial screening. A second subset of punishment therapy model procedures, designed to suppress or discourage the occurrence of aberrant behaviors, involves the contingent removal of various positive events and includes those of time out from positive reinforcement and response cost (e.g., potential sources of positive reinforcement are removed for a period of time following physical aggression) (Matson & DiLorenzo, 1984).

Variations of this punishment therapy paradigm have gained some popularity among behavioral researchers and clinicians for a variety of reasons, one of which is the relative efficacy of such procedures. As noted, this is especially evident in treatment of intense problems of long standing presented by the more severely mentally retarded person. Also, as noted earlier, some clinicians have a tendency to select these procedures designed to suppress excessively occurring problem behaviors in the absence of an adequate individual assessment of the factors that may be contributing to the client's problem. In fact, punishment (contingent presentation of aversive consequences or removal of positive consequences) as a therapy procedure frequently is based on the supposition that the aversive properties will be sufficient to suppress the problematic behavior by overcoming the effects of whatever may be producing or maintaining (i.e., causing) the behavior. Again, as is well known, there are a number of pragmatic and ethical/legal difficulties associated with excessive reliance on such intervention methods (LaVigna & Donnellan, 1986).

In my view, there is no justification for the use of the more intrusive punishment therapy procedures, except perhaps in carefully selected cases of symptoms that are highly dangerous to the client and for which there are no effective alternative treatments. Nor is there any justification for the use of any punishment therapy procedures, however mild these may appear, when used as the only or major treatment approach. Why then do these procedures continue to occupy the attention of a number of researchers and clinicians involved in treatment of the mentally retarded with significant mental health difficulties? A brief glance at the historical context in which punishment therapy procedures developed should prove beneficial in offering at least partial answers to this concern.

## Historical Context of Behavior Therapy

Some 30 years ago as a young psychologist who had been awarded a traineeship supported by the National Institute on Mental Health to specialize in mental retardation, I vividly recall my first visit to the back wards of a residential facility serving the mentally retarded. There were 30 to 35 men herded into a room with wooden benches around the walls and a tile floor slanting toward the center drain. These men, mostly severely and profoundly involved, perhaps neurologically impaired and autistic, currently would be provided a diagnosis both of mental retardation and mental disorder. Many were engaging in stereotypic activities, including self-abuse. Some were pacing aimlessly up and down the room, while others were sitting and staring blankly into space. A few would suddenly scream out as if in pain. Most were in jumpsuits. Some were without clothing due to their stripping, even though staff were attempting to keep them dressed. Many were wet with their own urine or saliva or soiled with their defecation. I observed instances of pica and even coprophagy. Occasionally, staff would wash the tile floors with a hose.

I naively inquired about the diagnosis of these people. I was informed that they were mentally retarded, had brain damage, and thus could not help themselves. I asked about the treatment programs available to them. I was informed that most stayed in the locked day room area throughout the day because their behavior problems precluded program attendance and participation. Occasionally, recreational activities were provided, but this was conducted on the living area because of the frequent occurrence of aggression, property destruction, toileting accidents, and the like.

Within the following few years, a dramatic change occurred in the training, treatment, and care of these and similar developmentally disabled individuals residing in institutional facilities across the nation. This change was significantly influenced by an assumption held by a group of behavior theorists and practitioners that the mentally retarded, regardless of the degree of cognitive or neurological impairment, could develop a range of behavioral skills if provided appropriate learning experiences. Dr. Sidney Bijou (Chapter 27) was one of the influential members of this group. His paper, published in the 1960s, entitled "A Functional Analysis of Retarded Development," continues to be widely read (Bijou, 1966).

In the early 1970s, I summarized these advances in training and treatment in a book entitled *Behavior Modification in Mental Retardation* (Gardner, 1971). Also, in a chapter that appeared in Dr. Frank Menolascino's book entitled *Psychiatric Approaches to Mental Retardation*, I noted the following (Gardner, 1970):

Recent reports of the application of various behavior modification techniques provide illustration of positive behavior change of a range, degree, and rate that most psychiatric, psychological, educational, and residential staff had not thought possible due to the presumed limitations inherent in the mentally retarded. It has been demonstrated that at least a significant degree of the behavioral limitations of the retarded may well reside in an inappropriate or limited learning environment rather than being unalterable manifestations of the person's retardation. Severely and profoundly involved persons who for years were beyond help or hope have, as a result of treatment programs using the systematic application of behavior modification procedures, developed language, motor, perceptual, cognitive, and social skills that have rendered them more capable and able to experience a meaningful and productive personal and social existence. (p. 251)

Thus, even in the early 1970s, behavior therapists, whether psychologist, psychiatrist, nurse, social worker, or educator, had the basic technology to teach the mentally retarded to dress themselves, toilet themselves, groom themselves, feed themselves, and generally to care for their own personal needs. Another contributor to this book, Dr. Travis Thompson, documented the feasibility of institutional-wide implementation of these procedures (Thompson & Grabowski, 1972).

Although improved somewhat by these new experiences, there remained, nonetheless, that group of individuals who continued to engage in prolonged periods of such problem behaviors as self-stimulation, self-injury, pica, psychogenic vomiting and rumination, property destruction, aggression and tantrums, agitation, excessive screaming, stealing, stripping, and general negativism.

As the behavioral approaches had been successful in providing training programs for teaching self-help, social, and communication skills, it was natural for administrators with large residential populations and limited budgets and staff resources to seek comparable success in dealing with the more visible psychological disorders that remained. The behavior therapist, most frequently a psychologist, was challenged to provide solutions. In fact, in many institutional settings, the behavior therapist was provided major responsibility for solving these most difficult behavior problems. However, in my opinion a strategic mistake was made by too many of these clinicians. Instead of making major use of the concepts and procedures of the skill development therapy approach that had served them well in teaching self-help and related skills, punishment therapy procedures were used too frequently. These tended to be used as easy immediate solutions for complex problems. This treatment selection perhaps was understandable, however, in the context in which the therapist functioned. In addition to limited staff resources, psychiatrists and other medical staff seldom were present to lend diagnostic and treatment alternatives. The physician who was on the institutional staff, while cognizant of the severe behavior problems of many residents, usually had no alternative treatment suggestions to offer.

Thus, in this context of limited resources and the relative absence of opportunity to interact with other mental health professionals in developing alternative effective intervention procedures, the behavior therapist all too frequently used punishment therapy procedures that produced results even though these typically were short-lived when used in isolation.

## Current Practices

Currently, as skill development therapy approaches have gained empirical, ethical, and legal support, a number of guidelines have developed that, while not negating the use of punishment procedures, do ensure that such procedures are properly used in the context of acceptable clinical practice (Favell, 1982; Gardner & Cole, 1984a, 1984b; Johnson & Baumeister, 1981). The following are suggested as minimal guides:

1. The behavior therapy program should be based on client assessment that serves as a basis for hypotheses concerning the functionality of the problem behavior.
2. The behavior therapy program should reflect client-specific assessment data concerning possible relationships between the problem behaviors and (a) external stimulus control events and (b) various client characteristics.
3. The behavior therapy program should include robust procedures for developing, strengthening, and/or maintaining specific prosocial skills that will replace the problem behaviors.
4. The behavior therapy program should initially use and evaluate the least intrusive procedures prior to use of more intrusive ones.
5. The behavior therapy program should use those procedures that offer the most promising long-term benefits to the client.
6. When intrusive procedures are used to suppress excessively occurring behaviors, the selection of these procedures must be based on hunches concerning factors that currently are influencing the problem behaviors.
7. Intrusive procedures using aversive consequences should never be used in isolation. Rather, when deemed essential because of the severity of the problems and the absence of suitable alternatives, such procedures should represent only one aspect of a program based predominately on skill development therapy procedures.
8. Although any behavior therapy program should be data-based, programs using aversive procedures should be monitored closely through ongoing analysis of objective behavioral data. Both specific positive effects and potential negative side effects should be monitored.
9. The aversive components of behavior therapy programs should be removed as soon as possible.

## Recommendations for the Future

To summarize, our focus as researchers and clinicians in work with the mentally retarded with severe and chronic behavioral and emotional disorders has been somewhat concerned with demonstrating immediate results—thus the early, and continuing, interest on the use of aversively based deceleration procedures. This is especially evident with problems presented by the more severely and profoundly handicapped. As noted, in cases of severe, chronic, and physically harmful self-injurious behavior, the treatment of choice, as reflected in the current professional literature, is the use of contingent aversive consequences (Favell, 1982). This is not to imply, however, that future research will continue to support this as the most efficacious procedure. We must turn our attention to explanatory models that dictate other treatment approaches, and that will lend direction to the thorny problems of generalization and maintenance of therapeutic gains.

Even in view of the success of behavioral approaches in treatment of a number of the more frequently occurring behavior disorders, it is overly optimistic, and perhaps simplistic, to believe that the behavior therapy of the past, or even that of the changing present, represents adequate approaches for effective treatment of the array of mental disorders presented by the mentally retarded. There is need for integrated models of psychopathology and mental health that entail behavioral, psychosocial, pharmacological, neuropsychiatric, and related physical medicine concepts. This development can best be fostered in the context of interdisciplinary clinical and research settings that have the resources to seek solutions in a systematic and thoughtful manner. To accomplish this, the following recommendations are presented for discussion:

1. Development of regional centers specializing in mental health difficulties presented by the mentally retarded. These centers not only should have a commitment to research but also should be designed to provide and demonstrate exemplary models of service, technical assistance, and professional training. This recommendation could be realized through designated expansion of current University Affiliated Facilities and research centers devoted to mental retardation.

2. As each center could not specialize in all mental disorders presented by the mentally retarded, it is further recommended that specific centers or groups of centers assume responsibility for developing a research focus in specific areas. For example, one center or consortium may focus on schizophrenia, another on depression, another on aggression and related conduct difficulties, and another on the range of behavior disorders such as self-injurious behavior, stereotypy, and pica that occur predominately among the more severely retarded. Although the centers could be generalists in clinical service, technical assistance, and training, the research focus could remain more specialized.

## References

Barrett, R.P. (Ed.). (1986). *Severe behavior disorders in the mentally retarded*. New York: Plenum.

Bellack, A.S., Hersen, M., & Kazdin, A.E. (Eds.). (1982). *International handbook of behavior modification and therapy*. New York: Plenum Press.

Bijou, S.W. (1966). A functional analysis of retarded development. In N.R. Ellis (Ed.), *International review of research in mental retardation* (Vol. 1, pp. 1–19). New York: Academic Press.

Favell, J.E. (Task Force Chairperson). (1982). The treatment of self-injurious behavior. *Behavior Therapy, 13*, 529–554.

Gardner, W.I. (1970). Use of behavior therapy with the mentally retarded. In F.J. Menolascino (Ed.), *Psychiatric approaches to mental retardation* (pp. 250–275). New York: Basic Books.

Gardner, W.I. (1971). *Behavior modification in mental retardation*. Chicago: Aldine/ Atherton.

Gardner, W.I., & Cole, C.L. (1984a). Aggression and related conduct difficulties in the mentally retarded: A multicomponent behavioral model. In S.E. Breuning, J.L. Matson, & R.P. Barrett (Eds.), *Advances in mental retardation and developmental disabilities* (Vol. 2, pp. 41–84). Greenwich, CN: JAI Press.

Gardner, W.I., & Cole, C.L. (1984b). Use of behavior therapy with the mentally retarded in community settings. In F.J. Menolascino & J.A. Stark (Eds.), *Handbook of mental illness in the mentally retarded* (pp. 97–153). New York: Plenum Press.

Gardner, W.I., & Cole, C.L. (1985). Acting-out disorders. In M. Hersen (Ed.), *Practice of inpatient behavior therapy: A clinical guide* (pp. 203–230). New York: Grune & Stratton.

Johnson, W.L., & Baumeister, A.A. (1981). Behavioral techniques for decreasing aberrant behaviors of retarded and autistic persons. In M. Hersen, R.M. Eisler, & P.M. Miller (Eds.), *Progress in behavior modification* (Vol. 12). New York: Academic Press.

LaVigna, G.W., & Donnellan, A.M. (1986). *Alternatives to punishment: Solving behavior problems with non-aversive strategies*. New York: Irvington Publishers.

Matson, J.L., & Barrett, R.P. (Eds.). (1982). *Psychopathology in the mentally retarded*. New York: Grune & Stratton.

Matson, J.L., & DiLorenzo, T.M. (1984). *Punishment and its alternatives: A new perspective for behavior modification*. New York: Springer Publishing.

Menolascino, F., & Stark, J. (Eds.). (1984). *The handbook of mental illness in the mentally retarded*. New York: Plenum Press.

Sigman, M. (Ed.). (1985). *Children with emotional disorders and developmental disabilities*. New York: Grune & Stratton.

Sovner, R., & Hurley, A.D. (1986). Managing aggressive behavior: A psychiatric approach. *Psychiatric Aspects of Mental Retardation Reviews, 5*, 16–21.

Thompson, T., & Grabowski, J.G. (Eds.). (1972). *Behavior modification of the mentally retarded*. New York: Oxford University Press.

Whitman, T.L, Scibak, J.W., & Reid, D.H. (1983). *Behavior modification with the severely and profoundly retarded: Research and application*. New York: Academic Press.

# 15
# Mental Health of Persons with Mental Retardation: A Solution, Obstacles to the Solution, and a Resolution for the Problem

C. Thomas Gualtieri

The problem, as suggested by the title, does in fact have a solution. Technical developments in modern neuropsychiatry are capable of alleviating most of the mental health problems of persons with mental retardation. There is a technology available to treat these problems wisely and well; there are cogent methods for developing treatments for the few problems that remain intractable.

The second problem is that there are structural barriers to the development of neuropsychiatry as a practical specialty available for the benefit of retarded individuals. There are formidable obstacles to professional development and research. It is an irony that the problem of mental health for persons with mental retardation already has a solution; the second problem, structural obstacles to this solution, is more formidable than the first. It is necessary to describe these obstacles bluntly and in a forthright fashion. If they are fairly described and carefully mapped, they will no longer be obstacles at all. To raise this second problem is to introduce the possibility of a solution. If the issue is ignored, it will never be resolved.

The first problem is the abysmal lack of neuropsychiatric care for mentally retarded people, especially for the severely retarded. This is the major neglected area in mental retardation today. However, it is not correct to attribute this problem to the divorce of mental retardation from mental health that occurred about a generation ago. For mental retardation, the separation from psychiatry was part of a revolutionary movement that deemphasized the "medical model" and redefined treatment as habilitation. A distinct class of professionals to serve mentally retarded people grew up who were capable of meeting their social and educational needs. The locus of care moved away from medical units and into the community, and the locus of training moved into a relatively free-standing system of University Affiliated Facilities (UAFs). These were, in the main, important and necessary changes. But this new class of professionals in mental retardation had no training or interest in applied neuroscience. The mental health requirements of mentally retarded people were not likely to be met as long as neuropsychiatry was absent from the multidisciplinary team assembled around this new movement.

There are some people who think that it was a mistake to separate psychiatry from mental retardation, but I don't think it was a bad idea at the time. The advantages of deemphasizing the medical model and of cultivating developmental, community-based models were abundant and are still readily apparent. More pertinent, however, is the fact that psychiatry had little to offer the severely mentally handicapped person 30 years ago.

Psychiatry had abandoned, or at least neglected, mental retardation long before the divorce occurred. Forcing the couple to live together would not have done much good. First, the development of modern neuropsychiatric technology is a comparatively recent development. Practitioners, capable of exercising these skills, have only recently come available in substantial numbers. Second, psychiatry's disinterest in mental retardation in particular has been paralleled only by its disinterest in chronic mental illness in general. Psychiatry has spent the last quarter century pursuing the medical model with the same ardor with which mental retardation, as a field, has run away from it. Its ideal has been that of the rest of medicine; a focus on acute care medicine for comparatively advantaged individuals, who happen to have third-party coverage. The appropriate slogan of modern medicine, indeed of modern psychiatry, is this: If a patient doesn't have third-party coverage, he has no right to be a patient. So, even if psychiatry and mental retardation had stayed together, psychiatry would not have had much to contribute to the relationship — no more than it has had for the chronically mentally ill, for severe epileptics, for the demented, or for head-injury patients.

The problem restated is the neglect of the mental health of severely retarded individuals by psychiatry. It is part of a larger problem of neglect of seriously handicapped individuals by medicine in general. It is an enormous problem, too — in terms of the number of patients, the extraordinary severity of their problems, and the degree of ignorance with which they are treated when they do come to medical attention.

It is appropriate to reflect on the reasons why mentally retarded people have such a high prevalence of psychiatric disorders, why their disorders are so severe, and why their prognosis, when they have a mental disorder, is so poor. Two reasons are traditionally given, well known, and widely accepted:

1. Persons with mental retardation, by dint of endowment and training, have limited capacity to cope with the pressures and demands of day-to-day life.
2. Day-to-day life challenges retarded persons to an extraordinary degree. A person with mental retardation rarely experiences what might be called a developmentally appropriate environment.

These two points have been the main area of concern by professionals and advocates for the mental health of persons with mental retardation. It is necessary to underscore and emphasize these two issues, because they probably account for most of the mental health problems retarded persons have. But they do not account for all the psychological problems of retarded people. It is necessary to pay deference to these two points, but it is not sufficient. The solution to the problem of mental health in severely mentally retarded people requires, in addition, careful attention to the following two points:

1. Moderate, severe, and profoundly retarded persons have sustained major malformations or damage to the brain. A substantial part of the behavior problems of mentally retarded persons is inextricably connected to a disorder or malfunction of brain. *Neuropathic damage* predisposes mentally retarded people to certain kinds of behavior problems that do not occur in individuals of normal intelligence. It renders treatment more difficult and its outcome less predictable. On the other hand, by one of those fatal ironies, it does not confer any degree of immunity to the psychiatric conditions to which people of normal intelligence succumb.

2. Mentally retarded people who develop psychiatric disorders, behavior problems, or seizures obtain, as a rule, very poor treatment from physicians or psychologists who are all too often ignorant, incompetent, overworked, or inattentive. Certain forms of drug "treatment," for example, can actually cause behavior problems, psychiatric disorders, or seizures, if clumsily prescribed or poorly monitored. Neuropsychiatric treatment for persons with mental retardation is, as a rule, nonexistent, clumsy, or inept.

It is not surprising that the mental health of severely handicapped individuals, taken as a group, is not very good; considering that they spend their lives in a world that neither welcomes nor succors them; that they have limited capacity to cope with the challenges and disappointments of life; that their brains are poorly developed, malformed, or damaged; that behaviors which are developmentally appropriate are frequently identified as pathological, while manifest neuropsychiatric syndromes may be overlooked or misdiagnosed; and that when their behavior is identified as pathological, the patients are treated ineptly, if at all. It is surprising that a large number of retarded people do *not* have severe mental illness. Proofs of the basic strength and goodness of the human spirit are not found too often. But the fact that perhaps half of the persons with severe retardation are psychologically healthy, in spite of such obstacles, is one such proof.

It is a reasonable estimate that half of the population of severely handicapped individuals have severe behavior problems. At the same time, they are systematically denied the provision of modern neuropsychiatric care. The regional residential center (RRC) has become an assemblage of persons with mental retardation who exhibit severe neuropsychiatric conditions. The RRCs have become, in effect, psychiatric hospitals, with no psychiatric administrators, no psychiatric nurses or social workers, no psychologists trained in neuropsychiatry, no psychiatrists, and no research. The circumstances of persons with mental retardation in community dwellings are perhaps less dire, since disturbed individuals in their midst tend to return to institutions. But even in well-endowed communities, their access to well-trained neuropsychiatrists is limited.

It is impossible to continue like this. There has to be a solution to the problem and a reintegration of the field. It is not only for the benefit of this population that I hold this belief; it is for the integrity of our profession.

## Neuropsychiatry

The solution is in the development of neuropsychiatry, a technology that is concerned specifically with the treatment of neurobehavioral symptoms in severely involved individuals: people whose behavior or emotional problems are attributable not only to a developmental disability, such as mental retardation, but also to other severe, chronically handicapping brain disorders, such as schizophrenia, severe forms of affective disorder, severe intractable epilepsy, Alzheimer's disease and other dementing conditions, and closed head injury. These individuals are all underserved or ill-served. They all have severe, brain-based disorders that have been considered hopeless for treatment. In a sense, that is true, since none of these problems can be "cured." But they can be treated effectively.

Neuropsychiatrists treat a diverse group of patients whose behavioral symptoms are as diverse and heterogeneous as their cognitive deficits. However, their symptoms and deficits are interchangeable. Aggression or withdrawal, hyperactivity or anergia, psychosis or head banging might be a neurobehavioral symptom in any of these conditions. A specific mix of symptoms may characterize one group more than another, but the range of problems has an almost perfect overlap. Thus, the skills acquired in working with one such group of patients are readily transferable, with only small modifications, to representatives of the other groups.

Neuropsychiatry is defined not only by a certain class of patients but also by an integrated evaluation and treatment technology. It is a new field that incorporates elements from psychopharmacology, behavioral neurology and epileptology, behavioral psychology, and neuropsychology. Neuropsychiatry includes representatives from all these disciplines, although they do not necessarily call themselves neuropsychiatrists. They have in their clinical work (but not in their training, because one cannot find formal training neuropsychiatry) acquired skills and knowledge from each of the parent disciplines. Good neuropsychiatrists represent a professional integration of the best, most salient elements of applied neuroscience.

Neuropsychiatry is defined by a patient population, by a specific technology, and by an integrated if not eclectic approach to diagnosis and treatment. The patients treated by neuropsychiatrists are generally people who cannot be treated by conventionally trained neurologists, psychologists, and psychiatrists. Issues in neuropsychiatry that are especially germane to mental retardation are psychopharmacology, behavior neurology and epileptology, behavioral psychology, and neuropsychology.

### Psychopharmacology

Most of the recent emphasis on psychopharmacology for the retarded has been to reduce or eliminate it entirely. This speaks to the history of overuse and misuse of neuroleptic drugs, especially in residential institutions for persons with mental retardation in the 1960s and 1970s. This pattern was finally interrupted in the past few years with (1) the discovery of very high rates of tardive dyskinesia in mentally retarded people (Gualtieri, Schroeder, Hicks, & Quade, 1986) and (2) the development of civil rights and tort litigation over neuroleptic misuse (Gualtieri, Sprague, & Cole, 1986). The most recent survey of psychotropic drug administration by Hill, Lakin, and Bruininks (1987) revealed that 20 to 30% of the institutionalized retarded are on chronic neuroleptic treatment, down from 50% 10 (Cohen & Sprague, 1977) and 20 years ago (Lipman, 1970). Considering the increased concentration of mentally retarded residents with severe behavior problems in institutions, especially in recent years, this represents a remarkable decline.

Dull-witted psychopharmacology has probably declined from 1968 to 1986, but intelligent psychopharmacology has not necessarily increased. There are only three centers (to the author's knowledge) where creative, intelligent, clinical psychopharmacologists work with retarded individuals. This is a shameful state of affairs, because clinical psychopharmacology has some powerful methods for alleviating behavioral symptoms and stabilizing the emotional state, even of severely handicapped individuals. Although there has not been any creative psychopharmacological research with retarded patients, there is sufficient knowledge from other patient groups to guide intelligent treatment. Nevertheless, it is unfortunate that the scientific community has not taken the opportunity to explore the new frontiers in psychopharmacology such as:

1. The diagnosis and treatment of major affective disorders in the retarded.
2. Subgroups of self-injurious patients and the pharmacotherapy of SIB.
3. Carbamazepine and lithium in the treatment of aggression and hyperactivity.
4. Diagnosis and treatment of panic attacks, phobias, and other anxiety states.
5. The proper use of neuroleptics and the proper diagnosis of psychosis and schizophrenia.
6. Stimulant and MAO treatment for dementia in Down's syndrome.
7. The contribution of preexisting brain damage or neuropathology to the development of tardive dyskinesia.

A whole new technology around the systematic evaluation of psychopharmacology in the retarded needs to be developed. Issues of instrumentation and research design have to be worked out. Reasonable hypotheses have to derive from the day-to-day work of gifted clinicians, not from academics who never see a patient but who argue about the "literature." Without a sound base of experience and practice to guide one's intuition, research in psychopharmacology is irrelevant. Good clinical practice improves the care of individuals, but, at the same time, it generates creative ideas for the proper course of research. When there is a "critical mass" of psychopharmacologists who work with mentally retarded persons, there will be new research ideas and good research. Until there is such a group, research will tend to be methodical but uninspired.

## Behavioral Neurology and Epileptology

It is amazing that neurology as a field has escaped criticism for the problems of excessive and inappropriate anticonvulsant treatment in the mentally retarded, which at this point probably surpasses the excesses of neuroleptic misuse. Every survey that has ever been done on the topic shows very high rates of anticonvulsant drug use in mentally retarded populations in community [11% (Gadow & Loney, 1981)] or residential [34% (Aman, 1983)] settings. The most sedating anticonvulsants like dilantin, phenobarbital, and primidone are still favored. Anticonvulsant polypharmacy is the rule, and routine screening for toxic effects and blood level variations is rare to nonexistent (Aman, Paxton, Field, & Foote, 1986). There is an extremely high rate of behavioral and cognitive toxicity with anticonvulsants that may be more important to developmentally disabled individuals than to the nondisabled. However, a few anticonvulsants may have promise as psychotropes, at least in certain clinical circumstances (Evans & Gualtieri, 1985).

An effective neuropsychiatric consultant to a mental retardation program knows how to monitor anticonvulsant drug treatment, how to measure behavioral and cognitive toxicity, and how to affect good seizure management with a minimum of medication. But he or she has learned to do so without any initiative or direction from the leadership in neurology toward clinical research for the retarded or for effective technology transfer from university-based neurologists to community practitioners.

Presumably, neurology has escaped critical scrutiny because anticonvulsants are "medical" treatments while psychotropes are "behavioral." This division is as artificial as it is absurd, and it is dangerous to patients. Anticonvulsants have the potential for behavioral toxicity or for behavioral improvement. They may improve learning or impair it. Inappropriate anticonvulsants may be overused and new, effective anticonvulsants may be underused. In any event, there is no escaping the need for sound professional judgment, careful monitoring, and a familiarity with the wider, habilitative environment of the disabled patient. And there is no escaping the need for national initiatives to promote good clinical care and relevant research.

Although there is said to be a surfeit of neurologists in the nation, there is an egregious imbalance when professional care is rarely afforded to individuals with the severest conditions. It is not unreasonable to require some degree of accountability from the neurological profession and from its national institute.

To an increasing degree, neuropsychiatrists are stepping into the void that has been left by traditional neurologists. Perhaps that is not so bad. After all, there are epilepsy syndromes with clear psychiatric consequences, like so-called temporal lobe epilepsy. *Absence* is part of the differential diagnosis of attention deficit disorder; partial epilepsy may be confused with Tourette's syndrome; anticonvulsant-induced dyskinesia may resemble tardive dyskinesia. It might be a good idea to centralize psychotropic and anticonvulsant drug treatment in one specialty, since so many psychotropic drugs can influence the seizure threshold, and every anticonvulsant has the capacity either to improve behavior and cognition or to impair it. Some neurologists are (finally) taking an interest in psychopharmacology; at the same time, many more psychiatrists are taking a responsible interest in anticonvulsants and epilepsy. There is a coming together of the two fields although it is slow, unorganized, and has received no encouragement or support from the national leadership.

## Behavioral Psychology

Behavioral psychology and applied behavioral analysis (in its practical, not theoretic, form) have contributed more to the understanding and treatment of behavior disorders in persons with mental retardation than any other discipline. Behaviorism has made four signal contributions: (1) a new technology for the measurement of behavior; (2) practical success in managing and shaping behavior; (3) a cadre of energetic and devoted clinical scientists, a growing force in mental retardation and neuropsychiatry; and (4) a refreshing liberation from theoretical bias (if, of course, one can ignore the theoretical biases of behaviorism itself).

It is no longer possible to practice effective neuropsychiatry in a mental retardation facility without reliable behavioral analysis or without some familiarity with behavioral programming. The definition and measurement of target behaviors are essential for the proper analysis of drug effects; establishing the inevitable limits of behavioral treatment is essential for determining the indication for drug treatment. Behavior analysis represents an alternative to traditional psychiatric diagnosis on the one hand and, on the other, a suitable technology for gauging the efficacy of a psychiatric intervention. It is an indispensable tool.

There are two major problems with behavioral psychology, though. One is external and the other internal. The external problem, over which behaviorists have little control, is the limited degree to which their discipline is integrated into the curriculum in medical schools, departments of psychiatry, and UAFs. Thus, the field remains spotty and isolated—strong in some areas and nonexistent in others. This is a tragedy, since behavioral technology is essential to good clinical practice.

The second problem may be causative to the first. Behavioral psychology is neither cheap nor prescriptive. There has to be work in the direction of developing inexpensive but accurate technology for behavioral analysis. And there has to be a promulgation of readily usable behavioral instruments. Behaviorism would do well to be more prescriptive—to adopt more of a medical model, if you will excuse the term. For example, which behavioral interventions are specifically indicated for which class of patients? What patient elements predict the response to a specific intervention? For a given disorder, what is the most effective behavioral remedy? (Behaviorists shudder at the utterance of a word like "disorder," but it is a young field and somewhat given to ideological purity; that will change as behaviorists achieve success and win acceptance.)

## Neuropsychology

The potential contributions of neuropsychology and cognitive psychology are less apparent to clinical research for mentally retarded people. The contributions of developmental psychology, in contrast, have been more important in the past than they will probably be in the future, as the mentally retarded population grows progressively older and the limitations of the developmental model, especially to account for the totality of behavior disorders in mentally retarded people, becomes apparent. Nonetheless, developmental psychology will continue to make a contribution, perhaps as strong as that of cognitive psychology, but probably not as important as neuropsychology.

Neuropsychology has given us an extraordinary new assessment technology that has finally grown cheap and reliable (Evans, Shear, & Gualtieri, 1985). It is also an enthusiastic young field with a preoccupation with brain–behavior relationships all too long neglected in mental retardation. The definition of specific brain syndromes like Klüver-Bucy, temporal lobe epilepsy, and the frontal lobe syndrome represent important conceptual advances in neuropsychology. It contributes strongly to psychopharmacology since certain neuropsychological measures turn out to be exquisitely drug sensitive (Gualtieri & Evans, 1985). The same is true of certain cognitive measures from psychophysics and cognitive sychology.

## Obstacles to the Solution

When elements from all these disciplines are joined, they comprise a powerful technology that transcends in range and salience the individual disciplines operating alone, out of a limited point of view. The differential diagnosis of neuroehavioral phenomena is much wider and likely to succeed when a formulation may be made in alternative vocabularies with reference to different conceptual structures and frames of reference. The potential for therapeutic success is much wider when the tools of several treatment-oriented disciplines are pooled. The whole is much greater and more effective than the sum of its parts.

Well, if the solution described here is indeed so fabulous, and if it is so effective in reducing or ameliorating the mental health problems of mentally handicapped patients, why is it such a well-kept secret? If the new field of neuropsychiatry is so promising for treatment and research, why aren't academic departments and the national instituted developing new programs in the area? If neuropsychiatry is the solution, why does the problem still exist?

There are three reasons: (1) professional jealousy, (2) institutional penury, and (3) a senium in academe.

The development of a new, integrative discipline will always be threatening to individuals whose focus is narrow and traditional. This is especially true of academia, where professional structures and academic boundaries are guarded jealously. There is also a kind of generation gap in academia, since universities have grown top-heavy with tenured, older faculty and opportunities for advancement for bright young people are seriously limited. People who are old but influential and well entrenched may not appreciate or accept the importance of a new, integrative specialty.

Or they may be preoccupied with other things; the same things they have always done, for example. Research directions are notoriously hard to shift in midcareer (or end-game). Staying in the lab is so much more comfortable than reaching out to the day-to-day struggles of research in a clinical setting. There is more lucre in grants for established areas of research than there is in opening new ones; there is more to be made from the treatment of high-prevalence, low-severity disorders like depression. That is not a trivial point, or a mean one. Medical schools survive on grants and patient income, and the latter comes only from patients who have insurance. Academia, in turn, influences the national institutes.

So the second problem is the existence of structural obstacles to the development of neuropsychiatry (applied neuroscience) for patients with severe neuro-behavioral disorders. Here again there is a solution, or perhaps two. But before considering what these solutions might be, permit me to tell you about a few interesting encounters I had in preparation for this chapter. In the 1969s, it was fashionable to talk about personal experiences that "radicalized" an individual. If my point of view appears to be radical, or excessive, please understand that it has arisen out of some extraordinary experiences.

One such experience had to do with our research in tardive dyskinesia. The research on the development of this severe neuroleptic side effect in children and persons with mental retardation occurred in the context of widespread neuro-leptic overuse and misuse. The pattern had persisted for 30 years, since the introduction of neuroleptics in 1953, in spite of draconian admonitions from George Crane (Crane, 1973) as early as 1968. But Crane's warnings had no influence on actual practice. In *1983*, it was estimated that no fewer than three million Americans were on chronic neuroleptic treatment (Singer, 1983). (If you ask me, they were the *wrong* three million Americans.) Virtually every survey that was done revealed that neuroleptics were applied for patients who did not really require drug treatment, that doses were excessive, polypharmacy was common, monitoring for drug side effects was rare, and informed consent for treatment was nonexistent. This situation continued, not only among the mentally retarded but also in children with behavioral or emotional problems and in the nursing home elderly. It continued in spite of journal reports, scientific articles, consensus conferences, guidelines, and task force reports (Gualtieri, Sprague, & Cole, 1986).

Now the pattern has changed. As I mentioned earlier in this chapter, there has been a perceptible decrease in neuroleptic prescription for retarded individuals. Psychiatrists are increasingly conservative in their use of neuroleptic drugs without compromising the care of patients who really require these medications. Finally, after 30 years, research into the severity, epidemiology, and prognosis of tardive dyskinesia is underway. The American Psychiatric Association has taken the leadership in promoting more intelligent use of these important, but potentially dangerous, medications. All this is a sanguine change. But let me assure you, it took some doing. The solution had to do with individual initiative; it did not come from the national leadership.

The second story has to do with a case of scientific fraud, which Robert Sprague (at the University of Illinois) and I discovered in December 1983. This involved the most prominent psychopharmacology researcher in the field of mental retardation. I won't name this person, but those readers who are familiar with the field must know that he is conspicuous by his absence in this book. While he promulgated an extensive body of methodologically perfect but completely fabricated research, he was an assistant professor at a large northeastern university, which incidentally, was the second largest recipient of NIMH extramural research dollars in 1983 (Gualtieri & Keppel, 1984). His fabricated data were published in the *American Journal of Psychiatry, Archives of General Psychiatry, Journal of Nervous and Mental Disease, Journal of the American Association of Mental Deficiency, Journal of Applied Research in Mental Retardation*, and *Psychopharmacology Bulletin*. His career was subsequently reviewed by no fewer than three university committees, one special investigator, and one NIMH committee. Soon after our discovery, he resigned his university post with honor. Now, more than four years after our discovery, it is sad to report that not one of his papers has been retracted. He is still writing articles for medical journals, and his citation index, after taking a plunge in 1984, is now rising to prediscovery levels (see Figure 15.1). This person is giving workshops around the country, and I am told that he holds a state contract to educate professionals in the proper use of psychopharmacological drugs for mentally retarded individuals.[1]

The third story has to do with fenfluramine in the treatment of autism. In 1982, a brief report appeared in the *New England Journal of Medicine* (Geller, Ritvo, Freeman, & Yuwiler, 1982) that suggested that a rational treatment for infantile autism was at last at hand. The atypical stimulant, fenfluramine, a serotonin inhibitor, was said to improve the behavior and adaptive functioning of autistic children and was even reported to "double the IQ" of one autistic child. The scientists who wrote this report embraced fenfluramine with the same blind enthusiasm that is usually attributed to the promoters of fad diets, hair analysis, ecobehavioral treatment, and megavitamins. Now it is discovered that the medication is relatively ineffective. Its neurochemical effects have nothing to do with whatever (dubious) clinical efficacy it may have and its long-term safety in the treatment of children is a question mark. In fact, there is concern within the neuropsychiatric community that the medication may be neurotoxic (Gualtieri, 1986). Twenty-eight years after the first description of tardive dyskinesia, parents and pediatricians found themselves victims of a media blitz promoting a medication that may, in the long run, effect a similar kind of neural damage. The sources of this mischief were a respected university with enormous funding from the national institutes and a medical journal that is normally endowed with probity and sound scientific judgment.

---

[1]The gentleman in question, Stephen R. Breuning of the University of Pittsburgh, was finally exposed after an NIMH investigation that lasted 3½ years (NIMH Report, 1987).

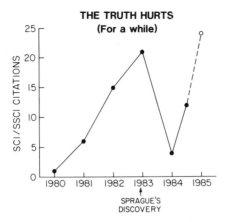

FIGURE 15.1. "The truth hurts (for a while)." The fabricated research of the individual in question was cited in scientific and social science journals with increasing frequency from 1980 to 1983. In 1984, his citation index took a sharp plunge – as the few researchers who knew of his fraud no longer cited his work. However, in 1985, his citation index began to rise again, as new writers learned of his work but remained ignorant of its fraudulent nature. As of October 1986, almost three years after our discovery, not one of his articles had been retracted.

Within the context suggested by the incidents I have recounted, the funding patterns illustrated in Figures 15.2 and 15.3 should come as no surprise. At NIMH, the major target of extramural research funds is research in the treatment of affective disorders. Now no one can maintain that affective disorders are trivial or that they are unworthy of investigation and research. They are a high-prevalence disorder. But they also happen to be the *only* psychiatric disorders that can be treated effectively, or cured if you will, and in some cases prevented. If one had to wish a serious psychiatric condition on oneself or a loved one, it would be an affective disorder. Why then is there such emphasis on research for a condition that is eminently treatable? No index of severity or human misery would represent depression to be twice as grave a disorder as schizophrenia. But it is the bread-and-butter of "modern" psychiatry. It is an acute illness, one that can be treated, and a disease of comparatively advantaged patients who usually carry third-party coverage.

Figure 15.2 clearly shows where the mental health needs of persons with mental retardation stand in the eyes of the NIMH, at the far right and at the bottom of the list.

From NICHD (Figure 15.3), there is a massive emphasis on basic biochemical and genetic studies, which is not unreasonable; but very little in the way of prevention, education, and treatment research. There continues to be massive expenditure for diagnosis and evaluation – as if the only thing we can do for a retarded person is evaluate, evaluate, evaluate. The families of developmentally

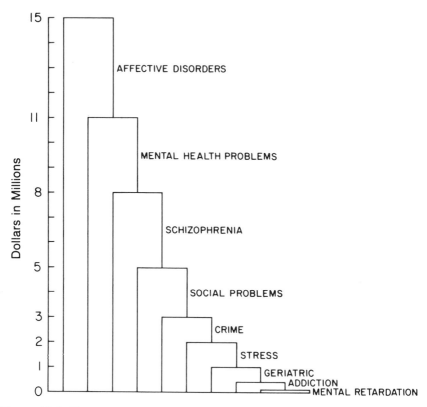

FIGURE 15.2. Extramural research dollars from the NIMH went largely to the study of affective disorders, the most eminently treatable of all psychiatric conditions. Although the NIMH is responsible for psychiatric research in mental retardation, hardly any money goes into this area. The pattern has not changed since 1983.

handicapped children do not need so much in the way of evaluations; they could use at least a bit in the way of treatment.

These are the obstacles to the development of modern neuropsychiatry and the development of modern, innovative approaches to the treatment of severely handicapped individuals. We have developed in mental health and in mental retardation an enormous structure around research, teaching, and policy implementation. But that structure is old and creaking. It is inflexible and responds reluctantly, if at all, to new initiatives. Its capacity for self-correction and change is extremely limited. Its accountability is really only to itself. The constituencies of national organizations like NIMH and NICHD are not the afflicted people whose medical conditions are their proper concern, or their families. Their constituency is the academics who set policy, sit on study sections, and receive

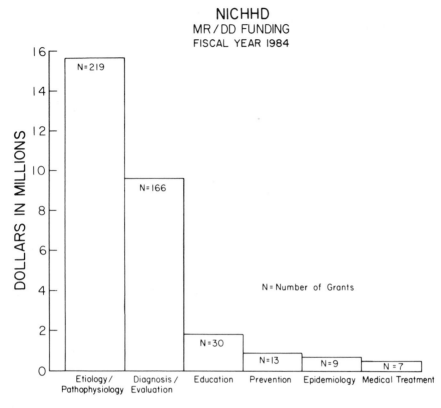

FIGURE 15.3. Extramural research dollars from the NICHHD go mainly to two traditional areas: basic medical studies and diagnosis/evaluation. Treatment research has a very low priority.

grant funds. It is a truism that the bureaucratic mentality gives the priorities of bureaucrats precedence over the needs of the citizens they serve. It must be understood that, in our field, the priorities of professionals are placed over the needs of patients; the priorities of teachers are placed over the needs of their students; and the priorities of scientists may take precedence even over science itself and the discovery of truth.

## Resolution for the Problem

I am not sure that the current structure of the national institutes and of academia is really capable of responding in an effective way to the challenge that this book is committed to address. From the national leadership, we may expect more consensus conferences, more professional meetings, a book, and perhaps a cosmetic grant or two. It is more likely that the solution to this problem will have to come from the development of new structures, perhaps at the state and local level, or perhaps in the private sector.

I mentioned that there might be two solutions to the second problem. One could be a solution at the national level. If there were a commitment at the national level, this is what it would have to comprise:

1. A special study section for neuropsychiatry, comprising representatives and funds from the National Institute of Mental Health, the National Institute of Child Health & Human Development, the National Institute of Neurology, Communicative Diseases and Stroke, and the National Institute of Disability and Rehabilitation Research.
2. Regional treatment centers for the development of treatment technologies, clinical research, and teaching.
3. Mental Health Research Centers and Mental Retardation Research Centers should be expected to show at least some interest in clinical research for the chronically mentally ill or the mentally retarded. It is not unreasonable to expect that at least a few of these "centers" should show some interest in this area of concern; at the present time, none does. Similarly, training funds from the national institutes should go only to program that have a credible commitment to patients with severe and chronic handicaps.
4. By manipulating parameters of third-party coverage, licensure, and accreditation, one could require private psychiatric hospitals to reserve at least some portion of their beds for patients who are indigent, chronically mentally ill, or mentally retarded. Psychiatric hospitals and general hospitals beyond a certain size should be required to devote at least a few inpatient beds to mentally retarded and chronically mentally handicapped patients.
5. I am not one to recommend more meetings, but there has to be a monitoring group of professionals and advocates who can work out the technical details implicit in these recommendations, who can monitor developments in the field, and who can press for quality control and accountability around the four points listed above.

On the basis of my experience, which you must allow has been unique, I have serious doubts that any such initiative will be taken on a national level. The talents of the national and academic leadership seem most suited to holding meetings, writing articles that no one reads, and supporting irrelevant research that looks good to editors and politicians but serves really as no more than a welfare program for middle-aged, white men. It may well be that the proper solution to the problems that I have outlined lies in the development of a different structure with alternative models for treatment, research, and training. These might best occur on the state level and within the private sector. There, one can hope for the development of new leadership and new ideas, especially around issues of quality control and accountability, the development of new treatment paradigms for severely involved individuals, and at least a partial commitment to research in applied neuroscience. To the degree that my colleagues and I in North Carolina are involved in such work, I am proud and hopeful.

The issue confronting this movement as reflected in this book does not really have to do with the mental health of the mentally retarded people. In no small part, it has to do with the integrity and the relevance of the national institutes and the research universities. Their performance in the recent past casts serious doubts on their capacity to provide national direction or leadership. They deserve to be held accountable.

With or without national leadership and support, the job will be done. We are doing it, and we shall continue to do it well. Our agenda has been written by developmentally disabled individuals and their families. Their needs and concerns will define a new national priority for research and treatment.

## References

Aman, M.G. (1983). Psychoactive drugs in mental retardation. In J. Matson & F. Andrasik (Eds.), *Treatment issues and innovations in mental retardation*. New York: Plenum Press.

Aman, M.G., Paxton, J.W., Field, C.J., & Foote, S.E. (1986). Prevalence of toxic anticonvulsant drug concentrations in mentally retarded persons with epilepsy. *American Journal of Mental Deficiency, 90*, 643–650.

Cohen, M.N., & Sprague, R.L. (1977). *Survey of drug usage in two midwestern institutions for the retarded*. Paper presented at the Gatlinburg conference on Research in Mental Retardation, Gatlinburg, TN.

Crane, G.E. (1973). Clinical psychopharmacology in its 20th year. *Science, 181*, 124–128.

Evans, R.W., Gualtieri, C.T. (1985). Carbamazepine: A neuropsychological and psychiatric profile. *Clinical Neuropharmacology, 8*, 221–241.

Evans, R.W., Shear, P.K., & Gualtieri, C.T. (1985). *Neuropsychological test manual: Description of measures in use*. Chapel Hill, NC: Biological Sciences Research Center, University of North Carolina.

Friedhoff, A.J., Conners, C.K., Shader, R.I., Vaughn, H.G., & Zigler, E.F. (1987). Final Report: Investigation of Alleged Scientific Misconduct on Grants MH-32206 and MH-37449. Published by the National Institute of Mental Health, Department of Health & Human Services, April 28.

Gadow, K., & Loney, J. (1981). *Psychosocial aspects of drug treatment for hyperactivity*. Boulder, CO: Westview Press.

Geller, E., Ritvo, E.R., Freeman, B.J., & Yuwiler, A. (1982). Preliminary observations on the effect of fenfluramine on blood serotonin symptoms in three autistic boys. *New England Journal of Medicine, 307*, 165–169.

Gualtieri, C.T. (1986). Fenfluramine and autism: A careful reappraisal is in order. *Journal of Pediatrics, 108*(3), 417–419.

Gualtieri, C.T., & Evans, R.W. (1985, October). *New developments in pharmacotherapy of attention deficit disorder*. Annual Meeting of the American Academy of Child Psychiatry, San Antonio, TX.

Gualtieri, C.T., & Keppel, J.M. (1984). *NIMH funding priorities fiscal year 1983*. Unpublished manuscript.

Gualtieri, C.T., Schroeder, S.R., Hicks, R.E., & Quade, D. (1986). Tardive dyskinesia in the mentally retarded. *Archives of General Psychiatry, 43*, 335–340.

Gualtieri, C.T., Sprague, R.L., & Cole, J.O. (1986). Tardive dyskinesia litigation, and the dilemmas of neuroleptic treatment. *Psychiatry and the Law, 14, Spring/Summer,* 187–216.

Hill, B.K., Lakin, K.C., & Bruininks, R.H. (in press). Trends in residential sources for mentally retarded people: 1977–1982. *The Journal of the Association for People with Severe Handicaps.*

Lipman, R.S. (1970). The use of psychopharmacological agents in residential facilities for the retarded. In F. Menolascino (Ed.), *Psychiatric approaches to mental retardation* (pp. 387–398). New York: Basic Books.

Singer, C. (1983). *CBS News,* personal communication of information obtained from FDA Drug Use Analysis Branch, prescriptions written to retail pharmacies only.

# 16
# Orthomolecular Principles in Treatment of Persons with Mental Retardation and Mental Illness

RICHARD A. KUNIN

## Introduction

Orthomolecular psychiatry has been identified primarily with megavitamin therapy. This is an overly narrow definition that has been obsolete since even before 1968 when Linus Pauling (1968) identified orthomolecular psychiatry as the treatment of mental disorders by varying the concentrations of substances normally found in the human body or as Dr. Pauling states, "The right molecules in the right amounts" (p. 265).

## The Standing of Orthomolecular Psychiatry

The variety and complexity of orthomolecular treatments and their relation to demonstrable physiological mechanisms lead us to the realization that orthomolecular psychiatry represents one major professional stream of interest in the return to the medical model of mental illness. Osmond and Sigler (1974) have written extensively on the important psychological benefits that this medical approach brings to patients and their families.

The medical model provides diagnostic benefits as well, for the process of differential diagnosis is broadened and the examination and testing procedures are more comprehensive than in conventional psychiatry. Several recent studies have shown that the frequency of undiagnosed medical illness in psychiatric patients is higher than had been suspected. Gardner and Hall (1980) found that 80% of 105 consecutive voluntary admissions to a state psychiatric hospital had at least one previously undetected physical illness that required medical treatment. In 42% of the cases, previously undiagnosed medical illnesses were found to be causing the presenting psychiatric symptoms. The psychiatric disorder improved in almost half the patients when the medical illnesses were treated. A combination of history and physical examination, multiple chemistry panel (SMA-34), electrocardiogram, urinalysis, and sleep-derived electroencephalogram identified over 90% of all medical illnesses.

The return of the medical model in orthomolecular psychiatry restores the psychiatrist to the role of a complete physician. In addition, the orthomolecular identity confers a sense of respect for medical nutrition and thus prompts a higher quality of medical care than is currently practiced, even in many general hospitals. In fact, several studies (Butterworth, 1974) have shown that more than half of typical general hospital patients are likely to be suffering from hospital-induced malnutrition and a third exhibit some iatrogenic symptom caused by medication.

Progress in orthomolecular psychiatry has paralleled progress in neurochemstry, particularly the research into neurotransmitters and neuromodulators. Of the neurotransmitters, acetylcholine, serotonin, norepinephrine, and dopamine have been most heralded, but gamma-aminobutyric acid (GABA) is implicated in the anxiety disorders and is clearly related both to niacinamide and the benzoiazepines, which share the same receptor. Taurine, glutamic acid, glutamine, choline, inositol, adenosine, and aspartate are among the other recognized transmitters now under scrutiny as therapeutic agents. On the other hand, the physician must keep in mind that dose-dependent nerve cell damage has been observed with aspartate, glycine L-tryptophan, and monosodium glutamate.

There is now available information to assist in establishing specific diagnoses and an allied rational basis for the treatment of mental disorders. There are laboratory tests to identify nutrient and metabolic factors and at lower expense than was possible even a few years ago. It is possible to measure serum and urine levels of vitamins, minerals, and their related enzymes and urinary metabolites. Hair can be used as a biopsy material for detection of heavy metals, and the recent introduction of amino acid and essential fatty acid profiling promises to open new horizons in clinical practice and research (Kunin, 1986).

## Major Principles of Orthomolecular Psychiatry

The development of orthomolecular medicine and this author's experience in the field would seem to indicate that there are a number of basic principles in orthomolecular psychiatry that have a number of implications for this dually diagnosed population:

1. Good medicine requires careful attention to nutrition; it is the basis of sound and effective medical practice. Therefore, diagnostic screening of nutrient levels is justified in order to develop effective treatment programs.
2. If drug therapy needs to be used, clinicians need to be aware of adverse effects and the role that orthomolecular mechanisms may offer as both an antidote and a prevention approach.
3. Clinicians need to be knowledgeable about neurotoxins. The environmental pollution of food, water, and air is common, and a diagnostic search for eurotoxins is justified.

4. Do not judge central nervous system nutrition by blood levels of nutrients because they do not always match. Diagnostic indices may not always be sensitive enough to identify CNS nutritional levels via blood analyses.
5. The Recommended Daily Allowance designated by the Food and Nutrition Board may not be correct for the dually diagnosed individual. Each family and person is unique. In essence, we have no accepted standards of RDA for developmentally disabled individuals.
6. Nutrient-related disorders are usually reversible and amenable to treatment.
7. Orthomolecular approaches may also prevent, delay, or significantly ameliorate hereditary disorders.

## Model of Molecular Medicine

The diagram in Figure 16.1 presents Rudin's concept of *the fundamental reaction in nutrition*. Rudin views the syndrome of deficiency disease in a biochemical matrix of substrate, catalyst, and modulator, which produce structural and reactant products. Defective or deficient production of cellular constituents, including enzymes, membrane lipids, and prostaglandin hormones, accounts for illnesses.

Most of the illnesses have overlapping symptoms that can be viewed as mixtures of beriberi and pellagra; only the extreme cases look like the "classical" syndromes. The diagram clarifies why similar syndromes may respond in one case to substrate protein or lipid substance and in another to supplemental vitamins or minerals.

Extensive research has revealed a typical pattern of four basic abnormalities that occur as a result of a defective or deficient enzyme: (1) increased metabolites proximal to the block; (2) decreased metabolized distal to it; (3) increased metabolites via alternate pathways; and (4) increased requirement for vitamins (to deal with the abnormal biochemistry that is present).

## Nutritional Supplementation and the Mentally Retarded Individual

Recent research by Springer (1987) focused on 82 mentally retarded individuals who were transferred from a residential institution to foster care homes and were provided nutrition services as part of their individual program plans. Findings of the nutrition assessment and intervention were analyzed to document the impact of deinstitutionalization and nutrition services. Nutrition-related problems identified were closely associated with the medical problems. More than half of the clients were diagnosed as having seizures and cerebral palsy and were therefore at high nutritional risk because of feeding problems and anticonvulsant-induced malnutrition. Forty-three of these 47 individuals who were reassessed showed

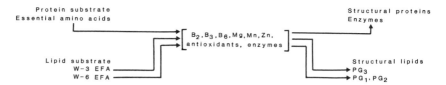

FIGURE 16.1. Rudin's concept of the fundamental reaction in nutrition.

positive changes in height, weight, triceps, skinfold thickness, dietary adequacy, and/or biochemical indices.

In a double-blind study, Harrell et al. (1981) treated children with mental retardation or Down's syndrome with megavitamins. Her findings were especially dramatic because the improvements were tangible, including improvement in vision, growth, and IQ test performance. Controversy has persisted over these findings and though some reported studies fail to confirm them, Bennett et al. (1983) asserted that compliance with nutrient supplements in these failures was not monitored.

## Neurotoxicity and Neurobehavioral Effects

The National Research Council estimates that human beings are exposed to some 53,000 distinct chemicals in the form of pesticides, drugs, food additives, cosmetics, and commercial substances each year. Almost none are tested for their neurobehavioral effects. The federal government through its National Institute for Occupational Health and Safety has set occupational standards for only 588 chemicals. Of these, only 167 (or 28%) are regulated because of the effects they have on the central nervous system, often discovered after they have produced significantly disabling side effects.

Most disturbing about this entire process is that we seem to react rather vigorously to chemicals that cause physical deformities, yet we seem to be remiss in our efforts to develop an effective program to alleviate toxins that lead to subtle neurological damage over decades of exposure. For example, studies have shown that children exposed to moderate levels of lead score 5 IQ points lower than children exposed to little or no lead. Although this may not seem like much, statistically, this would represent a decrease by almost 50% of those individuals with an IQ of 130 or above who are considered to be in the gifted classification range (i.e., 2 standard deviations above the mean).

The awareness that chemicals can poison our nervous system has been known for a long time. For example, the neurotoxic effects of lead have been documented before the time of Christ and the side effect of mercury ingestion was noted over four centuries ago. Despite this knowledge, it was not until the early 1970s that the federal government began to reduce the level of lead allowed in gasoline. Because of these adverse findings on the research of children's intellectual functioning, the level of lead in gasoline has dropped by 90% in 1987. It is well known from the studies of David et al. (1976) that hyperactivity and learning disability in children without an obvious diagnosis is caused by lead toxicity in at least half the cases.

Needleman and Barrett (1979) have provided convincing evidence that low-level lead exposure is more toxic than had originally been believed. The generally recognized toxic blood level has been lowered from 80 μg per 100 ml to less than half that, and intellectual impairments are now recognized at under 20 μg per 100 ml. The hair test for heavy metals and lead should be a standard procedure in every pediatric evaluation, particularly up to age 6 years.

Many studies confirm the fact that childhood undernutrition, particularly low intake of iron, calcium, and protein, permits greater damage from lead exposure. It is comforting to review Papaioannou, Sohler, and Pfeiffer's study (1978) of orthomolecular treatment of industrial lead exposure: The administration of zinc and ascorbic acid was followed by a lowering of blood lead in workers in a battery plant—despite continued exposure to lead. Pyridoxine has demonstrable antilead activity. Regunathan and Sundoresan (1983) found that lead reduced rat brain synthesis of GABA and glutamine. However, when pyridoxal phosphate was administered with lead, synthesis of these amino acids was increased over the control level in the cerebellum and brainstem but not the cerebral cortex. When given without lead, $B_6$ increased GABA, glutamic acid, and glutamine in the cerebral cortex as well. Further research on toxic effects of such pollutants as lead, cadmium, mercury, and their nutritional implications for individuals with mental retardation can be found in a comprehensive chapter by Davis (1987).

## Clinical History

An example of orthomolecular treatment involves the case of Liz, who was 15 years old when her parents first brought her for orthomolecular consultation in 1975. She had been severely mentally retarded since here first year of life. After an uneventful pregnancy and normal vaginal delivery here parents suspected abnormality when she couldn't crawl at 6 months, had cupping of her right hand, and did not look normal. She said only one word at 15 months and had a vocabulary of about 50 words at age 4, at which time she was also found to have seizures consisting of staring and eye blinking. The electroencephalogram was abnormal, with three per-second spikes, and she was treated with various anticonvulsants and finally maintained on diazepam (20 mg/day). On psychometrics, she tested between 45 and 80 IQ, and she was at the third-grade level in reading and math at age 15 years.

The administration of simple multivitamin supplements was followed by improved concentration and cooperation. She was better able to sit still, and she seemed more cheerful according to her parents' report. Niacin at low dose (i.e., under 100 mg and sufficient to cause a skin flush) made here tantrums worse. Higher doses, however, up to 1000 mg which suppressed the flush response, seemed to relax her. Carbohydrate restriction was beneficial, and she seemed best at an intake of only 15 to 30 g of carbohydrate per day. In ketosis she had no seizures and her speech improved.

After three months, she was observed to be better at school and more affectionate at home. Tantrums completely stopped, and she began talking all the time and participating in conversation for the first time in her life. Her menstrual period also became regular for the first time.

A relapse of tantrums and overaggressive behavior occurred when her mother mistakenly served her a quart of orange juice daily, thus raising her carbohydrate intake to well over 100 g. When this was lowered, she again regained her improvement and, in the course of the next year, graduated the special education program and began to work as a teacher's aide in the program. At this point, the addition of low-dose lithium (150 mg twice a day) seemed to cap the orthomolecular regimen. We claim lithium as an orthomolecular treatment, although it is used clinically as a megadose therapy in the affective disorders. Lithium is a trace mineral, at microgram levels in nature, although it is not used at microgram levels in the therapeutic approaches of modern psychiatry. Indeed, we are all participants in "megamedicine:" Strong agents and larger doses are commonly used. In any case, the lithium yielded further improvements in calmness and control in this case.

Liz also had a hereditary anemia, which was diagnosed as thalassemia minor. Her initial hemoglobin was 10.3 g, and the mean corpuscular volume (MCV) was 62 (normal would be 83 to 95 or 100, depending on the lab normals). A hair test for minerals was performed, and it was low in copper, manganese, folic acid, and cyanocobalamin. After three months of treatment, her mean corpuscular volume increased to 76 micra and her hemoglobin went to 11.7 from 10.2 g. So here is a hereditary disorder that was sensitive to the nutritional status and measurable not only as behavioral improvement but also as improvement in the hematological indices.

Hemoglobin electrophoresis demonstrated a 5% abnormal hemoglobin Type A-2, typical of thalassemia minor. Her father was tested and found to have the same 5% abnormality, yet he did not exhibit cognitive deficits, which was probably caused by a hemolytic crisis in her infancy, with microemboli, free radical damage owing to the release of unbound iron, and poor oxygen transport owing to the anemia. Why was her father spared and she afflicted? After carefully reviewing her history, I conclude the crucial factor is that she was a formula-fed baby, on condensed milk, corn syrup, and canned baby foods from birth. Since she was a 1960 baby, she was probably low in Vitamin E and $B_6$ as well as taurine and alpha linolenic acid (a prime source of Omega 3 fatty acids), which we now know are essential to brain development. Her father was an Italian, first-born son, nursed on human breast milk, and grown to be a brilliant and successful consultant on the doctoral level.

I think this brief case history exemplifies several orthomolecular principles: (1) that hereditary disorders are often responsive to nutrient support and (2) that no medicine is good medicine without serious attention to nutrition.

# Tardive Dyskinesia

An excellent example of the role of orthomolecular psychiatry in the treatment of dually diagnosed individuals can be found in tardive dyskinesia. Tardive dyskinesia is a movement disorder, frequently caused by the toxic effects of psychotropic drug therapy. In 1975, I reported good results in the treatment of 15 cases of tardive and withdrawal dyskinesia by the use of manganese and/or niacin. Although this series lacked a control group and blind design, it did have validity in that most of the patients had failed to recover normal extrapyramidal movement function for months or years preceding treatment with manganese. In 13 of the 15 cases (87%), treatment benefits were seen within five days and recovery was complete in seven cases—that's about half—in that time. Only one of these original cases out of the 15 was totally unresponsive to manganese. There were four cases of literally overnight cure.

At the advice of Dr. Abram Hoffer, I reviewed the manganese levels in my first 15 cases and found that in eight cases of prompt recovery, the average manganese in the hair was 0.52; in six cases that were merely improved the average of manganese was 0.4; and in the one case that was unimproved after manganese treatment, the hair test showed 0.2. This seemed to verify a relationship between the lack of manganese in the hair and increasing severity of dyskinesia.

There are real grounds to hypothesize that manganese administration might prevent or reduce the occurrence of dyskinesia of withdrawal or tardive dyskinesia, either or both. And the administration of manganese along with neuroleptics might prevent dyskinesia.

Much attention has been given to the use of acetylcholine precursors, such as deanol, choline, and lecithin, in treating drug-induced dyskinesias. However, these are cumbersome and expensive, and they require large doses. Manganese treatment is probably at least as effective and considerably cheaper. Divided doses of 10 to 30 mg of elemental manganese are usually adequate. It is safe by the oral route, and larger doses may be tried up to 100 or 200 mg. Human manganese toxicity is rare because of the carrier protein, transmagnin. If more extensive and better-controlled studies confirm these initial observations, it may be that nontoxic manganese is the treatment of choice in the neuroleptic drug-induced dyskinesis.

I might add that phenothiazines are chelating agents for manganese and copper. Manganese, in particular, forms a complex with acetylcholine and is an integral part, through its valence changes, in the storage and release of acetylcholine. In other words, the dyskinesia may be due to a localized deficiency of manganese, induced by chelation in situ by the phenothiazine.

# Conclusion

There is no need here to review and debate the merits of megavitamin therapy in psychiatry, in general, or mental retardation, in particular. Whether or not we can agree that benefits are demonstrable by statistical evaluation of double-blind control studies, the fact is that individual cases, albeit anecdotal, are well known to give evidence of treatment benefits. I do not think that any of us who are experienced clinicians want to deny any possible benefits to our patients.

In conclusion, we need far more research with nutrients in treating mental retardation and mental illness. I do not believe there is a disagreement over the fact that some retarded and mentally ill patients do respond favorably to orthomolecular treatment. The pressing need is to identify the responders. Hence, diagnostic search and therapeutic trial of various orthomolecular treatment strategies are indicated.

## References

Bennett, F.C., McClelland, S., Kriegsmann, E.A., Andrus, L.B., & Sells, C.J. (1983). Vitamin and mineral supplementation in Down's syndrome. *Pediatrics, 72*(5), 707–713.

Butterworth, C.E. (1974). Malnutrition in the hospital. *JAMA, 230,* 879.

David, O.J., Hoffman, S.P., Sverd, J., Clark, J., & Voeller, K. (1976). Lead and hyperactivity: Behavioral response to chelation. *American Journal of Psychiatry, 133,* 1155–1158.

Davis, D. (1987). Nutritional therapy in the prevention and reversal of mental retardation. In F.J. Menolascino & J.A. Stark (Eds.), *Preventive and curative intervention in mental retardation.* Baltimore, MD: Paul H. Brookes Publishing Company.

Gardner, E.R., & Hall, R.C.W. (1980). Medical screening of psychiatric patients. *Journal of Orthomolecular Psychiatry, 9,* 207–215.

Harrell, R.F., Capp, R.J., Davis, D.R., Peerless, J., & Ravitz, L.R. (1981). Can nutritional supplements help mentally retarded children? An exploratory study. *Proceedings of the National Academy of Sciences, USA, 78*(1), 574–578.

Kunin, R.A. (1986). Orthomolecular psychiatry. In R. Heumer, *The roots of molecular medicine.* New York: W.H. Freeman Company.

Needleman, H.L., & Barrett, P. (1979). Lead toxicity: Deficits in psychologic and classroom performance of children with elevated dentine lead levels. *New England Journal of Medicine, 300,* 689.

Osmond, H., & Siegler, M. (1974). *Models of madness, models of medicine.* New York: Macmillan.

Papaioannou, R., Sohler, A., & Pfeiffer, C.C. (1978). Reduction of blood lead levels in battery workers by zinc and vitamin C. *Journal of Orthomolecular Psychiatry, 7,* 94–106.

Pauling, L. (1968). Orthomolecular psychiatry. *Science, 160,* 265–271.

Regunathan, S., & Sundoresan, R. (1983). Incorporation of $^{14}C$ from glucose into amino acids in brain in vitro. *Life Sciences, 33,* 2277–2282.

Springer, N.S. (1987). From institution to foster care: Impact of nutritional status. *American Journal of Mental Deficiency, 91*(4), 321–327.

# 17
# Balanced Treatment and Assessment Approaches

JOHNNY L. MATSON

The issue of emotional disorders in mentally retarded persons, like many problems in this group of persons, has only recently begun to receive the attention it deserves. There have been periodic pleas for assessment, treatment, and program development for some time. There are a few programs, notably those at the University of Nebraska, University of Illinois at Chicago, and Louisiana State University, which emphasize both training and clinical service. Given the small number of programs available, however, little in the way of practical results has occurred on a national scale (Matson, 1985b). Having said this, it is also worth noting that sufficient research has been done to suggest the serious nature of the problem. A few examples should be sufficient to exemplify the situation. Pollock (1944) found that among 444 mentally retarded persons admitted to New York State hospitals in 1942, over 40% were deemed to be psychotic. Similarly, Dewan (1948) reported that 47% of the Canadian army recruits diagnosed as mentally retarded were also suffering from emotional problems. These two studies involved adult populations, but children have also been identified in large numbers. Rutter, Graham, and Yule (1970) found that the incidence of emotional problems in children was five to six times that observed in the general population in their now classic British study, the Isle of Wight. Similarly, Chazan (1964), who assessed mildly mentally retarded children, found the rates of emotional problems to be considerably greater than that seen in the overall population of children. One could argue the methodology of particular studies, or specific rates noted in the various studies mentioned and others that have been performed. However, the serious and widespread nature of the problem cannot be denied. Given these findings, there is no doubt that a great deal of empirical research is warranted. It becomes crucial, given limited resources, as to what some of the areas for study might be.

It is argued that one area worthy of attention is depression of mentally retarded children and adults. So far, the primary focus of research on depression in the mentally retarded has been on adults. Depression is called the common cold of emotional disorders given its frequent occurrence. Similarly, the topic has been a high priority of funding in NIMH, but not with persons who exhibit deficits in mental functioning that would characterize them as mentally retarded. It is suggested that further efforts with this group are certainly warranted, and the problem in mentally retarded children will be used to exemplify this situation.

This group is viewed as particularly crucial since early identification may head off even more serious episodes. Prevention has been a major focus of funding for mental retardation, particularly in NICHD, but primarily before birth, and certainly not with respect to mental health needs. With early detection, we may be able to treat emotional problems, such as depression, before the disorders become too well established in the person's daily living. And while little has been done on the topic until recently, the general child field, excluding mentally retarded children, has seen such an interest as to provide enough material for entire books on the topic, with most of this research having been done in the last 10 years (Cantwell & Carlson, 1983). Initially, a very broad list of symptoms had been used to describe the syndrome. Thus, symptoms such as dysphoric mood, irritability and weepiness, low self-esteem, self-depreciation, hopelessness, suicidal ideation, morbid ideas, disturbed concentration, social withdrawal, and fatigue were identified. Also, indirect symptoms, such as some types of aggression, were described as characteristic of childhood depression. Recent research suggests that a group of depressed children can clearly be delineated, particularly when a battery of measures including systematic structured interviews and standard evaluation methods are combined, at least with children of normal intelligence (Carlson & Cantwell, 1980; Kazdin, 1981; Matson & Nieminen, 1987; Petti, 1978).

Unfortunately, mentally retarded children have been almost completely ignored. This group constitutes approximately 3% of all children, and perhaps as much as 10 to 15% of the total population of emotionally disturbed children, given the much higher rate of emotional problems in mentally retarded children when compared to the population at large (Rutter et al., 1970).

While a proven and overwhelming need exists, no studies to date have been conducted that would establish viable treatments or methods of identifying depression in mentally retarded children. There are probably several reasons for this state of affairs. Briefly, a few possible explanations will be noted.

One hypothesis as to the general lack of study is the presumption by many mental health professionals that these handicapped persons did not have sufficient ego strength or cognitive ability to develop emotional problems. We now know that such a formulation was incorrect, given studies that show severe emotional problems in even the most profoundly mentally retarded individuals (Reid, 1980). Thus, genetic and environmental factors are most likely very important in accounting for many of the emotional problems of this group; these etiological variables probably account for many forms of emotional problems in these individuals (Matson, 1985a). Thus, biological precursors, chemical imbalances, environmental events, and chronicity of the emotional behavior might be factors better associated with the understanding of these problems.

A second factor that seems to be problematic is the general lack of interest shown by university faculty who are training the leaders in the mental health field. It is uncommon for child psychiatrists or clinical child psychologists to have any formal training within the area of mental retardation. As a result, many professionals are unaware of the serious nature or general lack of services with this group. Oftentimes, they even express surprise that this unique group of people requires specialized services. The fact that NIMH funds for mental retardation have been less than one-tenth of 1% of their total research budget further underlines this problem. This situation is compounded by the general perception that these persons are unlikely to change via therapy, that they somehow do not have feelings and emotions, or that existing technology and services are sufficient. A third and related issue is diagnostic overshadowing (Reiss & Szyszko, 1983). This term implies that many professionals are unable to diagnose differentially emotional disturbance and mental retardation. They are, in fact, likely to attribute many aspects of psychopathology to mental retardation, and, unfortunately, this phenomenon has been replicated across various professional groups. This latter point has most certainly led to an underidentification of this problem, further adding to the general assumption that nothing needs to be done.

Despite these factors, many concerned individuals in a number of professions have recognized the importance of treating this problem. Typical of this are self-injurious behavior, which many professionals incorrectly identify as being symptomatic of mental retardation rather than emotional disorder. It is now imperative that research program implementation for emotional difficulties of mentally retarded children begin. It is also important to recognize that mental health concerns with children are not merely a downward extension of emotional disorders with adults. Children have unique needs, and research is showing that the way emotional distress is exhibited may differ from that seen in adults, and even across age groups in children.

It is likely that depression in mentally retarded children is high, given what has been found regarding this emotional problem with the overall population of children (Cantwell & Carlson, 1983). Unfortunately, the available data tends to be indirect. *There are no assessment or treatment studies published on depression in mentally retarded children.* Rather, indirect support has been derived from research on depressed mentally retarded adults (Matson, Kazdin, & Senatore, 1984) and children without mental retardation (Cantwell & Carlson, 1983). However, in the latter case only one treatment study using a single-case research design with one child was published (Frame, Matson, Sonis, Fialkov, & Kazdin, 1982). Thus, research of this type with mentally retarded children is urgently needed. Suicide and severely debilitating affect are not unknown and should seriously be considered. Obviously, the provision of appropriate clinical services should also be a key issue. However, how can we provide treatment if we do not know how to identify the afflicted group or how to treat them effectively? Thus, assessment and related differential diagnosis research must be a first step.

Several issues need to be considered in future research if we are to learn how to deal effectively with the emotional problems of mentally retarded persons. Given that depression is a widespread problem in the general population and no research has been done with mentally retarded children evincing this problem, it would seem to be an important, even critical, area for study. What specifically do we need to know? First, a quantitative description of depression in these handicapped persons must be determined. We can establish this only by using a variety of tests of depression. These measures should cut across theoretical lines given that such behavior surely involved biological and social environmental factors.

This approach will not only help us understand what symptoms best characterize depression in these persons, but what instruments are best and most efficient in making this evaluation, and under what conditions. Work with the Psychopathology Instrument for Mentally Retarded Adults (Matson et al., 1984) is one example, albeit with adults, that would seem to encourage more work of this sort. Similarly, the DEX test and other chemical measures may prove to be useful, particularly with individuals with no or very poor verbal skills. Along these same lines, we need to know how age, sex, and intellectual ability result in differing patterns of depression and identifiable symptoms. This topic has been explained elsewhere on a psychosocial, biological model of psychopathology of the mentally retarded (Matson, 1985a). Other demographic variables such as the etiology of the person's mental retardation, the social support available, and other related factors may also prove to be very important. These are empirical questions, however, and can only be derived through extensive study. Several possibilities exist. The Child Depression Inventory (Kovacs & Beck, 1977) is one instrument that has had broad use. Other possibilities are the Child Depression Scale (Reynolds, 1981), Bellevue Index of Depression (Kazdin, French, & Unis, 1983; Petti, 1978), Kiddie SADS (Puig-Antich, Orvaschel, Tabrizi, & Chambers, 1980), and the Aberrant Behavior Checklist (Aman, Singh, Stewart, & Field, 1985) to name a few. Each of these instruments has been used successfully with the general population of children. Other procedures and instruments are also likely to prove beneficial but the instruments just noted have already been demonstrated to have some viability in various experimental trials with depressed children without mental retardation. An assessment study of this type to determine systematic ways of identifying the problem is a possible step.

Treatment research is also of paramount importance. It would be optimal, given a perfect world, if we could wait for the implementation of treatment protocols until adequate assessment procedures had been developed. Unfortunately, we do not have this luxury. With the development of effective differential diagnosis methods, treatment should definitely begin to be studied even more extensively. Some of the methods that are likely to prove effective (many of which are cited in the chapters in Section V and by Dr. Gardner, Chapter 14) are behavior therapy procedures of various types, particularly those that train parents as cotherapists so they could serve as active partners in the process. Such an approach should have the added advantages of decreasing the expense of treatment while involving parents as active collaborators and decision-makers. These procedures must include parent training components and assistance from school personnel to ensure the broadest possible generalization of treatment effects. Emphasis on enhancing these interactions will most certainly increase the generalization of treatment effects to the widest variety of persons and settings.

Furthermore, procedures of this sort have been shown to be effective with children in general, including those with developmental disabilities (Altman & Mira, 1983).

Antidepressant medications may also be called for, particularly if the children are approaching or in their teenage years. However, establishing drugs that are particularly safe at the minimum dosages would seem to be greatly needed. Furthermore, we know that learning to cope in one's environment is important and that drugs do not teach new behavior. Therefore, determining the best combinations of pharmacological and behavioral treatment is important. Studies of this issue have been rare indeed. Other treatments may also be useful, and if they seem plausible, they should be studied.

The description of the assessment and treatment procedures noted here suggest another important issue, better collaboration of professionals. Psychologists, psychiatrists, social workers, and other health professionals, regardless of theoretical orientation, must collaborate where possible (see also Gualtieri, Chapter 15). Efforts of this sort are long overdue and should prove to be of considerable value in improving the quality of life for many mentally retarded persons and their families. The leadership of noted professionals, advocates, and the major federal funding agencies are all needed if the effort is to be a successful one. It is time to look seriously at these neglected groups and begin to provide the types of services that may prove useful in enhancing the quality of life for these doubly handicapped persons, who have for so long been deprived of adequate care.

## References

Altman, K., & Mira, M. (1983). Training parents of developmentally disabled children. In J.L. Matson & F. Andrasik (Eds.), *Treatment issues and innovations in mental retardation*. New York: Plenum Press.

Aman, M.G., Singh, N.N., Stewart, A.W., & Field, C.J. (1985). Psychometric characteristics of the Aberrant Behavior Checklist. *American Journal of Mental Deficiency, 89*, 485–491.

Cantwell, D.P., & Carlson, G.A. (1983). *Affective disorders in childhood and adolescence: An update*. Jamaica, NY: Spectrum Publications.

Carlson, G.A., & Cantwell, D.P. (1980). A survey of depressive symptoms, syndrome and disorder in a child psychiatric population. *Journal of Child Psychology, Psychiatry and Allied Disciplines, 21*, 19–25.

Chazan, M. (1964). The incidence and nature of maladjustment among children in schools for the educationally subnormal. *British Journal of Educational Psychology, 34*, 292–304.

Dewan, J.G. (1948). Intelligence and emotional stability. *American Journal of Psychiatry, 104*, 548–554.

Frame, C., Matson, J.C., Sonis, W.A., Fialkov, M.J., & Kazdin, A.E. (1982). Behavioral treatment of depression in a prepubertal child. *Journal of Behavior Therapy and Experimental Psychiatry, 13*, 239–243.

Kazdin, A.E. (1981). Assessment techniques for childhood depression: A critical appraisal. *Journal of the American Academy of Child Psychiatry, 4*, 213–222.

Kazdin, A.E., French, N.H., & Unis, A.S. (1983). Child, mother and father evaluations of depression in psychiatric inpatient children. *Journal of Abnormal Child Psychology, 11*, 167–180.

Kovacs, M., & Beck, A.T. (1977). An empirical clinical approach towards a definition of childhood depression. In J.G. Schulterbrandt & A. Raskin (Eds.), *Depression in children*. New York: Raven Press.

Matson, J.L. (1985a). Biosocial theory of psychopathology: A three by three factor model. *Applied Research in Mental Retardation, 6*, 199–227.

Matson, J.L. (1985b). Emotional problems in the mentally retarded: The need for assessment and treatment. *Psychopharmacology Bulletin, 21*, 258–261.

Matson, J.L, Kazdin, A.E., & Senatore, V. (1984). Psychometric properties of the psychopathology instrument for mentally retarded adults. *Applied Research in Mental Retardation, 5*, 81–89.

Matson, J.L., & Nieminen, G.S. (1987). A validity study of measures of depression, conduct disorder and anxiety. *Journal of Clinical Child Psychology, 16*, 151–157.

Petti, T.A. (1978). Depression in hospitalized child psychiatric patients: Approaches to measuring depression. *Journal of the American Academy of Child Psychiatry, 17*, 49–59.

Pollack, H.M. (1944). Mental disease among mental defectives. *American Journal of Psychiatry, 191*, 361.

Puig-Antich, J., Orvaschel, H., Tabrizi, M.A., & Chambers, W. (1980). *The schedule for affective disorders and schizophrenia in school-age children: Epidemiological version (Kiddie-SADS-E)* (3rd ed.). New York: New York State Psychiatric Institute.

Reid, H.H. (1980). Diagnosis of psychiatric disorder in the severely and profoundly retarded patient. *Journal of the Royal Society of Medicine, 73*, 607–609.

Reiss, S.M., & Szyszko, J. (1983). Diagnostic overshadowing and professional experience with mentally retarded persons. *American Journal of Mental Deficiency, 87*, 396–402.

Reynolds, W.M. (1981). *Development and validation of a scale to measure depression in adolescents*. Madison, WI: University of Wisconsin. Unpublished manuscript.

Rutter, M., Graham, P., & Yule, W.A. (1970). *Neuropsychiatric study in childhood*. (Clinics in Developmental Medicine, Nos. 35/36.) London: SIMP/Heinemann.

# 18
## Issues Related to Applied
## Behavioral Analysis

JOHN J. McGEE

## Introduction

A fundamental challenge in the care and treatment of persons with persistent aggressive and self-injurious behaviors is to help them learn new means of interacting with others. Caregivers need to move away from the application of punishment and toward the teaching of bonding. Punishment is a common practice in the treatment of persons with severe behavioral challenges such as persistent aggression and self-injury (Baumeister & Rollings, 1976; Favell & Greene, 1981; Gardner & Cole, 1985). To move away from punitive practices, caregivers need to adopt a liberating posture toward persons with these needs and one that is based on a range of gentle teaching techniques. The goal of treatment becomes bonding rather than submission. This goal requires a substantive rejection of current behavioral practices and a critical analysis of how the values of the caregiver influence the behavioral change process. The challenge is not simply to eliminate maladaptive behavior, but to create new values in ourselves and the people whom we serve.

Bonding is the goal of gentle teaching. Punishment and submission are the antithesis of bonding. Bonding is the humanizing social attachment that must evolve between the caregiver and the person with severe behavioral problems. It is the establishment of reciprocal lines of communication between the caregiver and the person. Bonding results in mutually humanizing and liberating interactions. It develops affectional ties that lead to a mutual give and take between the caregiver and the person with special needs. The caregiver becomes a teacher of reward, and the behaviorally challenging person becomes a learner of new interactional behaviors.

## Role of Techniques

Techniques must be considered as secondary to human values (Freire, 1980). Techniques are tools and are generally neutral; their value and usefulness depend on our posture toward ourselves and toward others (McGee, 1984). If a caregiver wants to gain submission, any technique will do. Of if a caregiver has not questioned his or her beliefs and values, then techniques are seen as an end in themselves. But if a caregiver wants to teach bonding, it is important to select techniques coherent with our values and beliefs. How caregivers intervene is as important as why they intervene (Patterson & Reid, 1970). Punishment is a technique that is inherently corrupting for both the caregiver and the person with special needs.

A humanizing and liberating posture can give techniques life and meaning. They are the observable actions that reflect our values, ideals, and goals. In combination, they provide the responses to the moment to moment challenges that caregivers face and, as such, they communicate to the learner who we are and what we represent (Bijou & Dunitz-Johnson, 1981). As we focus on the interactions between the caregiver and the learner, intervention techniques should primarily serve to make mutually humanizing relationships possible. The underlying purpose of any intervention in the life of a person with severe behavioral problems should be to teach reward sharing, that is, to teach the person that human presence and participation have meaning. Techniques are therefore not only a reflection of our posture but also a representation of ourselves to the person as part of an interactional process. We call this process gentle teaching.

## Gentle Teaching Paradigm

In our work with over 540 mentally retarded persons with severe behavioral problems over the past 5 years, our basic pedagogical approach has been to teach value sharing (Casey, McGee, Stark, & Menolascino, 1985). We have used this approach with a range of severely disruptive and destructive behaviors, such as persistent aggression and self-injurious behaviors (Menolascino & McGee, 1983). In this process, there is a substantive emphasis on an ongoing questioning of the caregiver's posture and how this posture determines the goal of intervention. In observing the postures of caregivers, we have seen three typical types that require critical questioning. The first is an overprotective posture that victimizes the person and results in little growth. The second is an authoritarian posture that results in the punishment of a person in order to eliminate maladaptive behaviors. The third is a mechanistic posture that values compliance to rules but leaves the person devoid of any feeling of solidarity with the caregiver. It is the caregiver's posture that defines the type of intervention techniques to be used. A caregiver with an overprotective posture will place little demands on the person. At best, this results in a benevolent form of custodial care. An authoritarian posture might eliminate behavioral problems, but it leaves the person devoid of human feelings. A mechanistic posture is cold and values only conformity to rules and norms but does little to teach the giving and sharing of humanizing feelings. A posture of solidarity focuses on the interactional nature of human behaviors. It places the initial challenge of behavioral change on the caregiver and requires tolerance, warmth, and affection. It recognizes that the caregiver is, above all, a teacher of reward.

Our posture and goals mandate that reward must not only occur frequently, but that it be the primary focus of all interactions between the teacher and the learner. Ignoring, redirecting, and teaching reward enable a posture of solidarity to be expressed to the person. By using these techniques, maladaptive interactions can be rechanneled into rewarding interactions (see Fig. 18.1).

Reward is the primary focus for all techniques in gentle teaching because it allows us to teach the value of human presence and participation. The other components of the paradigm are secondary to reward in that they are used to make reward possible. In this sense, ignoring and redirection provide respectful, nonpunitive, and humanizing responses to maladaptive interactions and help refocus all interactions toward reward. Thus, the paradigm is used as our response to challenging behaviors. It helps direct both the teacher's and the learner's responses to more positive and mutually rewarding interactions.

The ignore–redirect–reward process is the most basic strategy used in gentle teaching. These three components are not separate steps or strategies that occur

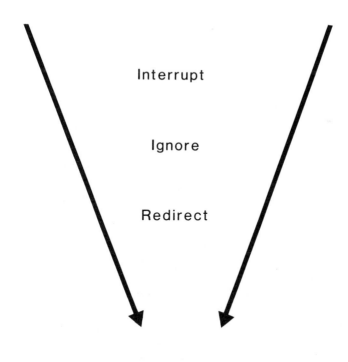

Interrupt

Ignore

Redirect

Reward

FIGURE 18.1. Gentle teaching paradigm.

TABLE 18.1. Components, purposes, and traits of gentle teaching.

| Components | Purposes | Traits |
|---|---|---|
| Ignore | To defuse | Act as if not occurring; no eye contact; minimal physical contact; continuation of teaching; do not increase proximity |
| Interrupt | To prevent harm | Minimally intrusive; nonreactive; continuation of teaching; ensuring safety; should defuse, not intensify |
| Redirect | To communicate options; to communicate reward is available | Nonverbal; reinstating interaction |
| Reward | To teach meaning, accepting, giving, sharing | Nonpunitive; respectful; active; leading to equity |

in isolation or in a rigid sequence. They are nearly concurrent steps that are best considered as a single process. They indicate that all caregiver interactions should lead to human valuing. In practice, it is often difficult to separate the specific components of a response into each of the three categories. The response is generally a fluid motion that accomplishes several purposes and has several characteristics and effects. The descriptions, purposes, and characteristics of each component should be viewed from this perspective (see Table 18.1).

## Ignore

In gentle teaching, "ignore" means avoiding or minimizing the attention, interaction, or other responses that occur after a maladaptive interaction. For example, if a person stands up at his or her desk in a classroom, the typical response might be to tell the person to sit down. If a person throws an object, most people feel it is necessary for that person to retrieve the thrown object. If a person says that he or she refuses to engage in a particular task, activity, or interaction, a frequent response is to try to verbally convince the person why he or she should engage in the activity (with severe consequences often following the frustration of such a debate). If a person swears, a verbal reprimand can be expected. If a person hits a caregiver, some form of negative consequence typically occurs and is often written into program policies and procedures—from loss of privileges to suspension or expulsion. These responses are typical. They consistently occur among caregivers and in all settings. By responding in this fashion, we give each of these maladaptive responses value and power; each occurrence of these behaviors results in a consistent response from us. The purpose of "ignore" is to defuse these and other undesirable responses and to take away their power in interactions between the caregiver and the person. The interaction and attention, the physical approach, and the increased eye contact and communication that typically occur after these responses need to be avoided or minimized, while at the same time continuing to bring about participation so that reward can be given.

There are several characteristics involved in ignoring maladaptive behaviors. These include withholding verbal responses, reprimands, threats, scoldings, and statements of rules or consequences that will occur. There are generally no positive, negative, or neutral verbalizations. Eye contact, physical contact, or other nonverbal communications or interactions are also avoided. The caregiver should avoid any physical, verbal, or gestural confrontation as a result of a maladaptive behavior. In effect, caregivers need to act as if the behavior has not occurred.

Ignoring does not mean that all interactions should stop. It is not synonymous with extinction, where all interaction stops until the behavior no longer occurs, or time-out, where the person is removed from the learning environment. Instead, the caregiver acts as if the response is not occurring and continues teaching. It does not mean that the caregiver does nothing (with an implicit corollary that the behavior is allowed to continue). Instead, the emphasis is on avoiding interactional responses to undesirable behaviors and redirecting the person to interactions that can be valued. At times, a reaction is impossible to avoid, such as when a person startles the caregiver by screaming. In these situations, the key is to minimize the reaction, avoiding emotional responses as much as possible and immediately returning to the teaching activity.

## Interrupt

Interruption is a corollary to the ignore phase of the paradigm since it is not always possible to withhold or minimize our attention and interaction after a person's undesirable responses. Occasionally, it is necessary to interrupt behaviors if they are potentially harmful. It is obvious that the caregiver must respond if a person is about to cause harm to self, to others in the environment, or even to property. In these situations, the person's responses are interrupted in as ignoring a manner as possible. The purpose of interruption should be to prevent harm or injury to the person or others or to prevent damage or destruction of property. Interruption has nothing to do with punishment or with the common practices reported under euphemistic terms such as "forced relaxation" or "overcorrection" (Foxx & Azrin, 1973). Its purpose is to prevent harm and to continue redirecting.

Most often, harmful behaviors can be prevented. Caregivers need to anticipate potentially dangerous responses before they occur. Interruption occurs not only to terminate injurious responses but also to prevent these responses before injury or damage occurs. When an object is thrown through a window the first time, it may not be possible to anticipate or interrupt this behavior. However, after the first occurrence, throwing can and should be anticipated and prevented. Most violence occurs after clear indications. Caregivers need to be alert and caring enough to pick up on these indicators, and redirect the person before violence or harm occurs. Many current practices result in violence. The goal is not to prevent harm, but to overcome the person who is attempting to harm themself or others (Watson, Owen, & Uzzell, 1980).

Interruption has several characteristics. First, it should be done in as minimally intrusive a manner as possible. Interruption should be carried out calmly with the idea of immediately redirecting the person toward a rewardable interaction. The caregiver must learn to control the typical emotional reactions of startle, fear, or anger, including all verbal and nonverbal communications that are a part of these reactions. As soon as potentially destructive behaviors decrease, the previous interaction should continue. Interruption should not terminate the teaching activities that were occurring prior to the interruption. The goal should be to refocus the interaction toward rewarding interactions. Preventive and interruptive actions should be terminated as soon as possible so that the balance of the interactions can be rewarding in nature. The caregiver should refocus the interaction on the teaching activity so that a rewardable response can occur. Finally, interruption should defuse the response and not intensify it. If negative consequences are given for negative behaviors, the caregiver is actually allowing those behaviors to change his or her posture and goal. Interruption involves a degree of interaction, and often includes minimal physical contact. Because of these characteristics, there is the potential that interruption may, in fact, reinforce the undesirable response, causing it to intensify and occur more frequently. As a result, the use of interruption requires sensitive monitoring and should be a rare event. It should be used only momentarily to avoid injury to and ensure the safety of the person. Other strategies should be used whenever possible. Interruption is not a technique that is used in isolation. It is a corollary component in the paradigm of ignore–redirect–reward in order to prevent harm.

When to use interruption is not always an easy decision. In some cases, it is difficult to decide whether to ignore a behavior or to interrupt it. Specific rules of application for specific types of behavior cannot be made; for example, always use interruption for head banging. Instead, this decision involves a judgment about the intensity of the behavior and whether harm will result. The caregiver must decide whether the person will cause harm, whether the behavior is increasing in intensity or will decrease if ignored and redirected, or whether the behavior can best be prevented using other methods such as environmental management. The caregiver's experience and posture must guide these judgments.

## Redirection

Redirection is the pivotal component in the gentle teaching paradigm. It is the key response of the caregiver that refocuses the interactional flow from undesirable to rewarding interactions. It is also a respectful alternative to the punitive approach that is so prevalent today.

The purpose of redirection is to communicate (often nonverbally) to the person alternate means of human interactions. It functions as a cue that communicates acceptable alternatives to the inappropriate responses that are occurring. It provides the person with information that indicates what other response is appropriate for the particular situation. In addition, it communicates that responses that previously terminated interactions or gained inappropriate or inequitable attention will no longer be effective or valued. Redirection breaks the maladaptive pattern of the interaction and defuses the power or effect of the person's undesirable response. By providing an unexpected response, the redirection communicates that previous patterns of interaction will no longer be in effect and that they will be replaced by reciprocally rewarding interactions. The third message communicated by redirection is not only that reward is available, but also how it can be gained. The unfortunate message that accompanies negative consequences is that the opportunity to gain reward has ended. The caregiver's tone of voice, facial expression, and body posture all indicate to the person that the chances of reward occurring are minimal. Redirection, on the other hand, is a response that communicates that the chances for reward have not ended and that reward is still available. More importantly, redirection communicates to the person what he or she needs to do to make reward happen. If necessary, the caregiver even helps the person participate so that reward can be received. It provides clear information about what response will result in a rewarding interaction with the caregiver. Redirection makes reward available and accessible to the person in spite of disruptive or destructive behaviors.

## Reward Teaching

The ignore and redirect components of the gentle teaching paradigm are all unified in their purpose; that is, reward giving and sharing are possible by directing all interactions toward human participation. Interruption prevents harm to the participants and others in the environment so that the interaction can be refocused elsewhere. Ignoring disruptive behaviors saves the caregiver's interactional responses so that responses can be used for valuing. Redirection refocuses the interactional flow toward mutually rewarding participation. The focus is to turn the direction of all interactions toward reward. In this manner, the goal of teaching the person the value of human presence and participation is continuously pursued.

The interactional restructuring that occurs as a result of this paradigm also defines the parameters of all interactions between the caregiver and the person. The goal of mutually rewarding interactions establishes the boundaries and limits of all interactions. All interactions become equitable to both parties. If an interaction is redirected toward a more equitable pattern of interaction, then mutual participation yields reward.

The most vital factor in the gentle teaching paradigm is reward (i.e., human valuing), not simply giving reward but literally teaching the goodness inherent in human reward. We assume that persons with these challenging behaviors do not know in any consistent way that human reward has value (that human presence, words, and touch have a mutually liberating power). It is therefore necessary to teach the value of human reward. From a behavioral perspective, we are assuming two critical factors. First, it is necessary to teach the person that human presence (the basic antecedent to all human behavior) needs to signal safety, consistency, and reward. The value inherent in human presence needs to be taught. Second, it is necessary to teach the person that human reward (the basic consequence of all human behavior) has a humanizing and liberating quality.

The unifying element in a bonded relationship is the reciprocal value that each person derives from the interactional process. Unfortunately, the person with challenging behaviors does not know and feel this reciprocal value. It must be taught. Caregivers initially have to superimpose this value on the person using tasks as the primary vehicle. By structuring the learner's day with a series of tasks, the caregiver creates a series of opportunities to redirect the person toward rewarding interactions. At first, the caregiver gives reward, but receives little or nothing in return. The person learns simply to accept reward through the ignoring and redirection process. Soon, however, the caregiver begins to ask for the reciprocation of reward. Gradually, mutual value sharing occurs. In order for this mutuality to evolve between caregivers and learners, the caregiver must first explicitly define, express, and teach the learner to accept, seek out, and finally reciprocate valuing human interactions. As this overt mutuality evolves, the presence of both persons comes to have implicit meaning and value. To initiate this process, the caregiver must highlight the meaning and value of human participation. Caregivers should not view the giving and receiving of human reward as a teaching or behavioral technique, but rather as a pedagogical purpose.

If a person fails to respond to human valuing, it becomes the caregiver's challenge to teach it. This assumption is critical. The failure to understand its importance is the primary reason why caregivers succumb to punishment practices or to make a referral for behavior they cannot or will not tolerate anymore (see also Szymanski, Chapter 11). Most caregivers start their intervention giving reward, but there is little or no consistently positive response. The use of punishment is inevitable unless caregivers realize that it is necessary to teach reward. An often heard refrain is, "We tried positives for a long time, but nothing worked." In gentle teaching, the challenge is to teach the humanizing and liberating meaning inherent in human presence and participation. The caregiver teaches the meaning of the most basic antecedent and consequences of human interactions (i.e., the value and goodness of human presence and human reward).

When the caregiver first gives reward to the person for any approximation toward participatory behaviors, it is likely that the learner will not respond in any positive manner. Indeed, praise might be reacted to with disdain. Yet, the caregiver must persist. At this point, it is important to remember that the task is the vehicle to give reward. The caregiver has to make participation happen. As the caregiver ignores the maladaptive behaviors and redirects the person to a task, reward is given for any movement toward participation. As this sequence occurs time after time, the learner begins to accept human valuing and the fact that the caregiver signals safety and human reward. The maladaptive behaviors might continue, but participation also begins to occur. The person begins to feel that participation has some meaning. Gradually, the maladaptive behaviors begin to decrease. The person begins to accept the caregiver's presence, words, and touch. Concurrent with this process, the caregiver begins to seek out for reward. The learner begins to reciprocate verbal or tactile praise, at first with assistance, and gradually in a natural, spontaneous manner. An environment of value-sharing then emerges.

# Conclusion

We have reviewed and analyzed the gentle teaching paradigm. It is not complex, but it requires an ongoing questioning of our posture, a continuous focus on our goals, creative teaching skills, and persevering effort. It is crucial to remember that the purpose of the paradigm is to create opportunities to give reward. Any endeavors that deviate from reward giving and eventually reward sharing are off-center.

The paradigm reflects a posture of solidarity with the person because its goal is to teach equitable interactions that lead to bonding. The first encounters often require a high degree of tolerance on the caregiver's part. The learner often will hit, kick, scratch, or scream as the caregiver attempts to direct the person to a task so that reward can be given. At these difficult moments, our posture must be at its strongest even though the common tendency is for our own emotions to become aggressive and retaliatory.

Gentle teaching is a pedagogy of liberation. It is an ongoing process that humanizes and liberates the teacher and the learner. Both become more. It challenges the caregiver to be the best teacher at the worst moments. It is based on a posture of human solidarity with the person. It requires warmth, tolerance, and affection and defines bonding as the goal of intervention. This posture and goal on the part of the caregiver help the caregiver to set aside punishment practices and discover a range of teaching strategies that teach the value inherent in human presence, participation, and reward.

# References

Baumeister, A.A., & Rollings, J.P. (1976). Self-injurious behavior. In N.R. Ellis (Ed.), *International review of research in mental retardation* (Vol. 8). New York: Academic Press.

Bijou, S.W., & Dunitz-Johnson, E. (1981). An interbehavior analysis of developmental retardation. *The Psychological Record, 31*, 305–329.

Casey, K., McGee, J., Stark, J., & Menolascino, F. (1985). *A community-based system for the mentally retarded: The ENCOR experience.* Lincoln, NE: University of Nebraska Press.

Favell, J.E., & Greene, J.W. (1981). *How to treat self-injurious behavior.* Lawrence, KS: H & H Enterprises.

Foxx, R.M., & Azrin, N.H. (1973). The elimination of autistic self-stimulatory behavior by overcorrection. *Journal of Applied Behavioral Analysis, 6*, 1–14.

Freire, P. (1980). *Educacao como a pratica da liberdade*. Rio de Janeiro: Paz e Terra.

Gardner, W.I., & Cole, C.L. (1985). *Selecting intervention procedures: What happened to behavioral assessment?* Unpublished manuscript.

McGee, J. (1984). *Gentle teaching*. Proceedings of the International Autism Conference of the Americas (pp. 253–264). San Antonio, TX.

Menolascino, F.J., & McGee, J.J. (1983). Persons with severe mental retardation and behavioral challenges: From disconnectedness to human engagement. *Journal of Psychiatric Treatment and Evaluation, 5*(2&3), 187–193.

Patterson, G.R., & Reid, J.B. (1970). Reciprocity and coercion: Two facets of social systems. In C. Neuringer & J.L. Michael (Eds.), *Behavioral modification in clinical psychology*. New York: Appleton-Century-Crofts.

Watson, L., Owen, J.R., & Uzzell, R. (1980). *Positive approach to managing disruptive behaviors*. Tuscaloosa, AL: Behavior Modification Technology, Inc.

# 19
# Ethical Issues in Interventions for Persons with Retardation, Autism and Related Developmental Disorders

Travis Thompson, William I. Gardner
and Alfred A. Baumeister

Jean Itard's remarkable effort to cure Victor, the so-called "Wild Child of Aveyron" (Itard, 1976), is the first documented case of the use of systematic teaching methods to overcome the disability of a severely handicapped youngster though it would be some 64 years before Seguin explicated the method in detail (Kanner, 1964; Rosen, Clark, & Kivitz, 1976; Scheerenberger, 1983). Itard's methods foreshadowed the technologies growing out of modern behavior analysis and intervention principles (Kazdin, 1978). Though effective educational methods for mildly and some moderately retarded children had been developed, residential services and educational methods for severely and profoundly retarded and autistic children and youth were largely custodial in the United States until the late 1960s. In the late 1950s and early 1960s, Bijou (1963), Orlando and Bijou (1960), Ellis and Pryer (1958), Barrett and Lindsley (1962), and Lindsley (1964) began to extend nonhuman behavior principles to laboratory research with mentally retarded children. These seminal studies led several brave practitioners working in large institutional settings to take the first serious steps to develop more adequate habilitative programming for retarded children and adults with whom no one else would even attempt to work seriously (Baumeister & Klosowski, 1965; Girardeau & Spradlin, 1964; Larsen & Bricker, 1968). Until that point, restraints, hydrotherapy, large doses of sedative-hypnotic and neuroleptic drugs, and prefrontal lobotomies or lobectomies were the primary treatments available. Following these initial demonstrations, several major institutional (Thompson & Grabowski, 1972, 1977) and educational (Haring & Bricker, 1976) programs emerged, revealing that self-help, vocational, social, and language skills could be taught and maintained in even severely-to-profoundly retarded individuals who had spent most of their lives in institutional settings and who displayed behavior problems (Gardner, 1971). The widespread availability of effective procedures, combined with strong pressure brought about through the early Right to Treatment Federal Court rulings (cf. *Welsh v. Likins*, 1974; *Wyatt v. Styckney*, 1972), dramatically changed services to severely and profoundly handicapped people. Men, women, and children who had been given up as "untreatable" suddenly began making their way into communities, and the primary habilitative modalities grew out of the behavior analysis and intervention methods developed in institutional settings in the late 1960s (cf. Brown, Nietupski, & Hamre-Nietupski, 1976; Thompson & Carey, 1980).

In the earliest programs, procedures that involved removing commonly available goods or services or that might produce discomfort were rarely useful because they were found generally unnecessary; when such methods were used on very unusual occasions, a furor arose (see Ulrich, Stachnick, & Mabrey, 1970). While the vast majority of practitioners behaved with a high degree of professionalism, a few poorly trained, untrained, and in several instances, trained professionals committed highly questionable acts while implementing parts of sound behavioral procedures under inappropriate circumstances, with inappropriate clients, or simply engaging in abusive practices and labeling them behavioral treatment. The most clearcut cases, which have been documented, have involved adult psychiatric patients (Cotter, 1967; Curran, Jorud, & Whitman, 1971). In both cases, psychiatrists having little training in behavior therapy principles or supervised training in behavioral procedures attempted to use elements of behavioral procedures, together with electroconvulsive shock, neuroleptic medications, or physical restraints, totally improperly. Although the procedures had little to do with behavior therapy, the fact that those doing the treating presented them as such created the misimpression that the procedures used were typical of behavioral intervention methods.

The technologies were new in the 1960s, and administrators, program supervisors, and school principals found themselves attracted to behavioral procedures that seemed to promise immediate results (which themselves were seldom used by most of the developers of modern behavioral procedures) because they wanted "quick fixes" at low cost for difficult programming problems. Some administrators avoided the cost of significant staff training, employed inadequate staff ratios, required little or no procedural or outcome documentation, and adopted aversive procedures all too readily, and often with little or no supervision. Many professionals worked diligently to develop protections for clients whose rights were clearly being violated by indiscriminate use of such procedures, some of which could be safe and effective under appropriate circumstances (Forehand & Baumeister, 1976; Johnson & Baumeister, 1981; Thompson & Grabowski, 1977; Thompson, Chapter 10). However, in a survey of policies in the 48 contiguous states, Thomas (1980) found few had anything approaching adequate safeguards in place in most jurisdictions concerning the use of such methods.

In attempting to understand the reluctance of states to regulate, it soon becomes clear that economics plays a major role. For example, in Minnesota, where efforts have been underway for the past 15 years to enact a Department of Human Services Rule specifically to regulate such procedures, several groups have consistently opposed the proposed draft rules during hearings. Institution administrators have typically opposed the draft rules as requiring too many highly trained staff, requiring too much paperwork, and as unnecessarily time consuming (and therefore costly). Employees' unions and residential provider organizations have opposed the regulations for similar reasons. Professional organizations have vacillated in support of various draft rules, in principle, as long as the rule did not alter professionals' freedom to do whatever they choose.

Only the advocacy groups have consistently supported development of adequate rules regulating procedures.

The difficulty in developing methods to regulate such procedures revolves around the effectiveness of the procedures, the available alternatives, and the public reaction of distaste at specific procedures. At various points in history, humankind rejected various medical procedures as violations of the sanctity of the body and akin to witchcraft (e.g., hypodermic injection and surgical procedures). However, as knowledge of anatomy and physiology progressed and medical information concerning the alternatives and efficacy of certain medical procedures became widespread, opposition waned. For example, surgical procedures often cause great discomfort, sometimes lasting for days or weeks, but the public has come to accept such discomfort as necessary. Although the details of surgical procedures may be distasteful to the layperson, they are usually willing to accept them as necessary. In the case of modern behavioral intervention procedures, the evidence suggests that in some instances (e.g., self-injury in nonautistic retarded individuals) a combination of positive reinforcement and aversive procedure is often the most effective approach in reducing or eliminating most self-injury (Baumtrog, 1985; Schroeder, Schroeder, Rojahn, & Mulick, 1980). The problem, however, is that we know little about either the durability of such treatment effects or precisely which people profit from such treatments and which people do not. The solution is to study, in a careful and far more systematic way, these basic issues: namely, how durable are the treatment effects and which procedures are most effective with which individuals and under what circumstances. While such information will not lead everyone who objects to some procedures as inherently distasteful to conclude they are acceptable, it will provide the basis for a gradual reassessment of what is and is not acceptable in the same way modern medical procedures are evaluated.

Finally, it is clear that any means does not justify a laudable end. The limits of society's adoption of procedures are dictated by numerous factors, not the least of which are the judiciousness of application of the procedure, the qualifications of those carrying out the procedures, and the alternatives. That treatment procedures involving limitations on material goods or services, or unpleasant experiences, are infrequently used by competent practitioners suggests that we need to examine very carefully the use of such methods by untrained, unsupervised, and unskilled staff. While doing so, however, it would seem unwise to rule out the use of entire classes of procedures of proven value, which are misused by some people, thereby eliminating the possibility of effectively treating the small number of individuals for whom those methods might be the treatments of choice (Thompson, 1984). We are reminded of a comment by St. Jerome who remarked in his letters: "It is no fault of Christianity that a hypocrite falls into sin."

## References

Barrett, B.H., & Lindsley, O.R. (1962). Deficits in acquisition of operant discrimination and differentiation shown by institutionalized retarded children. *American Journal of Mental Deficiency, 67,* 424–436.

Baumeister, A., & Klosowski, R. (1965). An attempt to group toilet trained severely retarded patients. *Mental Retardation, 3*, 24–26.

Baumtrog, C. (1985). *Effectiveness of behavior reduction procedures with individuals who are severely handicapped. A meta-analysis.* Unpublished doctoral dissertation, University of Minnesota, Minneapolis.

Bijou, S.W. (1963). Theory and research in mental (developmental) retardation. *Psychological Record, 13*, 95–110.

Brown, L., Nietupski, J., & Hamre-Nietupski, S. (1976). Criterion of ultimate functioning. In M.A. Thomas (Ed.), *Hey, don't forget about me!* Reston, VA: Council for Exceptional Children.

Cotter, L.H. (1967). Operant conditioning in a Vietnamese mental hospital. *American Journal of Psychiatry, 124*, 23–28.

Curran, J., Jorud, S., & Whitman, N. (1971). Unconventional treatment of treatment-resistant hospitalized patients. *The Psychiatric Quarterly, 45*, 186–208.

Ellis, N.R., & Pryer, M. (1958). Primary versus secondary reinforcement in simple discrimination learning of mental defectives. *Psychological Reports, 4*, 67–70.

Forehand, R., & Baumeister, A.A. (1976). Deceleration of aberrant behavior among retarded individuals. In M. Hersen & P. Miller (Eds.), *Progress in behavior modification* (Vol. 2). New York: Academic Press.

Gardner, W.I. (1971). *Behavior modification in mental retardation.* Chicago, IL: Aldine-Atherton.

Girardeau, F., & Spradlin, J. (1964). Token rewards in a cottage program. *Mental Retardation, 2*, 245–251.

Haring, N., & Bricker, D. (1976). Overview of comprehensive services for the severely/profoundly handicapped. In N. Haring & L. Brown (Eds.), *Teaching the severely handicapped* (Vol. 1). New York: Grune & Stratton.

Itard, J. (1976). *The wild boy of Aveyron* (H. Lane, Trans.). Cambridge, MA: Harvard University Press.

Johnson, W.L., & Baumeister, A.A. (1981). Behavior techniques for decreasing aberrant behavior of retarded and autistic persons. In M. Hersen, R.M. Eisler, & P.M. Miller (Eds.), *Progress in behavior modification* (Vol. 9). New York: Academic Press.

Kanner, L. (1964). *A history of the care and study of the mentally retarded.* Springfield, IL: Charles C. Thomas Publishers.

Kazdin, A.E. (1978). *History of behavior modification.* Baltimore, MD: Paul H. Brookes Publishing Company.

Larsen, L.A., & Bricker, W.A. (1968). A manual for parents and teachers of severely and moderately retarded children. *IMRID Papers and Reports, 5*(22). Nashville, TN: John F. Kennedy Center for Research on Education and Human Development.

Lindsley, O.R. (1964). Direct measurement and prosthesis of retarded behavior. *Journal of Education, 147*, 62–81.

Orlando, R., & Bijou, S.W. (1960). Single and multiple reinforcement schedules in developmentally retarded children. *Journal of the Experimental Analysis of Behavior, 3*, 339–348.

Rosen, M., Clark, G.R., & Kivitz, M.S. (Eds.). (1976). *The history of mental retardation* (Vol. 2). Baltimore, MD: University Park Press. [Reprinted from Seguin E. (1864). Origin of the treatment and training of idiots. In *Idiocy and its treatment by the physiological methods.*]

Scheerenberger, R.C. (1983). *A history of mental retardation.* Baltimore, MD: Paul H. Brookes Publishing Company.

Schroeder, S.R., Schroeder, C.S., Rojahn, J., & Mulick, J.A. (1980). Self-injurious behavior: An analysis of behavior management techniques. In J.L. Matson & M.R. McCartney (Eds.), *Handbook of behavior modification with the mentally retarded*. New York: Plenum Press.

Thomas, D. (1980, October). *Legal issues relevant to behavioral treatment of aggressive clients*. Paper presented at the Second Annual Behavioral Programming Symposium, Lincoln, IL.

Thompson, T. (1984). Review of Foxx, R., Increasing behavior of severely retarded and autistic persons and decreasing behavior of severely retarded and autistic persons. *Journal of Autism, 14*, 232–235.

Thompson, T., & Carey, A. (1980). Structured normalization: Intellectual and adaptive behavior change in a residential setting. *Mental Retardation, 18*, 193–197.

Thompson, T., & Grabowski, J.G. (Eds.). (1972). *Behavior modification of the mentally retarded*. New York: Oxford University Press.

Thompson, T., & Grabowski, J.G. (Eds.). (1977). *Behavior modification of the mentally retarded* (rev. ed.). New York: Oxford University Press.

Ulrich, R.T., Stachnick, T., & Mabry, J. (Eds.). (1970). *Control of human behavior: From cure to prevention*. Glenview, IL: Scott, Foresman & Co.

*Welsh v. Likins*, 353 F. Suppl. 487 (1974).

*Wyatt v. Styckney*, 344 F. Suppl. 387, 502 F.2d 1305 (1972).

# 20
# Ethical Issues of Aversive Techniques: A Response to Thompson, Gardner, and Baumeister

JOHN J. MCGEE

As the issue of the use of punishment as a treatment alternative emerges across the United States, several arguments have developed in defense of its application. In this response, I wish to question these arguments in a critical manner. Thompson, Gardner, and Baumeister (Chapter 19) encapsulated their reasons for supporting the use of aversive techniques. Their arguments center on the following: (1) the general contribution of the principles of applied behavioral analysis to the systematic teaching of persons with severe mental retardation with no mention made of punishment; (2) a harkening back to the crude types of psychiatric interventions used prior to the 1960s, such as hydrotherapy, prefrontal lobotomies, lobectomies, and the use of chemical restraint; (3) scapegoating those who use the principles of applied behavioral analysis incorrectly; (4) scapegoating the "system" for failing to develop adequate safeguards against the indiscriminate or undisciplined use of punishment procedures; and (5) advocating for the use of punishment as a research challenge, stating that more research has to be undertaken to validate the durability and effectiveness of punishment, especially in the area of self-injurious behavior. A constant refrain woven throughout all these arguments is the supposition that those who are daring enough to engage in the use of punishment are brave scientists performing the equivalent of behavioral surgery. The most common metaphor used in relation to the administration of punishment is that those who perform these deeds are akin to the physician who must cut in order to save.

## Contributions of Behaviorism

The literature over the past 20 years is replete with studies based on the effective use of the principles of applied behavioral analysis in the teaching of individuals with severe mental retardation. In the previous chapter, Thompson, Gardner, and Baumeister were correct in citing Itard's work with Victor, the Wild Boy of Aveyron (Lane, 1976) as one of the first documented cases in the use of systematic teaching methods to overcome the disabilities of a severely disabled youngster. However, they fail to remind the reader that Itard's work did not focus on the systematic use of punishment as is advocated in today's literature. Indeed, a very poignant vignette in Itard's account of Victor's life was his relationship with Madame Guerin. She was Victor's foster mother. It was with her that Victor bonded. According to Itard, she "treated him with the affection of a mother and the enlightenment of a teacher." It was toward her that Victor would run and fling himself, like a son, into his mother's arms. It is this spirit of bonding, mutuality, and human solidarity that the systematic use of punishment fails to recognize.

It is true that in the late 1950s and early 1960s, some practitioners began to work in large, custodial institutional settings in an attempt to apply the principles of applied behavioral analysis to mentally retarded persons who were considered to be "hopeless." Such early work in the United States was one of many phenomena that began to focus national attention on the validity of the developmental assumption (i.e., that all persons are capable of learning, regardless of the severity of any handicapping condition). Of course, concurrent with these seminal studies on the pedagogical use of the principles of applied behavioral analysis, there was also emerging a major national advocacy movement based on the dehumanizing conditions found in state institutions for persons with mental retardation.

Today's literature validates the developmental assumption and the effectiveness of applied behavioral analysis in the systematic teaching of persons with severe mental retardation (Berkson and Landesman-Dwyer, (1977).

There was a paucity of interest and research on punishment as an intervention method prior to the mid-1960s (Spradlin & Girardeau, 1966). However, after two decades of failed punishment-based research, Thompson, Gardner, and Baumeister now are advocating for a national focus on the same research questions raised by Gardner (1971) nearly 15 years ago: (1) How effective are punishment procedures? (2) Are such behavior changes temporary? and (3) What side effects are produced by punishment? The years have gone by. These questions have been raised and researched hundreds of times since the mid-1960s. Traditional punishment-based research has disregarded the nature and the value of the human person and the goal of intervention. The assumption has been that punishment works. Bucher and Lovass (1968) concluded that electric shock was the treatment of choice in dealing with the self-injurious behavior of retarded persons. Nearly all subsequent conclusions have simply been manipulated variations of Lovass' original false hypothesis. There has been little critical questioning of punishment as a procedure or of its immediate and long-term emotional impact. At best, traditional researchers have only invented variations of the original punishment theme. Electric shock is a far cry from Itard's admonition to intervene with the affection of a mother and the enlightment of a teacher. Likewise, it is unrelated to our colleagues' reminder to us of the positive benefits generated by the principles of applied behavioral analysis as a laudable teaching strategy. When critically analyzed, punishment can be seen as an authoritarian and mechanistic approach with a goal of submission.

# Medical Model

Proponents of the use of punishment set forth a dual argument centered on the medical model. On the one hand, they remind the public that in the days of old, hydrotherapy, straitjackets, and lobotomies were common medical intervention techniques. Their conclusion is that we surely do not wish to return to these antiquated and crude methods. On the other hand, they liken themselves to physicians who courageously perform surgery to save lives, even though it is temporarily necessary to harm the person in the surgical act of cutting. It is my contention that the systematic use of punishment is the emotional and spiritual equivalent of lobotomies. Advocates of punishment cannot have it both ways.

We have agreed with the contention that behaviorism has contributed much to the systematic teaching of skills to the severely retarded. However, Thompson, Gardner, and Baumeister fail to remind the reader of the parallel current in the professional literature that advocates for the use of punishment. Accepting their medical metaphor, I hold that the use of punishment is not a courageous and brave act, but rather it is the use of ill-conceived, poorly tested, and counterproductive methods. Indeed, the punishment practices cited in the literature since the 1960s are similar to pre-1960 methods, but under euphemistic names. Seclusion is now time-out. Chains have been replaced by forced relaxation. Lobotomies are replaced by grotesque practices such as squirting noxious substances in people's faces, eyes, and nostrils. Hydrotherapy is now water mist sprayed into the face. Punishment and neglect are now termed aversive therapy.

As previously stated, punishment-based practices embrace a 20-year time span. Lovass (1967) helped begin a punishment thrust by advocating for the need to control maladaptive behaviors through the use of punishment because "all behaviors are lawful and lawful implies control." This conclusion helped initiate a flood of research over the past two decades on the use of punishment. This theme remains a strong hypothesis up to today. Skinner, in defending the systematic use of grotesque forms of punishment for autistic behaviors, states: "Learning through the use of punishment has been recognized for centuries by governments and religions which threaten hell fire. . . . All use punishment to teach control" (Deitz, 1985). During the past 20 years, researchers have conducted a series of data-based projects based on the dehumanizing and enslaving assumption that punishment is a necessary and valid treatment method. Current reviews of the literature clearly point out this national trend (Gardner & Cole, 1984; Johnson & Baumeister, 1978). It is only recently that this assumption is being challenged owing to a deepening understanding of the communicative nature of aggressive and self-injurious behaviors and the interactional nature of all behavioral intervention (Donnellan, Mirenda, Mesaros, & Fassbender, 1984; Menolascino & McGee, 1983). The medical metaphor employed by Thompson, Gardner, and Baumeister equates maladaptive behaviors with a disease that has to be extracted and fails to value the holistic nature and value of the person.

# Incorrect Usage

The next argument scapegoats the staff who "incorrectly" use the range of punishment practices. This argument holds that it is not the systematic use of punishment that is in question, but rather those who use it incorrectly, partially, or indiscriminantly. This argument goes on to explain that when punishment does not work, it is because of poor staff training, inadequate staffing ratios, poor documentation, and poor supervision. This argument inevitably places the advocates of punishment above the common fray. While it is true that many who practice punishment are ill-trained and poorly supervised, it is also true that many who use it are highly trained and well supervised. Any analysis of punishment practices in our nation's institutions reveals that the planned, systematic use of punishment is common and based on propunishment literature and procedures.

At best, punishment results in submissive, obedient persons. More typically, after severe forms of punishment fail, the individuals are restrained or encased in helmets for the balance of their lives.

The fact of the matter is that in those places where punishment is used correctly and systematically, it is still repugnant and unnecessary. In a review of 543 persons with mental retardation and mental illness whom we have diagnosed and treated in the last 5 years, we served 82 children and adults with severe self-injurious behaviors. Their behaviors ranged from low-occurrence self-injuries, such as cutting a toe off or biting a finger off, to persistent and entrenched head banging, hair pulling, biting, slapping, or eye gouging (see Table 20.1). The sample includes a number of underlying psychiatric disorders. In no instance did we find it necessary to use punishment. A further analysis of these 82 individuals revealed that within an average treatment time of 28 days, all forms of self-injurious behaviors had decelerated to manageable levels and were maintained at that or even zero frequency up to a year later.

The review summarized in Table 20.1 shows that it is possible to treat those with the most difficult behaviors without the use of punishment and to maintain appropriate interactional behaviors in the mainstream of community-based alternatives.

# Inadequate Safeguards

If it is not ill-trained and poorly supervised direct-care staff, then it is the system that causes the inappropriate use of punishment. Thompson, Gardner, and Baumeister contend that few states have adequate regulations governing the use of punishment. This is simply not true. After 20 years of litigation in a myriad of class action lawsuits against the abuse and neglect found in so many institutions, there exist mammoth amounts of regulatory "safeguards" to the indiscriminate use of punishment. Yet, in reality, punishment abounds in our nation's classrooms, institutions, and group homes. We have conducted in-depth surveys in

Table 20.1. Descriptive analysis of patients served with self-injurious behaviors.

| Patient no. | Level of retardation | Age (yr) | Psychiatric diagnosis | Allied needs | Type of self-injurious behavior | Sequelae | Intensity before treatment | Intensity after treatment | Intensity at 1 year of treatment |
|---|---|---|---|---|---|---|---|---|---|
| 1 | Moderate | 28 | Personality disorder | Cerebral palsy | Breaks windows | Broken toes, scars on arms | High | Moderate | Low |
| 2 | Moderate | 36 | Adjustment disorder | Deaf, nonverbal | Bites self | Scars on hands | High | 0 | 0 |
| 3 | Mild | 25 | Schizophrenia | Seizures | Throws self | Scars on head and hands | High | Low | 0 |
| 4 | Moderate | 17 | Adjustment disorder | — | Slaps face | — | High | Low | Low |
| 5 | Severe | 22 | Depression | Nonverbal | Slaps face | Slaps face | High | Low | 0 |
| 6 | Moderate | 27 | Schizophrenia | Cerebral palsy | Bites self, bangs head | Scars on hands | High | Low | 0 |
| 7 | Mild | 26 | Schizophrenia | — | Bites self | Scars on hands and arms | High | 0 | 0 |
| 8 | Moderate | 23 | Adjustment disorder | Cerebral palsy | Slaps face | — | Moderate | Low | 0 |
| 9 | Mild | 15 | Premenstrual syndrome | — | Digs rectum, digs vagina | — | High | 0 | 0 |
| 10 | Mild | 30 | Adjustment disorder | Mute, nonverbal | Bites hands, breaks glass | Scars on arms and hands | Moderate | Low | 0 |
| 11 | Mild | 20 | Schizophrenia | — | Picks penis | — | High | 0 | 0 |
| 12 | Severe | 14 | Autism | Nonverbal | Slaps face | — | High | Low | 0 |
| 13 | Moderate | 14 | Autism | Nonverbal | Hits head | — | High | 0 | 0 |
| 14 | Moderate | 20 | Adjustment disorder | — | Slaps face | — | Moderate | 0 | 0 |
| 15 | Severe | 27 | Schizophrenia | Nonverbal | Bangs head | Scars | High | Low | 0 |
| 16 | Mild | 16 | Adjustment disorder | Stammers | Puts fist through windows | Scars on hands and arms | High | 0 | 0 |
| 17 | Moderate | 30 | Personality disorder | Cerebral palsy | Scratches face | Scars on face | High | 0 | 0 |
| 18 | Moderate | 35 | Personality disorder | Cerebral palsy | Slashes face | Scars on face | Low | Low | 0 |

| | | | | | | | | | |
|---|---|---|---|---|---|---|---|---|---|
| 19 | Moderate | 20 | Autism | — | Scratches face | — | High | 0 | 0 |
| 20 | Severe | 13 | Adjustment disorder | Nonverbal | Slaps face | — | High | Low | 0 |
| 21 | Severe | 16 | Autism | Nonverbal | Slaps face, bangs head | — | High | 0 | Low |
| 22 | Severe | 23 | Pervasive developmental disorder | Hodgkins | Bites hands, slaps face | Scars | High | Low | 0 |
| 23 | Mild | 18 | Schizophrenia | — | Bites self, slaps face | — | High | Low | 0 |
| 24 | Severe | 21 | Autism | — | Slaps face, bangs head, bites hands | — | High | 0 | 0 |
| 25 | Severe | 20 | Autism | Nonverbal | Bangs head, scratches body, bites self | Scars, cauliflower ears | High | Low | High |
| 26 | Severe | 2 | Autism | Nonverbal | Slaps face, bangs head | — | High | 0 | 0 |
| 27 | Mild | 17 | Schizophrenia | Seizures | Slaps face, bangs head | Scars on hands and head | Moderate | 0 | Moderate |
| 28 | Severe | 17 | Pervasive developmental disorder | Nonverbal | Gouges ears, slaps face, scratches self | Scars over body | High | 0 | 0 |
| 29 | Severe | 15 | Autism | — | Knees to face, bites self, bangs head, scratches self | Scars over body | High | Low | 0 |
| 30 | Moderate | 23 | Autism | Echolalic | Hits face, bangs head | Scars over body | High | Low | 0 |
| 31 | Moderate | 22 | Schizophrenia | Nonverbal | Pica, bangs head | Scars on head, spit fistula | High | Low | Deceased |
| 32 | Severe | 15 | Autism | Seizures | Slaps face, bangs head, pinches arms | Scars over body | High | 0 | 0 |

Table 20.1. (Continued).

| Patient no. | Level of retardation | Age (yr) | Psychiatric diagnosis | Allied needs | Type of self-injurious behavior | Sequelae | Intensity before treatment | Intensity after treatment | Intensity at 1 year of treatment |
|---|---|---|---|---|---|---|---|---|---|
| 33 | Severe | 18 | Pervasive developmental disorder | Nonverbal | Slaps face | – | High | 0 | 0 |
| 34 | Severe | 26 | Schizophrenia | Nonverbal | Pinches lips, scratches self, picks skin | Scars on arms and face | High | Low | 0 |
| 35 | Severe | 39 | Organic brain syndrome | Nonverbal | Bangs ears, hits face | Cauliflower ears | High | 0 | 0 |
| 36 | Severe | 24 | Schizophrenia | Nonverbal | Hits face | Scars on face, enucleation | High | 0 | 0 |
| 37 | Moderate | 27 | Adjustment disorder | – | Slaps face | – | High | 0 | 0 |
| 38 | Severe | 27 | Organic brain syndrome | Nonverbal, seizures | Gouges eyes | Detached retinas | High | Low | Low |
| 39 | Severe | 42 | Pervasive developmental disorder | Nonverbal, seizures | Slaps face, scratches face | Scars on face | High | 0 | 0 |
| 40 | Severe | 11 | Pervasive developmental disorder | Nonverbal | Hits self, picks skin | Scars on hands | High | Low | Low |
| 41 | Severe | 27 | Pervasive developmental disorder | Nonverbal | Bangs head, swallows tobacco | Rectal bleeding | High | 0 | Low |
| 42 | Severe | 36 | Pervasive developmental disorder | Nonverbal | Bangs head | Scars on head | HIgh | 0 | 0 |
| 43 | Moderate | 38 | Pervasive developmental disorder | Nonverbal | Bangs head, scratches self | Scars over body | High | 0 | 0 |
| 44 | Moderate | 28 | Adjustment disorder | – | Bangs head | Scars on head | High | 0 | 0 |
| 45 | Severe | 16 | Pervasive developmental disorder | Nonverbal | Bangs head, bites self | Scars on body | High | Low | 0 |

| | | | | | | | | | |
|---|---|---|---|---|---|---|---|---|---|
| 46 | Severe | 49 | Organic brain syndrome | Nonverbal | Bangs head, slaps self, scratches self | Scars | High | 0 | 0 |
| 47 | Severe | 20 | Pervasive developmental disorder | Nonverbal | Bangs head, slaps face, scratches body | Scars over body | High | 0 | 0 |
| 48 | Severe | 56 | Organic brain syndrome | Seizures | Bangs head, scratches self | Detached retina, scars | High | 0 | 0 |
| 49 | Severe | 34 | Organic brain syndrome | Nonverbal, blind, nonambulatory | Bangs head, bites self, gouges eyes | Scars over body | High | 0 | Low |
| 50 | Severe | 27 | Pervasive developmental disorder | — | Bangs head | — | High | 0 | Low |
| 51 | Severe | 28 | Pervasive developmental disorder | — | Bangs head, pulls out hair | Baldness, scars | High | 0 | 0 |
| 52 | Severe | 26 | Pervasive developmental disorder | Blind, nonambulatory | Gouges eyes, bangs head, bites self | Detached retinas, scars | High | Low | Low |
| 53 | Severe | 40 | Organic brain syndrome | Seizures, nonambulatory | Digs rectum, slaps face, eats feces | Scars | High | 0 | 0 |
| 54 | Severe | 46 | Pervasive developmental disorder | — | Bangs head, slaps face | Scars over body | High | Low | Low |
| 55 | Severe | 24 | Adjustment disorder | — | Picks skin, scratches self | Scars | High | 0 | 0 |
| 56 | Severe | 44 | Pervasive developmental disorder | Seizures | Bangs head | Scars on head and eyes | High | 0 | Low |
| 57 | Severe | 22 | Pervasive developmental disorder | Nonverbal | Bangs head | Scars on head | High | Low | 0 |
| 58 | Severe | 11 | Pervasive developmental disorder | — | Picks skin | Scars | High | Low | Low |

TABLE 20.1. (Continued).

| Patient no. | Level of retardation | Age (yr) | Psychiatric diagnosis | Allied needs | Type of self-injurious behavior | Sequelae | Intensity before treatment | Intensity after treatment | Intensity at 1 year of treatment |
|---|---|---|---|---|---|---|---|---|---|
| 59 | Severe | 30 | Pervasive developmental disorder | Nonverbal, seizures | Eats feces, slaps face, scratches face | Scars | High | Low | 0 |
| 60 | Severe | 46 | Pervasive developmental disorder | Blind, seizures | Gouges eyes, bangs head | Detached retina, scars | High | Low | Low |
| 61 | Severe | 16 | Pervasive developmental disorder | Nonambulatory, nonverbal | Scratches self, slaps face | Scars on hands and arms | High | Low | Low |
| 62 | Severe | 27 | Schizophrenia | Nonverbal | Bit finger off | Missing thumb | Low | 0 | 0 |
| 63 | Severe | 29 | Schizophrenia | — | Hits face, scratches self | Scars | High | Low | Low |
| 64 | Severe | 13 | Adjustment disorder | Nonverbal | Bangs head | — | High | 0 | 0 |
| 65 | Mild | 25 | Schizophrenia | — | Hits head | — | Moderate | 0 | 0 |
| 66 | Severe | 25 | Pervasive developmental disorder | Nonverbal | Gouges eyes, bangs head | Detached retina, scars | High | Low | Low |
| 67 | Severe | 18 | Pervasive developmental disorder | Nonverbal, nonambulatory | Gouges eyes, bangs head | Detached retina, scars | High | Low | Low |
| 68 | Severe | 42 | Pervasive developmental disorder | Nonverbal | Slaps face | — | High | 0 | 0 |
| 69 | Moderate | 27 | Adjustment disorder | — | Bangs head | — | High | 0 | 0 |
| 70 | Severe | 38 | Pervasive developmental disorder | Nonverbal | Scratches | Scars over body | High | 0 | Low |
| 71 | Mild | 20 | Personality disorder | Seizures | Suicide attempt | — | Low | 0 | 0 |
| 72 | Moderate | 26 | Depression | — | Suicide attempt | — | Moderate | 0 | 0 |
| 73 | Mild | 32 | Schizophrenia | — | Suicide attempt | — | Low | 0 | 0 |

institutions in five state institutions in the past 12 months in different geographical areas of the country and have found a consistent and persistent pattern of punishment in every institution. In each setting, there were more than sufficient regulations and procedures to eliminate the use of punishment, or at least dramatically decrease its use.

The issue is not regulations or even court mandates, but rather a revolutionary movement away from punishment practices just as our nation has moved away from the use of lobotomies and leeches. However, this revolution will require the shattering of the sophistic rationales adopted in current research literature.

## Research

The final argumentative bastion for proponents of punishment and blind defenders of behaviorism is to advocate for more of the same research that has filled professional literature during the last two decades. The punishment-based conclusions are well drawn. Over half of the literature on self-injurious behavior advocates the use of electric shock (Johnson & Baumeister, 1978). The vast majority of the literature on aggression is based on the use of punishment. No further propunishment research is needed. Punishment has been assumed as necessary and has thus been accepted as the treatment of choice. Of course, these specious conclusions are based on a view of the human person as merely a set of stimuli and responses and an unquestioned set of values. Most past and current research efforts disregard the interactional nature of human behavior, the liberating aspects of pedagogy, and the critical nature of our values toward the person.

Thompson, Gardner, and Baumeister would have our nation focus its resources on 20 more years of research on punishment—on its durability, its effects, and effectiveness. We reject this proposal because 20 years of research is enough. Punishment might sometimes work momentarily. But it inevitably results in submission. It disregards the interactional nature of teaching. It terminates in grotesque and torturous practices.

## Conclusion

As I stated in Chapter 18, the challenge is not more of the same, but the definition of a new pedagogy that precludes the use of punishment and focuses national attention on the dyadic nature of teaching, adopts the goal of teaching as bonding rather than submission, and generates the application of an array of mutually liberating intervention methods.

If we were to embark on this journey, we could eliminate the use of punishment in our nation over the next 10 years. But more importantly, we could create a new pedagogy that would harken us back to the time of Itard, a time in which his housekeeper, Madame Guerin, treated Victor with the affection of a mother and the enlightenment of a teacher and pedagogy that led Victor to fling himself into

Madame Guerin's arms like a son throwing himself into the arms of the one who gave him life.

## References

Berkson, G., & Landesman-Dwyer, S. (1977). Behavioral research on severe and profound mental retardation (1955-1974). *American Journal of Mental Deficiency, 81*, 428–454.

Bucher, B., & Lovass, I. (1968). Use of aversive stimulation in behavior modification. In M.R. Jones (Ed.), *Aversive stimulation* (pp. 77-145). Miami Symposium on the Prediction of Behavior, 1967. Coral Gables, FL: University of Miami Press.

Deitz, J. (1985). Psychologist B.F. Skinner comes to defense of autistic center leader. *The Boston Globe*, Thursday, October 17, 1985, p. 33.

Donnellan, A.M., Mirenda, P.L., Mesaros, R.A., & Fassbender, L.L. (1984). Analyzing the communicative functions of aberrant behavior. *Journal of the Association for Persons with Severe Handicaps, 9*(3), 201–212.

Gardner, W.I. (1971). *Behavior modification in mental retardation: The education and rehabilitation of the mentally retarded adolescent and adult.* Chicago, IL: Aldine-Atherton.

Gardner, W.I., & Cole, C.L. (1984). *Selecting intervention procedures: What happened to behavioral assessment?* Unpublished manuscript.

Johnson, H.G., & Baumeister, A.A. (1978). Self-injurious behavior: A review and analysis of methodological details of published studies. *Behavior Modification, 2*, 465–487.

Lane, H. (1976). *The wild boy of Aveyron.* Cambridge, MA: Harvard Press.

Lovass, O.I. (1967). A behavior therapy approach to treatment of childhood schizophrenia. In J. Hill (Ed.), *Symposia on child development* (Vol. 1, pp. 108–159). Minneapolis, MN: University of Minnesota Press.

Menolascino, F.J., & McGee, J.J. (1983). Persons with severe mental retardation and behavioral challenges: From disconnectedness to meaningful human engagement. *Journal of Psychiatric Treatment and Evaluation, 5*(2&3), 187–193.

Spradlin, J.E., & Girardeau, F.L. (1966). The behavior of moderately and severely retarded persons. In N. Ellis (Ed.), *International review of research in mental retardation* (Vol. 1, pp. 257–298). New York: Academic Press.

# 21
# Behavioral Psychopharmacology: A New Psychiatric Subspecialty

ROBERT SOVNER

After years of being viewed with distrust and challenged with medicolegal initiative (see reviews by: Aman, 1985; Aman & Singh, 1986; Plotkin & Gill, 1979; and Sprague, 1982), there has been a resurgence of interest in the use of psychotropic medications to treat behavioral and emotional disturbances in persons with developmental disabilities (Aman, 1983). This interest has been stimulated, in large part, by a growing awareness that the mentally retarded exhibit the full spectrum of mental disorders and can be treated with all types of psychiatric therapies (Corbett, 1979; Gostason, 1985; Lund, 1985; Reid, 1972a, 1972b; Reid, 1982; Sovner & Hurley, 1983; Wright, 1982).

Coincident with this increased interest in psychopharmacology has been a new demand for psychotropic drug therapy related services. Those residential facilities, forced by class action suits to implement habilitative service plans for their residents, have had to seek out psychiatrists who are knowledgeable about psychiatric diagnosis and psychotropic drug therapy in order to oversee the discontinuation of inappropriate drug regimens (usually long-term antipsychotic drug therapy) and the prescription of psychotropic medication for only drug-responsive disorders.

The demand for clinical services has been complicated by a change in the type of person who is now living in public residential facilities. As better-adapted individuals have left to live in "less restrictive settings," residential facilities have become reservoirs of psychopathology (Ballinger & Reid, 1977), increasingly populated by developmentally disabled adults whose disturbed behavior has prevented them from living in the community. This population often has severe organically based behavioral problems (Eyman & Call, 1977; Eyman, Moore, Capes, & Zachofsky, 1970; Reid, 1982; Reid, Ballinger, Heather, & Melvin, 1984) that are responsive to novel drug regimens. For example, the need to identify and treat propranolol-responsive rage attacks (Ratey et al., 1986) and lithium-responsive hyperactivity (Sovner & Hurley, 1981) has increased the demand for psychiatrists who can identify drug-responsive individuals and implement these innovative pharmacological regimens.

# Behavioral Psychopharmacology: A New Subspecialty

A consensus is now emerging that psychotropic drug therapy can play a positive role in the treatment of behavioral–emotional disturbances of mentally retarded persons (see also Gualtieri, Chapter 15). In selected individuals, psychotropic drug therapy must be viewed as the treatment of first choice (e.g., those persons suffering from an affective disorder). This is no longer as radical a statement as it might have been 15 years ago.

In addition, the demand for and interest in drug therapy has led to refinement of clinical psychopharmacological practice in order to meet the needs of developmentally disabled persons. It is my contention that this evolving expertise has coalesced to form the nucleus of a new psychiatric specialty which I have termed behavioral psychopharmacology.

Prescribing psychotropic drug therapy for developmentally handicapped adults requires clinical skills that are very different than those used to treat nonhandicapped persons. Although these skills resemble (with respect to diagnostic methodology and treatment monitoring) those used by child psychiatrists, the behavioral psychopharmacologist's patients are adults, and a background in child psychiatry is insufficient training for the task of treating these individuals.

1. *The behavioral psychopharmacologist must be able to differentiate psychiatric symptoms from maladaptive behavior secondary to developmental deficits and childhood onset pervasive developmental disorders.*

Adequate psychiatric diagnosis is an essential first step in psychotropic drug therapy. In general, treatment is not directed at behavior or symptoms per se, but at the underlying psychiatric disorder. Therefore, the behavioral psychopharmacologist must be able to differentiate between those maladaptive behaviors that represent the effects of operant conditioning (e.g., self-injurious behavior that serves as a demand avoidance function), or are best explained in a developmental context (e.g., the eye-poking behavior of a profoundly retarded person in a low-stimulus environment) (Menolascino, 1972, 1983), from behavior that reflects the presence of a psychiatric disorder (e.g., manic hyperactivity).

This differential diagnostic process requires a knowledge of normal behavior for mentally retarded people at all levels of developmental disabilities as well as an appreciation of the typical stress responses of this population.

Mentally retarded persons are exquisitely vulnerable to anxiety-induced behavioral decompensation (Hucker, Day, George, & Roth, 1979; Paniagua & DeFazio, 1983)—which I have termed *cognitive disintegration* (Sovner, 1986). During periods of stress, mentally retarded persons may appear quite bizarre and disorganized. Rather than being a specific sign of a psychiatric disorder, it may represent a nonspecific stress response with no diagnostic significance.

In addition, persons with childhood onset pervasive developmental disorders can develop psychiatric disorders (Wright, 1982). Thus, the behavioral psychopharmacologist must be able to differentiate the primary features of these disorders from the signs of superimposed psychiatric illnesses.

2. *The behavioral psychopharmacologist must be able to use diagnostic criteria that take into account the pathoplastic effects of mental retardation.*

The diagnostic process in mentally retarded persons is hindered by the lack of criteria that take into account the effects of mental retardation upon the presentation of psychiatric illness (Sovner, 1986). This is especially true for individuals with severe or greater disabilities.

The *Diagnostic and Statistical Manual of Mental Disorders*, 3rd Edition (DSM-III) was created for individuals of normal psychosocial development and intelligence. The DSM-III is difficult to use with mentally retarded persons because of the presence of four pathoplastic effects of developmental disabilities (Sovner, 1986).

The first effect, *cognitive disintegration*, has already been discussed. The second one, *intellectual distortion*, refers to the effects of developmental disabilities on the ability to identify internal feeling states and communicate them to others. This means that diagnostically critical information may not be elicited from the patient, and the diagnostic process must rely on longitudinal behavioral data collected by the family and/or direct caregivers. If intellectual distortion is present, it is virtually impossible to elicit information regarding the presence of hallucinations and delusions in individuals with an IQ of less than 50 (Corbett, 1979; Hucker et al., 1979; Reid, 1972b) because they lack the communication skills to report such symptoms in sufficient detail to be sure of their presence.

The third factor, *baseline exaggeration*, refers to the fact that premorbid maladaptive behaviors may increase in frequency with the onset of a psychiatric illness. This phenomenon is most likely explained on the basis of a nonspecific stress response. Therefore, the clinician must consider the exacerbation of pre-existing behavior as the important diagnostic variable, not just its presence.

The last pathoplastic factor is *psychosocial masking*. This factor reflects the impact of the limited life experience and expectations upon clinical presentation. For example, the delusional percepts of mentally retarded persons are often concrete and resemble the fears of young children. Therefore, the behavioral psychopharmacologist must be an expert in current diagnostic criteria for the various psychiatric disorders and be able to adapt them for use with mentally retarded persons.

3. *The behavioral psychopharmacologist must be able to employ appropriate assessment tools.*

The clinical interview is the principal treatment assessment mode in psychiatry (McHugh & Slavney, 1983). For outpatients, most clinicians rely on the face-to-face meeting with the individual to determine whether drug therapy has been effective. For inpatients, clinicians may also use staff reports and notes during treatment assessment. However, the reliance on the clinical interview is not possible when working with mentally retarded persons. Impaired communication skills, deficits in abstract thinking, and impoverished social skills all serve to render the clinical interview less than effective. Thus, the behavioral psychopharmacologist must depend on serial observations made by others rather than on his or her own perceptions. For this process, behaviorally based diagnostic and treatment evaluation methodologies, employing serial assessments by direct caregivers, are usually required (Aman & White, 1986).

4. *The behavioral psychopharmacologist must be able to employ innovative drug therapies in the treatment of maladaptive behavior syndromes.*

Maladaptive behavior is a heterogeneous phenomenon. Hyperactivity, self-injury, and aggressiveness can be the nonspecific expression of operant conditioning, many different neuropsychiatric syndromes, adverse drug reactions, and distress secondary to physical ailments (Matson, 1986; Sovner & Hurley, 1986). As such, there cannot be one effective intervention. The intervention of choice depends upon the cause of the behavior, not the behavior itself (see Figure 21.1).

The use of pharmacotherapy to treat maladaptive behavior is controversial within the developmental disabilities clinical community. It is usually claimed that the use of lithium or propranolol to treat behavior problems is "experimental" because these indications are not listed in the drug's package insert. However, in the United States this belief is erroneous since many drugs have what are termed "unlabeled" indications. This means that there is some evidence that the drug is effective for a specific disorder, but that the evidence is inconclusive.

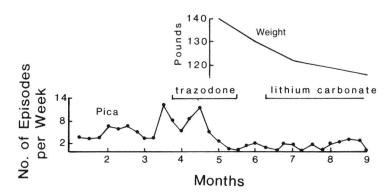

FIGURE 21.1. Treatment of pica associated with major depression. Patient was a 26-year-old woman with childhood onset pervasive developmental disorder and moderate mental retardation who was referred for treatment of pica and self-injurious behavior. Behavioral problems first developed at 7 years of age. Approximately 18 months prior to the evaluation she became apathetic, agitated, hypersomnic, and hyperphagic, and her work performance decreased. She also appeared depressed. A diagnosis of major depression was made. She developed an amphetamine reaction to imipramine and became sedated on trazodone. Once treated with lithium carbonate, she became more animated, her appetite decreased (with a 20-pound weight loss), and the frequency of pica greatly decreased.

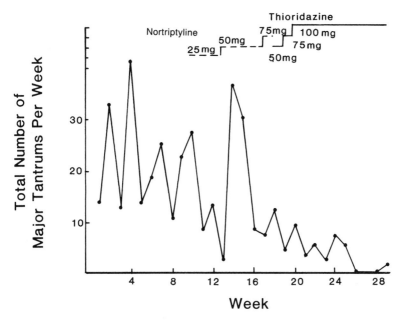

FIGURE 21.2. Treatment of irritability associated with childhood onset pervasive developmental disorder and epilepsy. Patient was a 29-year-old woman with a childhood onset pervasive developmental disorder, severe mental retardation, and a major motor seizure disorder who was referred for the treatment of tantrums characterized by irritable mood and head banging; tantrum frequency increased prior to seizures. She was taking carbamazepine and valproic acid. A diagnosis of organic personality disorder was made. She was first treated with nortriptyline (a depressive illness was suspected) and then with low-dose thioridazine. Upon use of this antipsychotic drug, there was a dramatic reduction in the frequency of her tantrums, which now occur only when she is physically ill and prior to a seizure.

Prescribing drugs for unlabeled indication has a long tradition in medicine and is neither illegal nor against sound medical principles (Archer, 1984; Kapp, 1981). The real conflict is between a medical tradition that is essentially empirical and a scientific one that is inductive and relies on experimental proof to demonstrate validity.

To date, the results of controlled studies have been equivocal, at best, because most of the studies have had crippling methodological flaws (Aman, 1985; Aman & Singh, 1980; Sprague & Werry, 1971). Thus, the evidence for the efficacy of psychotropic drug therapy in the treatment of maladaptive behavior comes largely from well-documented case reports and case series (vide infra) and is therefore largely empirical.

One of the most serious methodological problems in psychotropic drug research has been the failure to use a syndrome paradigm when selecting study subjects. Most drug trial participants share only a specific maladaptive behavior. There has usually been no attempt to select study subjects based on a predetermined set of clinical criteria that control for both neuropsychiatric and medical heterogeneity.

Given the absence of robust experimental data, the scientific issue of the efficacy of pharmacotherapy for maladaptive behavior syndromes cannot be resolved. Nevertheless, case report and anecdotal experience justify its use in selected cases in psychiatric practice, when the issues are clinical not scientific.

## Antipsychotic Drug Therapy

In the past, the use of psychotropic drug therapy, usually with antipsychotic agents, to treat maladaptive behavioral syndromes was heavy handed. Indiscriminate and high-dose antipsychotic drug therapy, without regard to diagnosis or response monitoring, has been the rule. This is unfortunate because antipsychotic drug therapy can produce significant therapeutic results as seen in Figure 21.2 (Aman & Singh, 1986; Mikkelson, 1986; Reid, 1982).

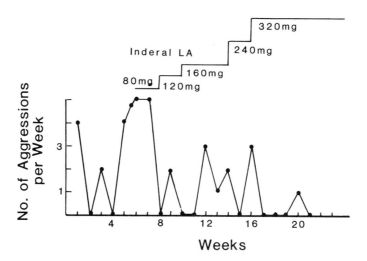

FIGURE 21.3. Treatment of rage attacks with propranolol. Patient was a 33-year-old woman with mild mental retardation and major motor and partial complex seizures. She was referred for the management of intermittent aggressive behavior. In response to any type of frustration, she would become destructive and assaultive. She was remorseful after an aggressive episode. There was no relationship between aggressive behavior and her seizures. At the time of treatment initiation, she was taking carbamazepine, phenobarbital, haloperidol, and benztropine. She was diagnosed as having an organic personality disorder and treated with long-acting propranolol. The treatment resulted in a decreased frequency and intensity of aggressive outbursts. Staff reported that she could now be redirected once an aggressive episode started.

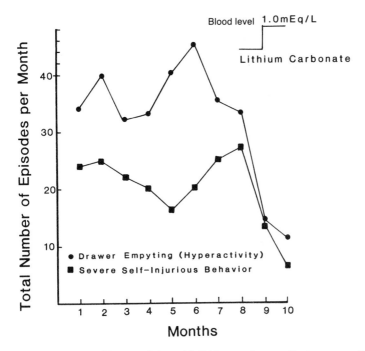

FIGURE 21.4. Treatment of hyperactivity with lithium carbonate. Patient was a 29-year-old man with profound mental retardation secondary to viral encephalitis at age 18 months and a major motor seizure disorder. He was referred for the management of severe hyperactivity associated with hyposomnia, face slapping, assaultiveness, and self-restraining behavior. He was taking thioridazine 400 mg/day at treatment initiation. He was diagnosed as having an atypical organic mental disorder (chronic hyperactivity). With lithium carbonate therapy, he began to sleep, the severity of his hyperactivity greatly diminished (as measured by the frequency of his opening and closing drawers at his residence), and the frequency of his self-injurious behavior decreased as well.

Despite the potential efficacy of antipsychotic drug therapy in selected cases, alternatives to it should be sought. Antipsychotic drugs carry with them the risk of tardive dyskinesia and other types of withdrawal reactions (vide infra).

## Beta-Adrenergic Receptor Blockers

Recent work by Ratey et al. (1986) has demonstrated global positive effects using nadolol and propranolol in mentally retarded individuals with a variety of behavioral problems. Beta-blocker responders appear to be suffering from an organic personality disorder in which they have difficulty modulating strong negative affect. The therapeutic effect seems to decrease the intensity of the rageful feelings, which allows the individual to remain in control (see Figure 21.3).

## Lithium Ion

Clinical experience with lithium in the treatment of hyperactivity and aggressive behavior is mixed. Case reports have documented a clear-cut response (Lion, Hill, & Madden, 1975; Sovner & Hurley, 1981) but clinical studies have reported mixed results (Dale, 1980; Tyrer, Walsh, Edwards, Berney, & Stephens, 1984; Worrall, Moody, & Naylor, 1975). Nonaffectively ill, mentally retarded lithium-responders often suffer from severe hyperactivity associated with hyposomia (see Figure 21.4). They also have a significant number of other maladaptive behaviors that can best be interpreted as secondary manifestations of their hyper-activity (Sovner & Hurley, 1982).

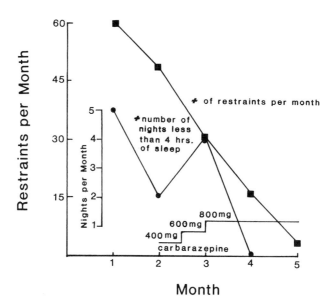

FIGURE 21.5. Treatment of organic personality disorder with carbamazepine. Patient was a 27-year-old woman with severe mental retardation and a major motor seizure disorder secondary to congenital rubella. She was referred for treatment of maladaptive behaviors, including intermittent hyposomia, negativism, self-injurious behavior, regurgitation of food, and self-restraining behavior. Chronic irritability was felt to be a significant problem, with many of her maladaptive behaviors serving a demand avoidance function. At the time of referral, she was taking haloperidol 20 mg/day, chlorpromazine 300 mg/day, phenytoin 200 mg/day, and phenobarbital 90 mg/day. A diagnosis of organic personality disorder (chronic irritability) was made and treatment with carbamazepine was initiated. Treatment response, measured by the number of four-point restraints needed each month, markedly decreased. Restlessness at night also decreased. Once stabilized on carbamazepine, the chlorpromazine, haloperidol, phenytoin, and phenobarbital were all tapered off without adverse effects.

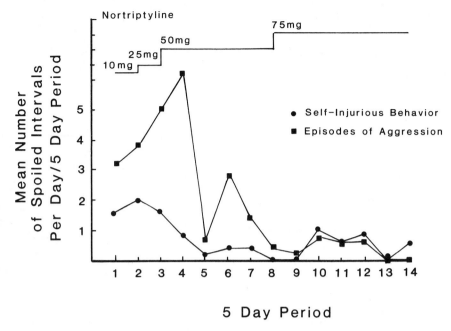

FIGURE 21.6. Treatment of self-injurious behavior associated with major depression. Patient was a 23-year-old woman with mild mental retardation and a major motor seizure disorder who was referred for the treatment of severe self-injurious and aggressive behavior. At the time of referral she lost interest in her usual activities, cried spontaneously, awoke in the middle of the night and banged her head, lost her self-care skills, and banged her head and grabbed other residents of her group home during the day. Her mother had been treated for recurrent depression. At treatment initiation she was being treated with thioridazine 200 mg/day and phenytoin 250 mg/day. A diagnosis of chronic major depression was made. She was treated with nortriptyline. This drug produced a dramatic decrease in the frequency of her self-injurious and aggressive behavior. However, she would engage in head banging whenever she experienced environmentally triggered emotional distress.

## Carbamazepine

Carbamazepine has been demonstrated to have significant psychotropic properties and may be as effective as lithium carbonate in the treatment of affective disorders (Ballinger & Post, 1980; Lerer, 1985). In addition, carbamazepine has been reported to have significant therapeutic effects in mentally retarded persons without the presence of a convulsive disorder (Kanjilal, 1977; Rapport, Sonis, Fialkov, Matson, & Kazdin, 1983; Reid, Naylor, & Kay, 1981). Carbamazepine is particularly effective in the treatment of chronic irritability in profoundly retarded persons (see Figure 21.5).

## Opiate Antagonists

Severe self-injurious behavior (SIB) is a major problem in residential facilities (Matson, 1986). To date, drug therapy has been effective in treating SIB only when it is secondary to a more primary disorder, for example, major depression (see Figure 21.6).

However, recent work has suggested that some types of SIB may be caused by an abnormality of central nervous system endorphin modulation (Richardson & Zaleski, 1986). Anecdotal reports (Gillman & Sandyk, 1985; Richardson & Zaleski, 1986) and a placebo controlled trial (Sandman et al., 1983) have supported the use of naloxone, an opiate antagonist, in SIB, but a recent double trial failed to replicate the efficacy of nalaxone (Beckwith, Couk, & Schumacher, 1986).

Clinical trials with nalaxone, while of significant theoretical interest, have limited treatment implications since the drug has to be administered parenterally. With the introduction of naltrexone, an oral opiate antagonist, the use of opiate antagonist therapy may have an expanded clinical role, especially in cases of severe treatment-resistant SIB.

5. *The behavioral psychopharmacologist must be able to monitor adverse drug reactions in mentally retarded persons, especially those without physical findings.*

Adverse reactions to psychotropic medication have been a principal reason why many clinicians have viewed drug therapy with distrust. In the past, psychiatrists have paid little attention to the potential costs of drug therapy (both psychological as well as physical) to their developmentally disabled patients.

Side effects are especially difficult to manage in mentally retarded persons who may lack the communication skills to report drug-induced distress. Adverse reactions such as constipation may produce serious discomfort without minimal objective findings. Other side effects that have no objective findings, for example, akathisia (Sovner & DiMascio, 1978) can be extremely unpleasant.

Therefore, side-effects management is an extremely important issue in behavioral psychopharmacology because of the possibility that drug therapy itself may exacerbate the problem being treated. Many behavioral problems can be viewed as a nonspecific response to stress. Thus, the presence of a drug-induced state of discomfort may result in the increased frequency of the maladaptive behavior being treated. Important behavioral side effects are listed in Table 21.1.

6. *The behavior psychopharmacologist must be able to implement drug withdrawal trials.*

In 1984, Gualtieri, Quade, Hicks, Mayo, and Schroeder described a behavioral syndrome that followed the discontinuation of thioridazine therapy in mentally retarded children and adolescents. It was characterized by agitation, irritability,

TABLE 21.1. Behavioral side effects of psychotropic drug therapy.[a]

| Behavior | Definition | Implicated drug classes |
|---|---|---|
| Aggression | Unprovoked rage | Benzodiazepines (except for oxazepam) |
| Akathisia | Involuntary motor restlessness | Antipsychotic drugs, amoxapine |
| Akinesia | Depression and muscle weakness | Antipsychotic drugs, amoxapine |
| Amphetamine reaction | Increased energy and racing thoughts | Monoamine oxidase inhibitors, tricyclic antidepressants |
| Carbohydrate craving | Urge to eat increased amounts of sugar and starches | Monoamine oxidase inhibitors, tricyclic antidepressants |
| Nightmares | Vivid and intensely frightening dreams | Antipsychotic drugs, tricyclic antidepressants |
| Urinary incontinence | Daytime and nocturnal enuresis | Antipsychotic drugs, benzodiazepines, lithium |

[a] See Sovner and Hurley (1982).

and insomnia. This syndrome developed in four subjects (out of 41 who were being withdrawn from thioridazine) and completely remitted within eight weeks of drug discontinuation. No data were presented regarding whether the reaction was related to the type of drug taper (slow versus rapid), treatment duration, presence of dyskinetic movements, or daily dose.

This withdrawal syndrome resembles an antipsychotic withdrawal reaction that has been reported to develop in chronic schizophrenics being tapered off low-potency antipsychotic drugs (Chouinard, Bradwejn, Annable, Jones, & Ross-Chouinard, 1984). It was characterized by "insomnia, anxiety, and tension restlessness." It occurred in 85% of patients (22/26) and did not appear to be related to cholinergic rebound effects, which can develop when drugs with anticholinergic effects are discontinued (Gardos, Cole, & Tarsy, 1978).

Despite the scarcity of attention that these withdrawal reactions have received in the clinical literature, they are almost universally reported in facilities carrying out drug withdrawal trials. In my experience, they tend to last several months, they are difficult to manage, and there appears to be no way to prevent them. A slow drug taper does not guarantee that a behavioral withdrawal reaction will not occur.

A complicating factor of this withdrawal reaction is that it may exacerbate preexisting behavioral problems (i.e., baseline exaggeration). This may make it very difficult to determine whether the client has relapsed or is experiencing a pure withdrawal reaction.

Consequently, the behavioral psychopharmacologist must be able to plan drug withdrawal programs which contain contingency plans for any withdrawal syndromes that develop. It is critical that such reactions are not misdiagnosed as a relapse secondary to the discontinuation of antipsychotic drug therapy. To do so may result in a patient receiving indefinite antipsychotic drug therapy.

# Conclusion

Psychotropic drug therapy can no longer be considered to be a second-class intervention to be used only when other "less restrictive" interventions have been unsuccessfully tried (Aman, 1985). While this belief was an understandable reaction by clinicians and advocates to past abuses, a refusal to acknowledge a role for drug therapy at the present time deprives some developmentally handicapped individuals of an enormously positive and prosocial intervention.

## References

Aman, M.G. (1983). Psychoactive drugs in mental retardation. In J.L. Matson & F. Andrasik (Eds.), *Treatment issues and innovations in mental retardation*. New York: Plenum Press.

Aman, M.G. (1985). Drugs in mental retardation: Treatment or tragedy? *Australian and New Zealand Journal of Developmental Disorders, 10*, 215–226.

Aman, M.G., & Singh, N.N. (1980). The usefulness of thioridazine for treating childhood disorders – Fact or folklore? *American Journal of Mental Deficiency, 83*, 331–338.

Aman, M.G., & Singh, N.N. (1986). A critical appraisal of recent drug research in mental retardation: The Coldwater studies. *Journal of Mental Deficiency Research, 30*, 203–216.

Aman, M.G., & White, A.J. (1986). Measures of drug change in mental retardation. *Advances in Learning and Behavioral Disabilities, 5*, 157–203.

Archer, J.D. (1984). The FDA does not approve uses of drugs (Editorial). *JAMA, 252*, 1054–1055.

Ballinger, J.C., & Post, R.M. (1980). Carbamazepine in manic–depressive illness. A new treatment. *American Journal of Psychiatry, 137*, 782–790.

Ballinger, B.R., & Reid, A.H. (1977). Psychiatric disorder in an adult training centre and a hospital for the mentally handicapped. *Psychological Medicine, 7*, 525–528.

Beckwith, B.E., Couk, D.I., & Schumacher, K. (1986). Failure of naloxone to reduce self-injurious behavior in two developmentally disabled females. *Applied Research in Mental Retardation, 7*, 183–188.

Chouinard, G., Bradwejn, J., Annable, L., Jones, B.D., & Ross-Chouinard, A. (1984). Withdrawal symptoms after long-term treatment with low-potency neuroleptics. *Journal of Clinical Psychiatry, 45*, 500–502.

Corbett, J. (1979). Psychiatric morbidity and mental retardation. In F.E. James & R.P. Snaith (Eds.), *Psychiatric illness and mental handicap* (pp. 11–25). London: Gaskell Press.

Dale, P.G. (1980). Lithium therapy in aggressive mentally subnormal patients. *British Journal of Psychiatry, 137*, 469–474.

Eyman, R.K., & Call, T. (1977). Maladaptive behavior and community placement of mentally retarded persons. *American Journal of Mental Deficiency, 82*, 137–144.

Eyman, R.K., Moore, B.C., Capes, L., & Zachofsky, T. (1970). Maladaptive behavior of institutionalized retardates with seizures. *American Journal of Mental Deficiency, 74*, 651–659.

Gardos, G., Cole, J.O., & Tarsy, D. (1978). Withdrawal syndromes associated with antipsychotic drugs. *American Journal of Psychiatry, 135*, 1321–1324.

Gillman, M.A., & Sandyk, R. (1985). Opiatergic and dopaminergic function and Lesch-Nyhan syndrome. *American Journal of Psychiatry, 142*, 1226.

Gostason, R. (1985). Psychiatric illness among the mentally retarded. *Acta Psychiatrica Scandinavica* (Suppl. 318), *71*, 1–117.

Gualtieri, C.T., Quade, D., Hicks, R.E., Mayo, J.P., & Schroeder, S.R. (1984). Tardive dyskinesia and other clinical consequences of neuroleptic treatment in children and adolescents. *American Journal of Psychiatry, 141*, 20–23.

Hucker, S.J., Day, K.A., George, S., & Roth, M. (1979). Psychosis in mentally handicapped adults. In F.E. James & R.P. Snaith (Eds.), *Psychiatric illness and mental handicap* (pp. 27–35). London: Gaskell Press.

Kanjilal, D.C. (1977). An evaluation of Tegretol in adults with epilepsy. In *Tegretol in Epilepsy Proceedings of an International Meeting* (pp. 55–57). London: Geigy Pharmaceuticals.

Kapp, M.B. (1981). Prescribing approved drugs for nonapproved uses: Physicians' disclosure obligations to their patients. *Law Medicine & Healthcare*, 20–23.

Lerer, B. (1985). Alternative therapies for bipolar disorder. *Journal of Clinical Psychiatry, 46*, 309–316.

Lion, J.R., Hill, J., & Madden, D.J. (1975). Lithium carbonate and aggression: A case report. *Diseases of the Nervous System, 36*, 557–558.

Lund, J. (1985). The prevalence of psychiatric morbidity in mentally retarded adults. *Acta Psychiatrica Scandinavica, 72*, 563–570.

Matson, J.L. (1986). Self-injury and its relationship to diagnostic schemes in psychopathology. *Applied Research in Mental Retardation, 7*, 223–227.

McHugh, P.R., & Slavney, P.R. (1983). *The perspective of psychiatry.* Baltimore, MD: The Johns Hopkins Press.

Menolascino, F.J. (1972). Primitive, atypical, and abnormal-psychotic behavior in institutionalized mentally retarded children. *Journal of Autism and Childhood Schizophrenia, 3*, 49–64.

Menolascino, F.J. (1983). Overview. Bridging the gap between mental retardation and mental illness. In F.J. Menolascino & B.M. McCann (Eds.), *Mental health and mental retardation.* Baltimore, MD: University Park Press.

Mikkelson, E.J. (1986). Low-dose haloperidol for stereotypic self-injurious behavior in the mentally retarded. *New England Journal of Medicine, 315*, 398–399.

Paniagua, C., & DeFazio, A. (1983). Psychodynamics of the mildly retarded and borderline intelligence adult. *Psychiatric Quarterly*, 242–252.

Plotkin, R., & Gill, K.R. (1979). Invisible manacles: Drugging mentally retarded people. *Stanford Law Review, 31*, 637–678.

Rapport, M.D., Sonis, W.A., Fialkov, M.J., Matson, J.L., & Kazdin, A.E. (1983). Carbamazepine and behavior therapy for aggressive behavior. *Behavior Modification, 7*, 255–265.

Ratey, J.J., Mikkelson, E.J., Smith, G.B., Upadhyaya, A., Zuckerman, H.S., Martell, D., Sorgi, P., Polakoff, S., & Bemporad, J. (1986). β-blockers in the severely and profoundly mentally retarded. *Journal of Clinical Psychopharmacology, 6*, 103–107.

Reid, A.H. (1972a). Psychoses in adult mental defectives: I. Manic depressive psychosis. *British Journal of Psychiatry, 120*, 205–212.

Reid, A.H., (1972b). Psychoses in adult mental defectives: II. Schizophrenic and paranoid psychoses. *British Journal of Psychiatry, 120*, 213–218.

Reid, A.H. (1982). *The psychiatry of mental handicap.* Oxford: Blackwell Scientific Publications.

Reid, A.H., Ballinger, B.R., Heather, B.B., & Melvin, S.J. (1984). The natural history of behavioral symptoms among severely and profoundly mentally retarded patients. *British Journal of Psychiatry, 145*, 289–293.

Reid, A.H., Naylor, G.J., & Kay, D.S.G. (1981). A double-blind, placebo controlled, crossover trial of carbamazepine in overactive, severely mentally handicapped patients. *Psychological Medicine, 11*, 109–113.

Richardson, J.S., & Zaleski, W.A. (1986). Endogenous opiates and self-mutilation. *American Journal of Psychiatry, 143*, 938–939.

Sandman, C.A., Datta, P.C., Barron, J., Hoehler, F.K., Williams, C., Swanson, J.M. (1983). Naxolone attentuates self-abusive behavior in developmentally disabled clients. *Applied Research in Mental Retardation, 4*, 5–11.

Sandyk, C.A., Datta, P.C., Barron, J., Hoehler, F.K., Williams, C., & Swanson, J.M. (1983). Naloxone attentuates self-abusive behavior in developmentally disabled clients. *Applied Research in Mental Retardation, 4*, 5–11.

Sovner, R. (1986). Limiting factors in the use of DSM-III criteria with mentally ill– mentally retarded persons. *Psychopharmacology Bulletin, 22*, 1055–1059.

Sovner, R., & DiMascio, A. (1978). Extrapyramidal syndromes and other neurological side effects of psychotropic drugs. In M.A. Lipton, A. DiMascio, & K.F. Killam (Eds.), *Psychopharmacology: A generation of progress.* New York: Raven Press.

Sovner, R., & Hurley, A.D. (1981). The management of chronic behavior disorders in mentally retarded adults with lithium carbonate. *Journal of Nervous and Mental Disorders, 169*, 191–195.

Sovner, R., & Hurley, A.D. (1982). Psychotropic drug side effects presenting as behavior disorders. *Psychiatric Aspects of Mental Retardation, 1*, 45–48.

Sovner, R., & Hurley, A.D. (1983). Do the mentally retarded suffer from affective illness? *Archives of General Psychiatry, 40*, 61–67.

Sovner, R., & Hurley, A.D. (1986). Managing aggressive behavior: A psychiatric approach. *Psychiatric Aspects of Mental Retardation, 5*, 16–21.

Sprague, R. (1982). Litigation, legislation, and regulations. In S.E. Breuning & A.D. Poling (Eds.), *Drugs and mental retardation* (pp. 377–414). Springfield, IL: Charles C Thomas.

Sprague, R.L., & Werry, J.S. (1971). Methodology of psychopharmacological studies with the retarded. In N.R. Ellis (Ed.), *International review of research in mental retardation* (Vol. 5). New York: Academic Press.

Tyrer, S.P., Walsh, A., Edwards, D.E., Berney, T.P., & Stephens, D.A. (1984). Factors associated with a good response to lithium in aggressive mentally handicapped subjects. *Progress in Neuro-Psychopharmacology & Biological Psychiatry, 8*, 751–755.

Worrall, E.P., Moody, J.P., & Naylor, G.J. (1975). Lithium in non-manic depressives: Antiaggressive effect and red blood cell lithium values. *British Journal of Psychiatry, 126*, 464–468.

Wright, E.C. (1982). The presentation of mental illness in mentally retarded adults. *British Journal of Psychiatry, 141*, 496–502.

# Conclusion

FRANK J. MENOLASCINO

In addition to the specific clinical treatment recommendations made by many of the authors within the eight chapters of this section, there are other global service recommendations that each of the authors feels will be required, if we are to carry out the treatment processes described within their individual approaches and programs.

1. We need to establish multistate regional treatment centers, where the dually diagnosed population will be provided service within a research and training setting. We also need to establish multidisciplinary service centers within each state to serve as satellite treatment programs that promote deinstitutionalization, prevent institutionalization, and provide an orderly transition from the schools into the community.
2. We need to use University Affiliated Facilities across the country to design model service programs to provide direct care to this population, as a vehicle for training and research activities in such areas as inpatient care, day hospitals, specialized outpatient treatment clinics, prevocational/vocational centers, parent and community support groups, and intervention techniques.
3. University Affiliated Facilities must reexamine their limited focus on children and exert additional efforts in training mental health personnel to meet the growing service needs of adults of all ages. Recent emphasis on transitional service, via administrative support from the Office of Special Education and Rehabilitation Services and the Administration on Developmental Disabilities, is an encouraging sign in this area.
4. We need to provide technical support and consultative services to community and institutional settings as they relate to the areas of diagnostic clarification and treatment options, as well as the establishment and maintenance of programs integrated into the community. Both vocational and residential components will be necessary in order for dually diagnosed individuals to live in the community.
5. We need further exploration into the diagnostic aspects of mental illness in the mentally retarded. We need to understand better how diagnostic instruments

can provide differential diagnoses between individuals who are mentally retarded/mentally ill and those who are mentally retarded and nonmentally ill. This will permit us a more valid comparison of treatment interventions and their overall effectiveness.

6. We need to study further the factors that make a person with mental retardation more at risk to develop concomitant mental illness (e.g., atypical developmental profiles and delayed language) and to separate biological and psychosocial parameters in order to understand these "at-risk" factors better.

# Section V: Program Models
## Introduction

PETER A. HOLMES

Treatment technology for the problems of mentally ill/mentally retarded (MI/MR) persons clearly exists. A survey of 463 agencies serving dually diagnosed persons found that the whole gamut of treatment techniques used with normal populations is used with MI/MR persons (Holmes, 1983). Implementing successful and comprehensive approaches to deal with the many problem areas identified in this book, however, is quite another matter. This section addresses pitfalls that occur when MI/MR persons are served in conventional treatment settings. Model programs and service strategies to overcome these pitfalls are discussed.

The chapters in this section use the label MI/MR broadly to refer to persons who are mentally retarded with serious functional problems of living – persons who function poorly in the environments they are in either because of the things they do or fail to do. This expanded functional definition covers the broad range of behaviors that puts persons with mental retardation at risk of more restrictive care or loss of opportunities for employment, mainstream schooling, or other community participation. For example, Steven Reiss (Chapter 23) has found that the greatest unmet need for mental health services for mentally retarded persons is to help adolescents and young adults adjust to community-based jobs, workshop programs, and residential placements. Although poor adjustment to living and working environments may not technically fit criteria for mental illness in DSM-III, treatment for such problems is certainly part of the activities normally carried out by mental health workers.

MI/MR persons are usually referred for treatment because they exhibit unwanted behaviors. Strategies to *eliminate* unwanted behavior frequently become the focus of treatment. Getting rid of behavior without identifying acceptable alternatives can lead to punitive consequences (as discussed in Section IV of this book).

Perhaps the debate over "aversive" control should be shifted to an analysis of the proper focus for treatment. Goldiamond (1974) distinguishes between eliminative and constructional treatment approaches. Eliminative approaches focus on reducing unwanted problem behaviors similar to a medical strategy to eliminate a rash by recommending a skin salve. On the other hand, constructional approaches focus on building a more appropriate behavioral repertoire. Successful programs make accomplishment of adaptive behaviors a higher priority than control of unwanted behaviors. The constructional approach is likely to lead to solutions that will have long-lasting effects (Cullen, Hattersley, & Tennant, 1981; Delprato, 1981). If unwanted behavior is our focus, we must design programs that educate – such as social skills training, communication, and money management.

Just as with individuals, treatment programs should be evaluated in terms of resident accomplishments, not just control of problem behavior. Unfortunately, most evaluation systems focus on *not* using certain procedures. Review agencies, such as the Accreditation Council for Mentally Retarded Developmentally Disabled (ACMRDD), mandate no seclusion and require that restraint, behavior-controlling drugs, and time-out devices be used as a last resort. This kind of pressure has reduced or eliminated restrictive and intrusive procedures, but this has not necessarily resulted in improved client functioning or adaptive behaviors. The Staffing Needs Assessment Plan (SNAP) actually reinforces agencies for reporting high rates of maladaptive behaviors that require "spontaneous intervention." SNAP bases future staffing levels on the number of inappropriate behaviors; agencies benefit from crises.

Accrediting review agencies could get away from this negative focus by scrutinizing the number of acquired, measurable, adaptive, self-care, socialization, vocational, and leisure skills achieved for residents of the programs they evaluate. Outcome success of service providers should become as important an index of program accountability as the lack of negative controls as demonstrated in the chapters in this section.

Much time and planning go into finding an ideal environment for MI/MR persons. Placement agencies often make assignments to living environments based on a behavioral history from an institutional setting, psychological reports, and clinical intuition. Unfortunately, likelihood of success predictors are woefully inadequate.

Robitscher (1980) carefully documents the failure of psychiatrists to predict dangerousness of mental patients. Steadman (1973) found that less than 3% of criminally insane patients acted dangerously during a four-year follow-up of their release; a release that was made despite psychiatrists' judgments that these persons were likely to commit violent acts. The American Psychiatric Association has gone on record citing that "study after study has shown" that the psychiatrist "is ill-equipped to undertake ... the prediction of his patient's potential dangerousness" (American Psychiatric Association, 1976).

Postdischarge adjustment data from an adolescent treatment program show similar problems with predictive success for MI/MR persons (Minnesota Learning Center, 1982). For youngsters given a planned release from the program, 70% made a satisfactory adjustment to reentry to their home and school setting. For youngsters given an unplanned release (persons not considered ready for a return to the community), 45% made a satisfactory readjustment to the home and school and another 12% made a satisfactory adjustment to at least one of these two environments. Few programs collect as much information about clients or carefully plan for graduation of clients as the Minnesota Learning Center (MLC) program. Despite careful assessment and planning, almost half of the participants not considered ready for discharge made a successful transition back to the community. Other programs that pay less attention to resident behavior and graduation planning are likely to have even lower predictive success than the MLC.

It is important to recognize the limitations of placement success predictors. It is especially important to give institutionalized persons the benefit of the doubt and attempt to place them in as normal an environment as possible. It is only then that a MI/MR person's ability to adjust to community living can be assessed fairly.

Many other chapters in this section also refer to how MI/MR persons fall through the cracks of mental health systems. Programs designed for MI/MR persons easily become a dumping ground for all the clients no one else wants. Rehabilitation for this kind of problem can only be handled in natural settings (Brown et al., 1979, 1981) and through a developmental process as described in Chapter 26 by Bijou and Chapter 27 by Stark, Kiernan, and Goldsbury. Highly individualized plans that estimate the level of "ultimate functioning" are necessary if we wish to help these individuals become more independent and return to society. Just as with treatment focus, our vocational and living plans for MI/MR persons will determine their future success. If we plan special program sites for them, they will end up in sheltered workshops, behavior treatment units, and day treatment programs. If we plan for them to be integrated into community settings, they will, at a minimum, end up in supported work, transitional community programs, and semi-independent living environments.

Another failure of transition has been this population residing in state mental institutions. For example, an actual count of patients in Michigan mental hospitals has determined that 8% of long-term institutionalized patients meet AAMD's criteria for mental retardation and DSM-III criteria for some form of mental illness. This is undoubtedly a low estimate since many low-functioning adult patients did not have IQ records before the age of 18. A common theme throughout not only this section but the entire book is that this dual diagnosed population is probably the most underserved population cared for in America. Efforts to move these dually diagnosed persons out of mental health settings and into mental retardation settings in the community should be a top priority for every state mental health system that has not already done so.

## References

American Psychiatric Association. (1976). *Amicus Curiae Brief, Tarasoff v. Regents of University of California*, 551 P. 2d 334.

Brown, L., Branston, M.B., Hamre-Nietupski, S., Pumpian, I., Certo, N., & Gruenewald, L. (1979). A strategy for developing chronological age appropriate and functional curricular content for severely handicapped adolescents and young adults. *Journal of Special Education, 13*(1), 81–90.

Brown, L., Pumpian, I., Baumgart, D., VanDeventer, P., Ford, A., Nisbet, J., Schroeder, J., & Gruenewald, L. (1981). Longitudinal transition plans in programs for severely handicapped students. *Exceptional Children, 47*(8), 1–10.

Cullen, C., Hattersley, J., & Tennant, L. (1981). Establishing behavior; the constructional approach. In G. Davey (Eds.), *Applications of conditioning theory* (pp. 149–161). London: Methuen.

Delprato, D.J. (1981). The constructional approach to behavioral modification. *Journal of Behavior Therapy and Experimental Psychiatry, 12*, 49–55.

Goldiamond, I. (1974). Toward a constructional approach to social problems. *Behaviorism, 2*, 1–84.

Holmes, P.A. (1983). Final report dual diagnosis program study: MI/MR state-of-the-art service delivery. Available from DD Planning Council, Michigan Department of Mental Health (Lewis Cass Building), Lansing, MI.

Minnesota Learning Center. (1982). *Annual report and program description (fiscal year 1982)*. Brainard, MN: Author. Thomas D.R.

Robitscher, J. (1980). *The powers of psychiatry*. Boston, MA: Houghton Mifflin.

Steadman, H. (1973). Follow-up on Baxstrom patients returned to hospitals for the criminally insane. *American Journal of Psychiatry, 130*, 317–319.

# 22
# A University-Based Demonstration Program on Outpatient Mental Health Services for Mentally Retarded People

STEVEN REISS

The consequences of untreated emotional problems among mentally retarded people include intense suffering (Reiss & Benson, 1984), unemployment (Greenspan & Shoultz, 1981), placement in state institutions (Eyman, O'Connor, Tarjan, & Justice, 1972), suicide (Benson & Laman, 1986), and crime. For example, depression in mentally retarded people is associated with social isolation, ineffective social interactions, and inappropriate social behavior (Laman & Reiss, 1986). Aggression and conduct disorders are among the most frequently cited problems in providing adequate services for mentally retarded people. Schizophrenia and schizoid personality processes lead to withdrawal from the interpersonal environment and significantly impair the quality of the individual's life. Personality disorders lead to social problems and sometimes result in placement in restrictive residential facilities.

In 1980, Steven Reiss and Joseph Szyszko created a developmental disabilities mental health program at the University of Illinois at Chicago (Reiss & Trenn, 1984). This program, called the Illinois–Chicago Mental Health Program, has research, clinical, and educational activities. The program is jointly sponsored by the Illinois Department of Mental Health and Developmental Disabilities and the University of Illinois at Chicago.

Perhaps the best-known research conducted at the Illinois–Chicago Program concerned a phenomenon we called *diagnostic overshadowing*. This concept applies to instances in which the presence of mental retardation decreases the chances that an accompanying emotional disorder will be diagnosed. For example, psychologists tend to rate the same case description of schizophrenia lower on scales of psychopathology when the individual is mentally retarded versus intellectually average. Our first two experiments established that overshadowing occurs for cases involving schizophrenia, personality disorder, and debilitating fear. We also found that this overshadowing phenomenon can be demonstrated with psychologists who have had much professional experience with mentally retarded people. The results of these overshadowing studies may help to explain the inadequate level of mental health services for mentally retarded people. That is, the level of mental health services may be inadequate because professionals do not diagnose emotional problems as often as they should.

Another research project at the Illinois–Chicago program concerns the occurrence of depression among mentally retarded people. Depression is among the most frequently seen problems at our outpatient developmental disabilities mental health clinic; depression is especially common among lonely, adult women with mental retardation. In our initial studies, we found that depression in mentally retarded people is associated with low levels of social support and with poor social skills (Benson, Reiss, Smith, & Laman, 1985; Reiss & Benson, 1985). We also identified some of the specific social skill deficiencies that are associated with depressed mood in mentally retarded people (Laman & Reiss, 1986). These studies add to our understanding of depressed mood and provide a basis for future research. One hypothesis is that social skills training might prevent or partially cure some cases of depressed mood among mentally retarded people.

Dr. Betsey Benson, a research psychologist in our program, has been working on the development of a new therapy for the treatment of conduct disorders. This therapy, called Anger Management Therapy, is based on the principles of cognitive-behavior therapy (Benson, 1986; Benson, Rice, & Miranti, 1986). The program teaches mentally retarded people to identify social situations that make them angry, to stop engaging in self-talk that makes them angry, and to solve anger-provoking problems in socially appropriate ways. The results of the initial research on this new therapy have been encouraging. Mentally retarded adults like this therapy and it seems to have benefits in diminishing angry outbursts.

An Illinois–Chicago research team developed a screening test for emotional problems of mentally retarded people. The test, called the "Reiss Screen for Maladaptive Behavior," screens for 40 possible symptoms of emotional disorders (Benson & Reiss, 1984). The noteworthy features of the test are plain language definitions of psychiatric symptoms and the use of behavioral examples to help raters understand each symptom. Caretakers rate the extent to which each symptom is "no problem," a "problem," or a "major problem" for the person who is being rated.

Graduate student research projects at the Illinois–Chicago program include efforts to develop new methods for treating romantic loneliness in mentally retarded people, the development of a scale measuring stigmatization, and an evaluation of how mentally retarded and nonretarded people respond to stress.

# Clinical Services

The Illinois–Chicago program sponsors an outpatient developmental disabilities mental health program. The clinic serves all age groups on a "first come, first served" basis. It provides only mental health services for mentally retarded people and does not accept referrals for the diagnosis of mental retardation.

## Consumer Demand

The results of the Illinois–Chicago clinical study indicate a strong level of unmet consumer demand for mental health services for mentally retarded people (Reiss & Trenn, 1984). In the last five years, the clinic has received approximately 125 new referrals per year. The clinic has served between 50 and 75 clients per week, mostly on an individual basis. The demand for services has greatly exceeded the capacity of the clinic.

In addition to demonstrating a high level of consumer demand for services, the Illinois–Chicago clinic also provided data on the characteristics of the people seeking services. Benson (1985) studied a sample of the first 130 referrals to the Illinois–Chicago clinic. The clients ranged in age from 4 to 55 years, and males outnumbered females by about 70% to 30%. The sample consisted of 56 Blacks, 60 Caucasians, and 14 Hispanics. The demand for mental health services for mentally retarded people appears to be greater for adolescents and young adults than children. Reiss and Trenn (1984) reported that 63.8% of the clients were between the ages of 15 and 29. They suggested that the greater demand for this age group may in part be due to the loss of a major social support system (public schools) and to "aging out." Aging out is a process where mentally retarded people receive fewer services as they become older.

## Psychopathology

The Reiss (1982) and Benson (1985) surveys at the Illinois–Chicago clinic provided information on the types of emotional disorders for which mentally retarded people seek mental health services. On the one hand, the findings supported previous reports that mentally retarded people are vulnerable to the full range of psychopathology (Eaton & Menolascino, 1982; Philips, 1967; Sarason & Gladwyn, 1958). On the other hand, some emotional disorders were seen at the clinic much more frequently than others. Benson (1985) reported that about 85% of the referrals to the Illinois–Chicago clinic could be classified into one of three broad groups: schizoid–unresponsive and psychotic disorders, conduct disorders, and anxious–depressed withdrawal disorders.

## Therapy

The administrative philosophy of the Illinois–Chicago clinic has been to support qualified therapists regardless of theoretical orientation. The clinic has welcomed behavior therapists, cognitive therapists, psychodynamic therapists, art therapists, reinforcement therapists, family therapists, and drug therapists. The clinic has had success and failure with each of these therapies; much seems to depend on the individual case, the individual therapist, and the course of life circumstances beyond the control of the therapist. Generally, mentally retarded people are appreciative customers of psychotherapy. Many mentally retarded people with emotional problems respond well to therapists who show them concern and respect.

The experience of the Illinois–Chicago clinic suggests that we might need to pay special attention to the concept of therapy as a supportive service that is available when needed as opposed to the idea that therapy can "cure" mentally retarded people of "mental diseases." Every so often, a person with mental retardation might stumble in his or her effort to adjust to independent living. Unfortunate life events might occur that cause emotional problems or stimulate the recurrence of abnormal behavior. At such a point in the life of a person with mental retardation, mental health services can help support the individual until the difficult adjustment period has passed.

## Educational Activities

The Illinois–Chicago program sponsors a wide range of educational activities. Graduate education includes both professional and research training on a multi-disciplinary basis. The Illinois–Chicago program is affiliated with a clinical psychology training program approved by the American Psychological Association. The Illinois–Chicago program also is affiliated with the university's training programs in art therapy and social work.

The Illinois–Chicago program provides graduate and medical training for students from six Chicago-area universities. The list includes the Chicago Medical School, Illinois School of Professional Psychology, Loyola Medical School, Northern Illinois University, Northwestern University, and the University of Illinois at Chicago. Starting in 1987, the program will train graduate and medical students from the University of Seville.

The Illinois–Chicago program has demonstrated a strong level of consumer demand for continuing education about the mental health aspects of mental retardation. The program sponsors a sequence of three continuing education courses. Each course consists of eight weekly sessions lasting about three hours each. Each course is taught once per year with enrollment limited to 50 professionals working with mentally retarded people. Additionally, the Illinois–Chicago program provides workshops and lectures throughout the State of Illinois. These activities are provided by special arrangements at the request of agency and state administrators.

## Conclusions

We need to pay greater attention to the mental health aspects of mental retardation. We need to know more about the causes, nature, prevention, and treatment of mental health problems in mentally retarded people. We need to train professionals who are knowledgeable on this topic, and we also need to make state-of-the-art services available to more people. These services are especially relevant to supporting the movement toward community care of mentally retarded people. As has been demonstrated at the University of Illinois at Chicago, University Affiliated Facilities in mental retardation are well suited to develop needed demonstration programs on the mental health aspects of mental retardation.

### References

Benson, B.A. (1985). Emotional disturbance and mental retardation: Association with age, sex, and level of functioning in an outpatient clinic sample. *Applied Research in Mental Retardation, 6*, 70–85.

Benson, B.A. (1986). Anger management training. *Psychiatric Aspects of Mental Retardation, 5*, 51–56.

Benson, B.A., & Laman, D.S. (1986). *Suicide among the mentally retarded.* Unpublished paper, University of Illinois at Chicago.

Benson, B.A., & Reiss, S. (1984). A factor analysis of emotional disorders in mentally retarded people. *Australia and New Zealand Journal of Developmental Disabilities, 10*, 135–139.

Benson, B.A., Reiss, S., Smith, D., & Laman, D.S. (1985). Psychosocial correlates of depression in mentally retarded adults. II. Social skills. *American Journal of Mental Deficiency, 89*, 657–659.

Benson, B.A., Rice, C.J., & Miranti, S.V. (1986). Effects of anger management training with mentally retarded adults in group treatment. *Journal of Consulting and Clinical Psychology, 54*, 728–729.

Eaton, L.F., & Menolascino, F.J. (1982). Psychiatric disorders in the mentally retarded: Types, problems, and challenges. *American Journal of Psychiatry, 139*, 1297–1303.

Eyman, R.K., O'Connor, G., Tarjan, G., & Justice, R.S. (1972). Factors determining residential placement of mentally retarded children. *American Journal of Mental Deficiency, 76*, 692–698.

Greenspan, S., & Shoultz, B. (1981). Why mentally retarded adults lose their jobs: Social competence as a factor in work adjustment. *Applied Research in Mental Retardation, 2*, 23–38.

Laman, D.S., & Reiss, S. (1986). Social skill deficits associated with depressed mood in mentally retarded adults. Unpublished manuscript, University of Illinois at Chicago.

Levitan, G.W., & Reiss, S. (1983). Generality of diagnostic overshadowing across disciplines. *Applied Research in Mental Retardation, 2*, 23–38.

Philips, I. (1967). Psychopathology and mental retardation: *American Journal of Psychiatry, 124*, 29–35.

Reiss, S. (1982). Psychopathology and mental retardation: Survey of a developmental disabilities mental health program. *Mental Retardation, 20*, 128–132.

Reiss, S. (1985). The mentally retarded, emotionally disturbed adult. In M. Sigman (Ed.), *Children with emotional disorders and developmental disabilities.* Orlando, FL: Grune & Stratton.

Reiss, S., & Benson, B.A. (1984). Awareness of negative social conditions among mentally retarded, emotionally disturbed outpatients. *American Journal of Psychiatry, 141*, 88–90.

Reiss, S., & Benson, B.A. (1985). Psychosocial correlates of depression in mentally retarded adults: I. Minimal social support and stigmatization. *American Journal of Mental Deficiency, 89*, 567–574.

Reiss, S., Levitan, G., & Szyszko, J. (1982). Emotional disturbance and mental retardation: Diagnostic overshadowing. *American Journal of Mental Deficiency, 86*, 567–574.

Reiss, S., & Szyszko, J. (1983). Diagnostic overshadowing and professional experience with retarded persons. *American Journal of Mental Deficiency, 87*, 396–402.

Reiss, S., & Trenn, E. (1984). Consumer demand for outpatient mental health services for mentally retarded people. *Mental Retardation, 22*, 112–116.

Sarason, S.B., & Gladwyn, T. (1958). Psychological and cultural problems in mental subnormality. In R.L. Masland, S.B. Sarason, & T. Gladwin (Eds.), *Mental subnormality.* New York: Basic Books.

# 23
# A County Systems Model: Comprehensive Services for the Dually Diagnosed

ROBERT J. FLETCHER

## Issues and Problems

As the primary focus of care for the mentally retarded has changed from institutional settings to community environments, substantial numbers of these individuals need concomitant mental health services (Menolascino, 1983). A number of studies have demonstrated that mental illness is present in the mentally retarded (Chess, 1962; Eaton & Menolascino, 1982; Webster, 1971). Outpatient clinic studies have found a 20 to 35% prevalence of mental illness in the mentally retarded (Menolascino, 1965; Philips & Williams, 1975).

Yet, neither the field of mental retardation nor that of mental health is adequately addressing the needs of individuals who have the coexistence of mental illness and mental retardation. The mental health delivery systems for mentally retarded persons are unresponsive, utterly inadequate, and often nonexistent (President's Commission on Mental Health, 1978). Mentally retarded people who are also mentally ill may constitute one of the most underserved populations in the United States (Reiss, Levitan, & McNally, 1982). They frequently "fall through the cracks," as they are unidentified and undertreated — ergo, neglected.

There are a number of complex explanations for the neglect of mental health services for the mentally retarded. In the early twentieth century, the field of mental health and that of mental retardation began to diverge. The emergence of IQ testing, specifically the Binet Test, changed diagnostic procedures for the mentally retarded; the IQ measurement as a diagnostic tool replaced the traditional psychiatric assessment procedure. The first two decades of this century is the "tragic interlude," in which the interest of mental health involvement shifted away from mental retardation (Menolascino, 1983). Psychological testing helped to advance the national policy of institutionalization, in which mentally retarded persons were "warehoused" in large, impersonal, and dehumanizing institutions.

Another explanation is professional and community ignorance, bias, and negative attitudes toward the mentally retarded. Professionals are vulnerable to the same cultural biases and misconceptions regarding mental retardation that are held by society at large (Cushna, Szymanski, & Tanguay, 1980). Psychotherapists tend to view the retarded in the same way nonprofessionals view this popultion: as uninteresting and unattractive (West & Richardson, 1981). Many professionals do not perceive mentally retarded persons as being candidates for, or as benefiting from, mental health services. The lack of formal training regarding the mental health needs of the mentally retarded contributes to the misconception that mentally retarded persons are "eternal children and happy-go-lucky prince charmings." The mildly retarded have been characterized as worry-free and thus mentally healthy. The severely retarded have been considered to express no feelings and therefore do not experience emotional stress.

A third explanation is the recent changes in regulatory bodies. During the last decade, many state governments moved to restructure the delivery of mental hygiene services, which resulted in a separation of mental health and mental retardation systems. Each system developed its own policies, procedures, and funding mechanisms. Access into either system is based on diagnostic criteria. Simply stated, persons diagnosed as mentally retarded have access to services regulated by the state mental retardation and developmental disabilities system, while those diagnosed as having mental health problems have access to the state mental health system. The primary diagnosis is the leading—and usually the sole—criterion determining which of the two systems a person has access to.

The social policy of deinstitutionalization has focused attention on the mental health needs of community-based, mentally retarded persons. The move from institutions to community-based settings has not only been a physical change; the definition of normal and abnormal behavior has been revised (Menolascino, 1983). Some maladaptive behaviors observed in the institutions were viewed as manifestations of the condition of mental retardation and therefore were considered normal. The same behaviors manifested by a community-based, mentally retarded individual are viewed as abnormal, as related to allied mental health problems.

Although the relationship of maladaptive behavior in the mentally retarded to psychopathology has been noted in the literature for decades, only in recent years has there been a growing professional concern, reflected in the proliferation of publications and the founding of the National Association for the Dually Diagnosed. However, this population still is underserved. Significant policy issues need to be addressed on national, state, and local levels. Since there has been no national policy regarding the dually diagnosed population (those with the coexistence of mental retardation and mental illness), there have been no financial incentives for state levels of government to peruse program development for them. The wheels of government move slowly, and the problems cannot wait for a national solution. There is a crucial need to address these issues now, and the local level is best equipped to begin to do it. Although federal and state policy development and funding are essential in the long run, local government need not wait for them. Local initiatives can respond to the mental health problems of the mentally retarded.

## Local-Level Model

This chapter describes a program to address the holistic needs of dually diagnosed individuals administered by Ulster County, a rural area between New York City and Albany, New York. The county is geographically large and has a total population of 160,000. There are a sizable number of chronically mentally ill and mentally retarded persons living in Ulster County, partially because of the deinstitutionalization process.

The chapter describes the services that currently exist as well as those in the planning stages. Compositely, this represents a local-level systems' model of comprehensive services for the dually diagnosed population.

Although a limited number of services for the dually diagnosed client have existed for several years in Ulster County, a planned systems' development model toward providing a comprehensive service was not initiated until 1984. It is impossible to plan effectively or rationally without knowing how many individuals were inadequately served in the existing service system and what services were needed to fill the gaps. In early 1985, a survey instrument was developed and sent to all mental retardation and mental health agencies within the county. The data from the survey have revealed some interesting information. The following is a cursory review of some of the data.

There are approximately 200 dually diagnosed clients in the county (using DSM-III classification):

17% of the mentally retarded clients in Ulster County have a concomitant psychiatric disorder;
45% of the dually diagnosed clients in Ulster County live in unsupervised settings;
73.5% were between the ages of 18 and 44;
62% did not receive mental health service within the past 12 months;
82% were served through the mental retardation system, the rest by the mental-health-funded system;
54% of the study population did not receive services across disability lines.

These figures, as well as the analysis of other data from the survey, suggest that there is a large number of individuals in Ulster County who have the coexistence of mental retardation and mental illness and that the majority of these individuals are not receiving adequate services. The analysis also suggests that there is a need for the mental retardation system and mental health system to work in a more coordinated manner toward the development of an appropriate delivery service system. The plan involves six service components for providing a comprehensive service system:

Outpatient mental health services
Day treatment services
Inpatient psychiatric care
Appropriate community-based residential services

Vocational training and employment
Staff training and systems coordination

The following will describe each of these service provisions and its stage of development.

## Outpatient Mental Health Services

Outpatient mental health services are currently provided by Ulster County Community Mental Health Services. Currently, there are two full-time social workers and a part-time psychiatrist specifically designated to provide mental health services to the dually diagnosed citizens and their families.

A family systems' treatment model is frequently employed when the dually diagnosed individual resides with his or her natural family. Our experience has suggested that many problems occur as a result of dysfunctional family dynamics (see also Allin, Chapter 24). Individual therapy sessions tend to take an existential (here-and-now) approach. The focus is on helping the client to identify the problem(s) and to explore effective and appropriate ways to manage problem situations. In this way, the client learns problem-solving skills. Medication treatment and psychiatric consultation are also available. In addition to office visits, the two social work specialists go into the group homes and sheltered workshops to provide individual counseling and group therapy services. This outreach mobile treatment has helped to bridge the gap between the mental health and mental retardation system barriers.

## Day Treatment Services

Ulster County has had a day-treatment program for dually diagnosed persons since 1980. The program is operated by Beacon House, a large psychiatric partial-hospitalization service, under the auspices of Ulster County Community Mental Health Services. The dual diagnosis day-treatment program is administratively and physically under the umbrella of an existing day-treatment service, and therefore it has been cost effective. Concomitantly, this specialized service has developed its own unique clinical and programmatic perspective.

The age range of the recipients of this service is from 24 to 46 years and the IQ range is from 54 to 82. All the clients have a DSM-III psychiatric disorder reflected as the primary diagnosis. Most of the clients are referred to this program after they have been terminated by other provider agencies owing to behavioral problems, or they have not been accepted into the service offered by other agencies owing to the fact of their dual diagnosis.

Common threads found in the clients' case histories are dysfunctional family systems, failure in school, rejection by peers, and difficulty in establishing and maintaining appropriate interactional behaviors. The program uses a highly structured group method of treatment in a supportive environment. Individual therapy is also provided by licensed clinicians, and medication treatment is available. The program components within an interdisciplinary team approach include clinical services, creative art therapies, socialization, social skill training, and recreation. A salient aspect of this model is that one's active involvement in the program becomes the primary vehicle for treatment. The members have developed positive group identity, and a feeling of community has been the result. This sense of belonging to a peer group and being a member of a milieu community counteracts the feelings of isolation, defeat, and inadequacy that are characteristic of these individuals. Essential features of the model are the therapeutic relationships, bonding, and the quality of human interactions that occur between staff and clients. Mutual respect and dignity for one another are the philosophical cornerstones of the program.

Research that I conducted in 1983 (Fletcher, 1984), to measure the effectiveness of the program, demonstrated a significant improvement in the study population in areas of socialization skills, impulse control, self-esteem, and problem-solving skills. This day-treatment service is considered a model program and has been replicated by various agencies in the country.

The survey data indicated a top priority to expand the day-treatment service. However, Beacon House is not able to expand the day-treatment service for the dually diagnosed owing to both staffing and physical space limitations. To address this identified need, the mental retardation system has offered to license and operate the program as they have the resources to expand the service. This would enable 35 to 50 clients to be served on a five-day-a-week schedule, which began in 1986. Ulster County Mental Health Services intends to provide two psychiatric social workers and a psychiatrist to complement the staffing pattern of the new program. These mental health professionals have provided psychiatric assessments, individual, group, and family treatment services, as well as staff training and development. This is another example of how the mental health and mental retardation systems, at the local level, can use available resources in a cooperative manner toward planning and operating services.

## Inpatient Psychiatric Care

Accessibility into inpatient psychiatric care for this population has been a problem. Ulster County has two resources in the catchment area: a community-based hospital that has a psychiatric ward and a state psychiatric hospital. The problem occurs when a mentally retarded person manifests one or more of the following: acute psychotic symptoms, suicidal ideations, and/or assaultive behavior. Although these symptoms are commonly found in a nonretarded psychiatric client, when they are manifested in a mentally retarded person, they are seen differently by admitting physicians. Often they are viewed as symptoms of the condition of mental retardation, rather than as symptoms of existing psychopathology, and therefore perceived as untreatable. And, of course, we have the provincial boundary issue. Hospital doctors and administrators often take the "pass-the-buck" approach. A typical response would be, "Well, he is mentally retarded and therefore ineligible for psychiatric inpatient care at this facility." All too often, this results in the merry-go-round referral process.

A significant step that recently took place is an arrangement with another state psychiatric hospital that presently operates a specialized unit for the dually diagnosed population. Clients will have access to an appropriate inpatient service and receive treatment by trained and experienced professional mental health providers.

## Appropriate Community-Based Residential Services

At present, the local mental retardation system operates two community-based residences for mentally retarded adults who exhibit severe behavioral problems. They are regulated and operated by the Developmental Disability Service Office (DDSO) of Ulster County, a local arm of the New York State Office of Mental Retardation and Developmental Disabilities (OMRDD). Both are licensed as Intermediate Care Facilities (ICFs). One residence is for 12 adult males, the other is for 12 adult females. All clients have a primary diagnosis of moderate to mild mental retardation, and most have an identified psychiatric disorder. Common characteristics among the clients include marked and prolonged dysfunctional interpersonal relationships, antisocial behaviors, psychotic episodes, and a long history of institutionalization. The identification of these two community-based residences for the "mentally retarded with severe behavioral problems," rather than specifically designated for the dually diagnosed, is more of an administrative function of the mental retardation regulatory body than it is of the clinical characteristics of the clients. The treatment in the residence is structured and staff intensive. Each client goal includes the transition to a less-restrictive living arrangement.

The survey data indicated a need for further residential program development. To address this identified need, the DDSO of Ulster County is planning to develop two additional community-based residences specifically for the dually diagnosed client population. One residence will be for higher-functioning individuals: mildly retarded individuals who have mental health problems. The other will be for lower-functioning individuals, the moderately retarded with mental health problems. The development of these two community-based residences is an important step in meeting the residential needs of the dually diagnosed in Ulster County and will provide valuable resources toward a comprehensive service system.

## Vocational Training and Employment

Ulster County has two sheltered workshops. One is operated by the mental retardation system, the other by the mental health system. The former will not accept mentally retarded persons who manifest significant mental health problems, whereas the latter will accept a limited number of individuals who have the coexistence of mental retardation and mental illness. However, experience has demonstrated that these vocational programs are not usually suitable for this population. It is difficult for the dually diagnosed individual to perform a production activity such as benchwork assembly—in a sheltered workshop—for five hours per day, five days per week. Limited attention span, high distractibility, impulse control difficulty, and poor interactional skills contribute to a high rate of termination from the sheltered workshop setting for the dually diagnosed client.

The vocational services are limited and largely inadequate for this population. Combined services, encompassing both day treatment and vocational rehabilitation, are prohibited by bureaucratic and funding barriers.

## Staff Training and Systems Coordination

At present, there is no systematic formal training or educational service regarding mental health aspects of mental retardation. There have been inservice training programs dealing with this subject, but this has been on an agency ad hoc level rather than on a county-wide interagency basis. However, Ulster County Community Mental Health Services, in cooperation with other service providers, is in the early stages of developing a full range of consultation, educational, and training services addressing the multiple issues and problems concerning the dually diagnosed population. The comprehensive staff development training program will be designed for the professional community, for both mental health and mental retardation personnel. The areas to be addressed will include the following: (1) psychopathology in the mentally retarded; (2) assessment and diagnostic approaches; (3) individual, group, and family therapy techniques; (4) behavioral analysis; (5) techniques to deal with assaultive and aggressive behavior; and (6) psychosexual dysfunction and deviance, among others. Additionally, an educational program will be offered to the general public.

Ulster County Community Mental Health Services has appointed a coordinator charged with developing a dual diagnosis (MI/MR) task force. The task force consists of clinical and administrative staff from both the mental health and mental retardation provider agencies. The intended purpose is to develop coordinated, comprehensive services for the dually diagnosed citizens of Ulster County. The task force has the responsibility for the following: (1) clarify clinical and administrative goals; (2) develop cross-boundary, comprehensive treatment planning; (3) assist in the development of staff-training programs; (4)

develop a client tracking system; and (5) explore meaningful ways for cross-system integration of services. The task force has acted as a catalyst for stimulating research endeavors.

## Discussion

Persons who have the coexistence of mental retardation and mental illness are commonly referred to as the dually diagnosed population. The term *dual diagnosis* has generated a considerable amount of controversy over the last few years. Some have indicated that this new label is inappropriate, unnecessary, and potentially destructive (Szymanski & Grossman, 1984). Others, however, have reported that *dual diagnosis*, as a descriptive term, reflects mental retardation and allied signs of mental illness that require a variety of treatment–management interventions for those individuals who are affected by this multiple disability (Menolascino, McGee, & Casey, 1984). From a political and social policy perspective, the terms *dual diagnosis* and *dually diagnosed* focus national attention on the issues concerning individuals who have the coexistence of mental illness and mental retardation. These terms are not intended either to propose a third mental hygiene system or to define discrete clinical dimensions in an individual other than mental illness and mental retardation; they bring attention to the complexity of the needs and multiplicity of services necessary for this underserved population.

## Recommendations

The multifaceted problems concerning the dually diagnosed require a multi-dimensional approach to meet the holistic needs of this population.

One approach is for the local level of service delivery not to wait for national solutions. The local level has the potential to deal with the complex issues and gain a sharp perspective on local needs and resources. The establishment of a task force can be an effective vehicle in facilitating communication between the mental health and mental retardation systems, collecting data, and exploring meaningful ways to bridge the systemic, attitudinal, and training gaps in providing services to the dually diagnosed. The plan in Ulster County, as described in this chapter, can be viewed as a model for a local-level system for the dually diagnosed. There needs to be a willingness on the part of local-level policymakers, administrators, and clinicians to begin a dialogue, a forum of communication within which the representatives of mental health and mental retardation systems can identify the local problems and search for local and cooperative solutions.

Another approach is for educational institutions to be resources for training people to understand the clinical relationship between mental illness and mental retardation. For example, the University Affiliated Program (UAP) can be called upon to train professionals and paraprofessionals to meet the mental health needs of mentally retarded persons. The preparation of personnel will require a national commitment of the UAPs toward a realistic interface with the mental health and mental retardation system (McGee & Pearson, 1983).

Mental health issues in the mentally retarded should be in the curricula of undergraduate and graduate education in course subjects related to mental retardation, mental illness, or developmental disabilities. This subject material should be available across disciplines (i.e., psychiatry, social work, psychology); no single discipline has the knowledge base or the ability to cover all aspects required in the treatment and rehabilitation of the dually diagnosed. The interdisciplinary team approach has become mandatory because of the broad range of required services (Cushna, Szymanski, & Tanguay, 1980). This type of curriculum can be taught at the community college level for paraprofessional staff, and a more sophisticated curricula can be provided through postdoctoral studies. As an example of the gross deficiency of this type of education, Leaverton and Van der Heide (1975) reported that only about 50% of programs in child psychiatry included any training in mental retardation.

The third approach is for the federal government to take a visible stance with regard to the mental health needs of mentally retarded persons. This too can be multidimensional. The government should develop research funds through the National Institute of Mental Health (NIMH) and the National Institute of Child Health and Human Development (NICHHD) to create panels for mental retardation research. The Administration on Developmental Disabilities (ADD) could fund the establishment of a system for centralized information and dissemination that would assist units of government, provider agencies, and others in such technical areas as program development, staff training, systems' development, model programs, and resources. A federal agency could fund applied research on treatment approaches and on assessment of program models. Also, program and treatment models that have proved effective could be replicated with federal money as demonstration projects.

The fourth approach is for focusing national attention. The dually diagnosed need the attention of policymakers, administrators, clinicians, researchers, parents, and the general public. The issues, problems, and concerns are only beginning to be recognized by some in the professional community; the dually diagnosed need to be recognized as underserved by a larger group of professionals (Reiss et al., 1982). The National Association for the Dually Diagnosed: Mental Illness/Mental Retardation (NADD) has been instrumental in drawing national attention to the issues. NADD is a multidisciplinary and parent association designed to promote interest, stimulate appropriate resource development, and disseminate information. The organization was founded just seven years ago and has already sponsored five well-attended national conferences and five regional conferences; it also publishes a quarterly newsletter. NADD has emerged and is recognized as a leading national organization, spearheading national attention concerning the complex problems and solutions associated with the dually diagnosed population. This effort needs to be strengthened and widened. An alliance between NADD and other national organizations would broaden the attention that needs to be drawn from both the mental health and mental retardation systems.

## Summary

What is described in this chapter are the programs and plans, from a county-level perspective, in addressing the holistic needs of dually diagnosed persons. At the local level, there is a recognition of the specific needs of the dually diagnosed and an awareness of the service provisions required to meet these needs. These specialized services are intended to be short-term, transitional programs to enable a dually diagnosed person to return to the generic service delivery system. Discrete and time-limited programs for this population serve two important functions: First, they provide needed services for individuals who might otherwise fall through the cracks in the delivery of service systems. Second, these short-term programs serve as a diversion to institutionalization.

Limited service development for this population has been in effect in Ulster County with the highly successful day-treatment service since 1980, but only recently has there been a concerned effort toward developing a full range of services. There is now a design, a planned direction, toward bridging the gap between mental health and mental retardation delivery-care systems. The provision of a comprehensive service system for the dually diagnosed in Ulster County will emerge from a proactive stance spearheaded by concerned people.

## Conclusion

There are no simple solutions to the complex issues regarding the mental health problems of the mentally retarded. The problems will need to be addressed at all levels and with all the resources available. There is a need to respond to the social policy of deinstitutionalization, since society has not yet fulfilled the promise of community-based services. Neither transinstitutionalization nor being lost in the cracks of the delivery-care system should be the human cost of the deinstitutionalization process.

We have an ethical and social responsibility to provide the basic elements of life for those who need it the most. The systemic problems that impose barriers to the development of effective service systems for this underserved population are a major challenge and one that we must meet without delay.

### References

Chess, S. (1962). Psychiatric treatment of the mentally retarded child with behavior problems. *American Journal of Orthopsychiatry, 32*, 863–869.

Cushna, B., Szymanski, L.S., & Tanguay, P.E. (1980). Professional roles and unmet man-power needs. In L.S. Szymanski & P.E. Tanguay (Eds.), *Emotional disorders of mentally retarded persons*. Baltimore, MD: University Park Press.

Eaton, L., & Menolascino, F. (1982). Psychiatric disorders in the mentally retarded: Types, problems and challenges. *American Journal of Psychiatry, 139*, 10.

Fletcher, R. (1984). A model day-treatment service for the mentally retarded–mentally ill population. IN F. Menolascino & J. Stark (Eds.), *Handbook of mental illness in the mentally retarded*. New York: Plenum Press.

Leaverton, D., & Van der Heide, C. (1975, May). Paper read at the American Association on Mental Deficiency Annual Meeting, Portland, Oregon.

McGee, J., & Pearson, P. (1983). Role of the University-Affiliated Programs. In F. Menolascino & B. McCann (Eds.), *Mental health and mental retardation: Bridging the gap*. Baltimore, MD: University Park Press.

Menolascino, F. (1965). Emotional disturbance and mental retardation. *American Journal of Mental Deficiency, 70*, 248–256.

Menolascino, F. (1983). Overview: Bridging the gap between mental retardation and mental health. In F. Menolascino & B. McCann (Eds.), *Mental health and mental retardation: Bridging the gap*. Baltimore, MD: University Park Press.

Menolascino, F., McGee, J., & Casey, K. (1984). *Dual diagnosis: Direct implications*. Unpublished paper.

Philips, I., & Williams, N. (1975). Psychopathology and mental retardation: A study of 100 mentally retarded children. *American Journal of Psychiatry, 132*, 1265–1271.

President's Commission on Mental Health. (1978). *Report of the Liaison Task Force on Mental Retardation* (Vol. 4, Appendix, pp. 2001–2078). Washington, DC: Author.

Reiss, S., Levitan, G.W., & McNally, R.J. (1982). Emotionally disturbed mentally retarded people: An underserved population. *American Psychologist, 37*(4), 361–367.

Szymanski, L., & Grossman, H. (1984). Dual implications of dual diagnosis. *Mental Retardation, 22*(4), 155–156.

Webster, T. (1971). Unique aspects of emotional development in mentally retarded children. In F. Menolascino (Ed.), *Psychiatric approaches to mental retardation*. New York: Basic Books.

West, M., & Richardson, M. (1981). A statewide survey of C: MHC. Programs of mentally retarded individuals. *Hospital and Community Psychiatry, 32*(6), 413–416.

# 24
# Intensive Home-Based Treatment Interventions with Mentally Retarded/Emotionally Disturbed Individuals and Their Families

Robert B. Allin, Jr.

## Introduction

The unique problems of individuals with mental retardation and behavioral or emotional disturbances have generated interest in designing alternative programs to effectively address related needs. Trends toward deinstitutionalization and normalization, the paucity of professionals in this field, and the increased demands for alternative modes of service have stimulated research in this area.

One component that has been studied in programs designed for a variety of populations, though not specifically for dually diagnosed individuals, is parent involvement. Parents have not only been the target for therapy interventions but have also been therapeutic agents assuming the role of educator or trainer (Hawkins, Peterson, Schweid, & Bijou, 1966; Heifetz, 1977; Watson & Bassinger, 1974). The involvement of parents, caretakers, and significant others would appear to be of great value in programming efforts with dually diagnosed individuals.

Another component of interest in the design of this and other intervention programs for people with mental retardation is the type of theoretical orientation. Psychodynamic (Baum, 1962; Evans, 1976), informational (Berger & Foster, 1976), and behavioral (Berkowitz & Graziano, 1976; O'Dell, 1974) intervention strategies have all been attempted. Eclectic or combined approaches, however, appear to provide increased sensitivity to highly diverse individual, family, and situational demands—an important advantage that becomes limited by adherence to a single approach (Tymchuck, 1975, 1983).

The context for therapeutic intervention must become still another concern in the development of programs for dually diagnosed individuals. While typical settings for therapeutic assessment and intervention have been office, clinic, or institutional situations, a small body of research indicates that the home or natural environment can provide an excellent and even superior medium in which to assess problems and implement various modalities (Allin & Allin, 1984; Cianci, 1951; Hansen, 1968; Kinney, Madsen, Flemming, & Haapala, 1977; Wolfensberger, 1967).

TABLE 24.1. Components of the Home Intervention Program.

1. Services provided in the natural environment
2. Male–female therapist team
3. Eclectic approach to treatment
4. Flexible time scheduling (i.e., time of day and amount of time)

The Home Intervention Program (HIP) is an active and practical attempt to help fill the gap in services offered to individuals with mental retardation and behavioral or emotional disturbance. The program model represents the unique combination of several distinct components, which are presented in Table 24.1 and as follows: (1) services provided in the natural environment, (2) a male–female therapist team, (3) an eclectic approach to treatment, and (4) flexible time scheduling (i.e., time of day and amount of time).

The design of this program may be viewed as developing from and incorporating the work especially of the following: (1) Baker, Brightman, Heifetz, and Murphey (1976) and Heifetz (1977) on developing training manuals for parents of the retarded; (2) Watson and Bassinger (1974) on describing a parent training technology system; (3) Tymchuck's (1975, 1979) parent therapy model; and (4) the Kinney–Madsen–Fleming–Haapala (1977) model of the Homebuilder's Program.

The main idea of the HIP is for the staff team to work in the natural environment where problems occur and to work with supportive persons in that environment such as parents, teachers, group home counselors, and work supervisors or employers. Exposure to the home environment allows staff to observe and assess client problems first hand; then to design and implement an individually tailored treatment program according to situational demands. The involvement of parents and significant others is a main focus, because they are considered important agents for changing problem behaviors. They are an integral part of the treatment program in that they help to formulate the plan and are taught and shown skills that can help them take responsibility for managing problem behaviors when staff are no longer involved.

The HIP is a cooperative venture between the Mental Health and Mental Retardation Services of the Community Services Board in Chesterfield County, Virginia. The HIP is currently in its ninth year of operation. Historically, the program began in late 1978 with phases relating to research and design. Program implementation and data collection commenced in mid-1979; evaluative findings, early in 1982, supported the continuation of services. The project has been encouraged and funded by the Virginia Department of Mental Health and Mental Retardation and the Chesterfield County Board of Supervisors.

The program has an annual operational budget of $70,000: $65,000 for salaries and benefits for two staff; $2,500 for local travel expenditures, and $2,500 for office supplies, instructional equipment, staff training expenditures, publications, and so on.

# Description of Program

## Participants

Participants in the program include families, or other supportive persons, who have in their care a person, to be identified here as the client, who is mentally retarded and who presents problem behavior. The program serves clients of all ages and all ranges of mental retardation. Problem behavior typically overwhelms family members to the point where they no longer feel able to cope, and more restrictive placements may be under consideration. Frequently, problem behaviors of these individuals carry over into other environments such as school, work, and community programs where, in some instances, continued participation in those activities may be in jeopardy.

A wide range of problem behaviors has been addressed by the HIP; typically, problems are abusive or disruptive in nature. Examples of the types of problem behavior presented by HIP clients are shown in Table 24.2.

The bulk (approximately 70%) of clients served by the HIP live in their home with their natural family, while the approximate remaining 30% live in foster or adoptive homes, group homes or other supportive living situations, or institutional settings. In cases where individuals are in institutional settings at the time of referral, the HIP has facilitated the transition from the institution to the community by working closely with the appropriate support persons. The program has also worked with cases where the identified client has been the parent; that is, with persons who themselves have some degree of intellectual retardation and who have children. The focus of the HIP with this group is, of course, on enhancing their parenting abilities.

## Staff

As mentioned earlier, the program staff consists of a male–female therapist team who usually work together on each case. Occasionally, visits are made by one team member when the team approach is not necessary or clinically indicated.

TABLE 24.2. Random list of types of problems presented by HIP clients.

| | |
|---|---|
| Temper outbursts (major) | Somatic complaints |
| Physical aggressions toward others | Lying |
| Suicidal threats | Verbal abuse |
| Inappropriate sexual behavior | Toileting skills deficits |
| Temper tantrums (minor) | Obsessive–compulsive behaviors |
| General noncompliance | Child abuse/neglect |
| Depression | Parenting skills deficits |
| Shyness | Marital problems |
| Communication skill deficits | Sibling rivalry |
| Refusal to do chores | Alcohol abuse |
| Property destruction | Self-abusive behavior |

It may be of interest that originally the male–female team consisted of a husband and wife; a condition that was able to continue for six years (and successfully so, I might add, in terms of both the program's operation and the functioning of the marital relationship).

## Program Procedures

A planned aspect of the HIP is that the program procedures remain flexible enough to meet the needs of the participants and to be responsive to situational demands. Although the treatments are individualized in implementation, several phases or procedures are considered common to all cases. In temporal order they are listed in Table 24.3 and briefly described below.

### CLIENT SELECTION PHASE

The number of cases that the program can serve at any single point in time is limited by the small number of staff and the potential for an intensive commitment of time in each of these cases. A waiting list of referrals usually results, and therefore a selection process is used that determines the next recipient. This process involves rating eligible candidates in the areas of (1) risk of institutionalization or removal from less restrictive, undesirable situations; (2) need for immediate intervention; (3) potential to benefit from treatments; and (4) client–family motivation to receive and participate in services. The cases with the highest ratings are the next to participate in the program.

To assist in the selection of cases and to ensure that the family has occasion to learn about the HIP before making a commitment to work with the program, an

TABLE 24.3. Phases of program procedures.

1. Client selection phase
    (a) Introductory home visit
    (b) Rating of candidates referred
    (c) Selection of next case

2. Intensive involvement phase
    (a) Observation and problem assessment
    (b) Development of treatment plan
    (c) Implementation of treatment

3. Supportive involvement phase
    (a) Reduction in staff time
    (b) Increased expectation for family to take full responsibility for implementation of techniques

4. Termination phase
    (a) Continued phasing out of staff time
    (b) Termination issues addressed

5. Follow-up phase
    (a) Support given on an "as-needed" basis via occasional visits and/or phone contacts

introductory home visit is made prior to the rating process. The family has an opportunity to meet staff and to ask questions about having outsiders or strangers in the home. Program details and examples of techniques that could be expected are explained by staff. Family members are given an opportunity to discuss their specific problems and needs, and staff are able to make assessment as to the viability of the program in their particular situation.

INTENSIVE INVOLVEMENT PHASE

A major focus of this phase is *observation of the client in his or her natural environment*. Staff observations typically occur over a three- or four-day period and take place in a variety of settings, such as the home, the school, and the work or training center. Observation visits are planned during both "problem" and "no-problem" times and range in duration from one to five hours. In general, the role of staff during periods of observation is one of "casual observer." For example, it is explained to family members that their normal routine and responses to situations should continue and that staff will not make suggestions for handling problems differently at this time. Staff, in most cases, remain visible (e.g., in the same room or part of the house) so that clients and family members become more accustomed to their presence. The interactions of staff and family members during these observation sessions are limited by staff to the aims of (1) enabling staff to more clearly understand problems and (2) establishing increased levels of comfort and rapport between staff and family members.

Another major focus of this phase is the *development of a treatment plan* that is based on the information previously gathered. It is individualized for each case. Planning sessions between staff and family take place to establish the problem areas to be targeted for treatment. Staff then draft an initial treatment plan that is presented to the family and significant others for explanation, modification, and finalizing. A time schedule for the next several weeks is then discussed, and treatment goals (Goal Attainment Scales) for each problem area are established. Whenever possible, the client is involved in the treatment-planning process.

The third major focus is on *implementation of the treatment plan*. This aspect of program procedures is the most crucial and requires the greatest concentration of time and effort. It usually begins with teaching and explaining the technique that will be used in changing and coping with problem behaviors. Principles of behavior modification or effective communication, for example, are reviewed and discussed by staff during the initial sessions. No lengthy teaching of academic principles is attempted; emphasis is placed on the *application* of techniques: "teaching by doing" and modeling for parents are emphasized. As treatment progresses, staff increase their expectations that parents and other family members will take on more responsibility for implementing techniques with gradually decreasing staff assistance. Techniques are practiced in hypothetical situations when necessary, then gradually introduced into real problem situations. Practice (*fire drilling*, as we refer to it) is especially useful in situations where the behavior targeted for change is low in its frequency of occurrence and high in its problem intensity.

Throughout the implementation of the treatment plan, staff use various methods of assisting, coaching, or reminding the parents to employ the techniques in the treatment plan. These methods range from verbal prompting to passing written messages. Frequently, information and reminders are posted on the refrigerator or in some other highly visible location. In situations where behavioral techniques are used, the recording of data is often required to be done by one or two specific members of the family. These data records are also posted, and checks on their reliability are periodically made by staff. Also, in situations where clients have reading skills, information such as responsibility schedules or point systems is posted in tactful locations for their observation.

Ideally, throughout treatment plan implementation, the family members are highly motivated and active in their follow-through. However, this is not true in the majority of cases. Issues contributing to resistance or difficulty in carrying through aspects of the treatment plan require, and receive, special consideration from staff. Sometimes, the issue is easily identifiable and dealt with quickly. One set of parents, for example, were progressing nicely until the plan required that they ignore their daughter's crying in certain situations. The matter was explored with them, and it was found that both parents were feeling a sense of guilt for abandoning their child when the tantrum crying occurred. They were soon able to ignore this behavior, and consistently so, after discussing their feelings and receiving assurances from staff. In other cases, issues such as fear of being physically hurt by an offspring if the plan was implemented, unrealistically low expectations of client behavior, parental burnout, and overprotectiveness have required considerably more time and attention.

SUPPORTIVE INVOLVEMENT PHASE

This phase can be viewed as a continuation of the treatment plan implementation discussed above with two major changes. First, there is a reduction in staff–client contact time. Although visits occur more frequently and are usually of longer duration during the period of intensive involvement (e.g., a maximum of four visits per week; three to four hours per visit), both the number of visits and the time length of each visit are reduced during the supportive phase (e.g., a maximum of two visits per week; one to two hours per visit). Second, there are increased expectations that family members will take more responsibility for implementing aspects of the treatment plan. The teaching and learning of techniques are considered completed, and family members during this phase are encouraged to adjust to following through with the techniques with considerably less staff assistance. The staff role is one of providing support by encouraging consistency and follow-through, sharpening parents' abilities to use the techniques, and generalizing their abilities to use the techniques in similar or new problem situations. Factors that contribute to families' tendencies to be dependent on staff for plan implementation are identified and dealt with during this period.

TERMINATION PHASE

The final stages in the removal of regularly scheduled staff–case contact time occur during the termination phase. This phase also involves a reduction in staff contact time: Visits during this period usually occur one time per week for a one-hour to two-hour period. The family is expected to carry through with all areas of the treatment plan for which they have responsibility. During this phase, the issue of termination is addressed specifically in terms of its impact on the family system and the ability of the family members to continue their use and application of the learned skills.

FOLLOW-UP PHASE

The final aspect of the HIP involvement is the case follow-up. Contacts via phone or actual visits to the natural environment are made on an "as-needed" basis. These contacts are initiated by both staff and family members for the purposes of giving and receiving further assistance in carrying out techniques, problem solving in new or crisis situations, monitoring the continued use of program techniques, and checking on the extent to which the reduction or elimination of problem behavior has been sustained over time.

## Time Issues

The amount of time spent with each case in any given phase of the program procedures varies in accordance with individual needs and situational demands. The major concentration of time and visits occurs during the intensive phase of the program procedures. As the program progresses in each case, the families are in a sense "weaned," with increasingly smaller amounts of time spent during the final phases. New cases are accepted as soon as current cases reach the support and termination phases (see Table 24.4, for maximum time available to a case).

In general, there is no established or rigid plan for coordinating the time when visits will occur. Although tentative schedules for contact are discussed for each phase of program involvement, staff typically set up final schedules with the families on a weekly or daily basis to maintain flexibility in responsiveness to client needs. Scheduling frequently becomes a rather complex piece of business that takes into consideration such factors as the availability of the family members, "prime" problem times, and the schedules that staff have established with other cases concurrently receiving treatment.

## Program Evaluation

An important aspect of the HIP was the incorporation of an evaluation component to assess the effectiveness of the program model in reaching objectives specific to the client and the family (see Table 24.5). This evaluation was completed in 1982. Conclusions from this research indicated that, in regard to the client, the program was highly successful in eliminating or decreasing presenting

TABLE 24.4. Schedule of maximum time availability.[a]

| Phase of involvement | Time/visits per week | Duration of involvement | Totals |
|---|---|---|---|
| Intensive phase | 12 hours 3–4 visits | 4 weeks | 48 hours 12–16 visits |
| Supportive phase | 4–6 hours 2 visits | 4 weeks | 24 hours 8 visits |
| Termination phase | 2 hours 1 visit | 4 weeks | 8 hours 4 visits |
| | Totals | 12 weeks | 80 hours 28 visits |

[a] It is assumed that (1) the particular case requires intensive intervention and (2) this intervention will follow a three-month course, changing phases each month. Under these conditions, services are available to a maximum of three cases concurrently each in a different phase of intervention.
*Note:* It is important to note that all cases do not require the intensive time plan depicted in the table. The HIP has provided services concurrently for up to 12 cases. There is a flexibility to become intensively involved if necessary. Program statistics show that the total time spent per case has ranged from 16 to 130 hours, while total visits per case have ranged from 11 to 76. The mean amount of total direct time per case is approximately 60 hours, with a mean number of about 30 visits per case.

problem behaviors, the majority of which involved abusive–destructive temper outbursts, and in increasing skills focused on personal responsibility and independence. Increased self-control and self-esteem were also noted, especially among the higher functioning individuals in this group.

The research also indicated that, in regard to the family, parents who participated in the program clearly demonstrated, as a group, increased abilities to consciously, constructively, and effectively use behavioral skills with their son or daughter. It was interesting that these parents were able to apply behavioral skills and to implement successful behavior-change programs without significant increases in their tested understanding of theoretical behavioral principles. The program was also successful in reducing parents' overwhelmed feelings and tendencies to "overprotect." Parents also demonstrated positive changes in the area of sensitivity to others, indicative of increased abilities to communicate more effectively with their offspring.

While a major evaluative effort was made initially, evaluation of program effectiveness remains a concern and is currently done on an individual case basis through the use of behavioral data recordings and goal attainment scales, examples of which are presented in Figures 24.1 to 24.5.

# A Clinical and Administrative Perspective on the Advantages and Disadvantages of the HIP Model

The most distinct and powerful advantage of the HIP model is that the locus for treatment is based within the context of the client's natural environment. Our presence in vivo provides us with unique opportunities to observe problem

TABLE 24.5. Service delivery objectives.

Objectives specific to the client
1. To decrease or eliminate presenting problem behaviors (GAS, ABS, behavioral data).
2. To increase independence skills such as self-help, leisure, and communication skills when applicable (GAS, ABS, behavioral data).
3. To increase self-control (GAS, behavioral data).
4. To increase self-esteem (GAS, behavioral data).
5. To increase positive, constructive behavior in general (GAS, ABS, behavioral data).
6. To increase acceptability to other family members.
7. To live in the community.

Objectives specific to the parents or family
1. To increase knowledge of behavior modification principles (KBPAC).
2. To increase the conscious and constructive application of behavioral skills with son or daughter (behavioral data, GAS).
3. To decrease "overwhelmed" feelings and increase feelings of personal control (GAS, LOC).
4. To decrease overprotective behavior and foster independence and responsibility in son or daughter (GAS, behavioral data, STO).
5. To increase overall quality of interaction with son or daughter (STO).
6. To increase awareness of, and ability to deal with, feelings and attitudes relative to son or daughter.
7. To increase knowledge of mental retardation, if necessary.
8. To increase knowledge and understanding of emotional–behavioral component of problems presented by son or daughter.
9. To formulate, if necessary, realistic expectations of offspring's potential.
10. To increase acceptance of son or daughter as family member.

Key to dependent measures used to evaluate objectives:
ABS: American Association on Mental Deficiency Adaptive Behavior Scale.
Behavioral data: Recording of specific behavioral information.
GAS: Goal Attainment Scales.
KBPAC: Knowledge of Behavior Principles questionnaire.
LOC: Locus of control measure.
STO: Sensitivity to Others questionnaire.

situations ourselves. We are able to see problems as they typically occur in the settings where they normally occur. Initial observations allow us to understand the nature of the problems more completely and accurately. Frequently, our understanding of a situation as described to us verbally, by phone, or in other "out-of-context" settings is changed quite drastically once we are able to see the events occurring in the home environment. These observations produce valuable assessment data, which then are used in planning the course of the treatment intervention. For example, we are easily able to identify the antecedents and the consequences surrounding particular behaviors by being present; this is vital information for a trained, objective observer and not easily discernible to an overwhelmed parent.

It is important to mention that behavior demonstrated by family members during the early stages of HIP involvement is usually guarded and somewhat tempered in a positive sense as a function of staff presence. Although this "doing what the therapist would want me to" or "halo effect" can be considered a disadvantage of home-based treatment, its effects in each case are relatively short-lived and usually dissipate within one or two weeks time. Individuals may "temper" or

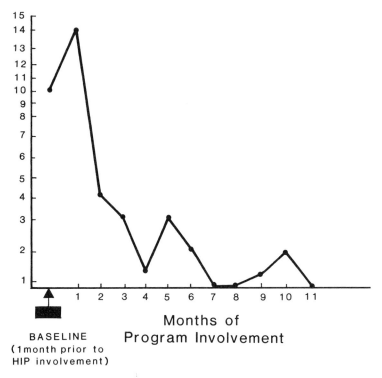

FIGURE 24.1. Temper outbursts per month of program involvement.

"tone down" particular behaviors, but general patterns of behavior, interactions, and coping responses are very obvious and are valuable pieces of information that we use to formulate the course of treatment.

The natural environment is also an excellent setting in which to implement treatment. Just as we learn and understand aspects of client–family problems more completely by being in the home setting, family members are able to benefit from our presence and close contact with them in the places where the problems occur.

The HIP provides opportunities to teach new behavior to clients *and* parents. We feel that underlying the majority of client problem behaviors are skills deficits. For example, deficits in communication skills lead to problems of expressing feelings or needs; too often abusive behavior results as a language, a means to communicate as one attempts to deal with the environment. This behavior may then become reinforced by parents or other caregivers. In addition, skills deficits exist on the part of parents who are too frequently unequipped to deal with a son or daughter who is mentally retarded. While the program deals with problem behaviors, the focus of treatment is linked closely with reducing the skills deficits—a skills deficit approach—and, by increasing skill levels of

| SCALE ATTAINMENT LEVELS | SCALE 1: Independence related to personal skills & work attendance. | SCALE 2: Self concept: self confidence, positive self image. | SCALE 3: Anger control (temper outbursts). | SCALE 4: Mother's feelings of being overwhelmed: Terrorized, unable to set limits, have own needs. | Scale 5: Mother's overprotectiveness (expectation level at home). |
|---|---|---|---|---|---|
| 0 — Most unfavorable treatment outcome thought likely | Takes on no personal responsibility for self-help skills or work attendance | Is deeply depressed and frequently exhibits self-destructive behaviors. | Continuously demonstrates temper outbursts which are of both high frequency and high intensity. | Is overwhelmed that son cannot live at home. She feels constantly threatened and terrorized, unable to set any limits. | Consistently does for son, not allowing him to do for himself at all. |
| 1 | (✓ pre) | (✓ pre) | (✓ pre) | (✓ pre) | (✓ pre) |
| 2 — Less than expected success with treatment | Takes on some personal responsibility for many self-help skills and work attendance | Is depressed and is exhibiting many negative self-statements but few self-destructive behaviors. | Frequently demonstrates temper outbursts which are of high intensity. | Mother often feels overwhelmed but wants son to remain in home. She is only occasionally able to set limits. Frequently feels threatened. | Mother able to entertain idea of doing less for son. Allows son some increased independence with staff support. |
| 3 | | (✓✓ post) | | (✓ post) | (✓✓ post) |
| 4 — Expected level of treatment success | Takes on responsibility for many self-help skills and work attendance. | Mood is variable. Is exhibiting no self-destructive behaviors and few negative self-statements. | Occasionally demonstrates temper outbursts that are of moderate intensity. Uses appropriate coping behaviors when reminded. | Mother able to set limits fairly regularly and feels threatened only occasionally. | Making effort to give son independence and such occurring most of the time. |
| 5 | (✓✓ post) | | (✓✓ post) | (✓✓✓ follow-up) | (✓✓✓ follow-up) |
| 6 — More than expected success with treatment | Takes on responsibility for most of self-help skills and work attendance. | Is usually in a positive mood and exhibits positive self-statements 85% of the time. | Rarely demonstrates temper outburst behavior. Will verbalize angry feelings and self-initiate appropriate coping behaviors most of the time. | Mother regularly able to set limits with minimal fear. | Mother only occasionally does for son when he is able to do for himself. |
| 7 | (✓✓✓ follow-up) | (✓✓✓ follow-up) | (✓✓✓ follow-up) | | |
| 8 — Best anticipated success with treatment | Takes on responsibility for all of self-help skills and work attendance within physical limitations. | Is a happy, positive person and exhibits positive self statements 95% of the time. | Does not exhibit temper outbursts. Handles anger appropriately at all times. | Mother not threatened at all by son and is able to set limits without any fear. | Mother always encourages son to be more independent and doesn't do for him if he can do for himself. |
| 9 | | | | | |

FIGURE 24.2. Goal attainment scales for Case 1: (✓) pre; (✓✓) post; (✓✓✓) follow-up.

CASE  2 (TS)

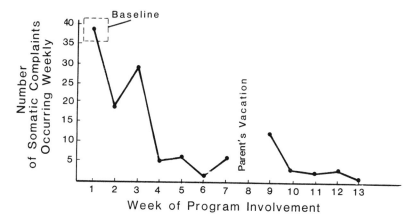

FIGURE 24.3. Number of somatic complaints made per week of program involvement.

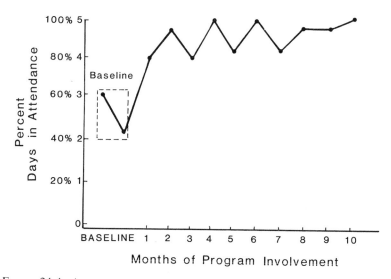

FIGURE 24.4. Average number of days in attendance at Adult Training Center.

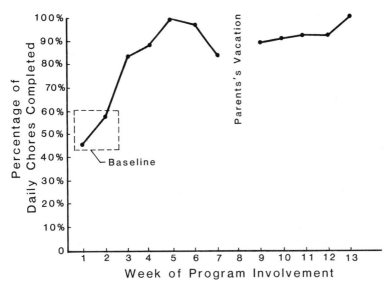

FIGURE 24.5. Percentage of daily chores completed per week of program involvement.

clients *and* parents, we see reductions in presenting problem behaviors.

Furthermore, we are able to teach skills and alternative coping responses in real, and often quite intense, problem situations. Parents are given the opportunity to observe and learn from us, from our behavior. Conveyed in this process of modeling are not only the basic aspects of a technique but the more subtle forms of information, such as attitude, intonation, physical movements, and body language, which would be most difficult to describe and so much more difficult to enact if the situation were not real. Our presence and our attempts to use techniques in the context of real problem situations also help us to understand and respond to the difficulties that the parents have in using the same skills themselves. We are able to make particular treatments more practical or to enhance their potential for continued use and success by modifying a single technique or by uniquely combining techniques for use in particular problem situations.

The effect of the therapists' presence in home settings also seems to be one that has great utility in helping to "break" firmly established and deeply seated patterns of events and interactions associated with problem situations. We are "there" to encourage and support families in their efforts to change—even in circumstances where emotions are peaked. We have the definite sense that if we weren't present during the initial and crucial stages when the parents begin to use the treatment techniques, the frustrations that typically accompanied the problems would probably discourage their efforts to follow through. (Indeed, some parents are inclined to give up on a new technique even in our presence!) HIP involvement in other aspects of the client's natural environment also has definite advantages. This broad and more inclusive focus enables treatment to span settings, and it provides consistency and continuity in treatment planning and implementation. Interprogram efforts clearly help to facilitate the treatment process.

Although the advantages of in vivo interventions are apparent to us, there are some disadvantages. One unavoidable limitation involves the issue of travel time. Although this factor would appear to reduce the overall availability and use of "productive" staff time, as we cannot "see" clients while driving to their homes, we do attempt to make efficient use of the time spent in transit. For example, travel time provides opportunities for us to prepare and plan for visits while on the way to them and to "process" visits as a team on the trip back. Also, the use of a portable tape-recording device while traveling enables us to make dictations of case-related information, thereby facilitating the completion of necessary paperwork while maximizing the use of travel time.

Another disadvantage of services offered in vivo is the fact that staff presence in the home can be too overwhelming, threatening, or distasteful for some families. At times, services are made available but are refused by a family. In these instances, the family members may express concern about having "outsiders" in their home. Some may state that their schedule is not conducive to people coming in. One skeptical foster father said that he did not want his personal life or the personal life of his family scrutinized by strangers. It is interesting to note that in a majority of these cases, client problems are enmeshed in other, serious family problems, such as alcoholism and abuse. Although in-home intervention is welcomed by and helpful to some families, it does have its limits of acceptability for others.

A "combination of efforts" on the part of staff in the HIP, who work as a therapist team, has many advantages. At the simplest level, working as a team enables us to share the work load. Thus, individual case assessments, the compilation of data bases, treatment plans, and so on are joint efforts. In addition, the team approach to working with families creates a climate within which we can support and reinforce each other. This circumstance is particularly advantageous in working with families' resistance to change, where a combined effort is useful for confronting, understanding, and working through issues that might block progress. At times, we are able to take on specified roles in a joint effort to facilitate treatment. Thus, for example, one of us can be the "heavy" (i.e., the confronter, the limit setter, the identifier of unpopular issues), and the other can assume the role of the "understander" (i.e., the empathetic listener). The fact that there are two of us also provides numerous opportunities to "role-play" together and to model the desired behavior. Finally, as members of a team, we are able to process feelings with each other regarding difficult cases and to maintain a high degree of enthusiasm for our client work.

One apparent effect of the male–female team approach is that it fosters relationship building with families. There are times when, quite simply, the females with whom we are working relate best to the female therapist, and the males to the male team member. At times, however, the opposite is true. Another important benefit of the relationships built between the male or female team member and the same-sexed parent is the establishment of identification bonds where mothers or fathers "identify" with the female or male therapist. This identification is manifested most explicitly in instances when the "desired behavior" is modeled by staff. It seems as if mothers can more easily or willingly model their behavior after that of the female team member. Similarly, fathers appear to exhibit the behaviors that they see demonstrated by the male therapist.

## Conclusion

The Home Intervention Program represents the unique combination of several distinct components: services provided in the natural environment, a male–female therapist team, an eclectic approach to treatment, and flexible time scheduling. The program uses this particular model with mentally retarded/emotionally disturbed individuals and their families. The program was designed to help fulfill a tremendous need for services, to provide useful information to others in the field, and to serve as a stimulus for the development of similar programs in other service systems.

In conducting the original research, it was generally hypothesized that the HIP model would promote the attainment of specific objectives that were directly related to changes in the behavior of the client and his or her family. The results, as presented on group and individual case bases, indicate that the hypothesis has withstood disconfirmation.

The program has shown that parents and families can make changes to alleviate problems and that the support of staff working in the natural environment is instrumental in this process. By giving parents a direction, some information, insight, and a practical approach, *they* are able to impact on a wide range of behavior that otherwise threatens family unity and client independence and places more demands on our community resources.

Although the program's focus is primarily on work with parents, the family, or caretakers to effect changes in problem behavior, there are situations where their capacities to make necessary changes are limited. In this regard, the ability of the program to focus on parents' or caretakers' feelings and attitudes, to be flexible in time and approach, and to involve the total environment in the treatment effort is instrumental in maximizing the potential for positive change. It is clear that these are fundamental requirements for any program intending to meet the needs of this particular population.

For the past several years, HIP staff have had the privilege of working closely with families. We have been exposed to portions of their lives, have witnessed their frustration and despair, joy, and love. While the program has offered skills and techniques, it has also provided opportunities for a powerful humanistic exchange that has fostered understanding, trust, and a mutual sharing of thoughts, feelings, and effort. Although it is not a panacea, the HIP does offer a way of alleviating frustration and hopelessness; and it enhances the quality of, and potential for, continued community living.

## References

Allin, R.B., Jr., & Allin, D.W. (1984). A home intervention program for mentally retarded-emotionally disturbed individuals and their families. In F.J. Menolascino & J.A. Stark (Eds.), *Handbook of mental illness in the mentally retarded* (pp. 313–344). New York: Plenum Press.

Baker, B.L., Brightman, A.J., Heifetz, L.J., & Murphey, D.M. (1976). *Steps to independence series: Intermediate and advanced self help skills; behavior problems; toilet training; training guide.* Champaign, IL: Research Press.

Baum, M.H. (1962). Some dynamic factors affecting family adjustment to the handicapped child. *Exceptional Children, April*, 387–392.

Berger, M., & Foster, M. (1976). Family-level interventions for retarded children: A multivariate approach to issues and strategies. *Multivariate Experimental Clinical Research, 2*, 2–21.

Berkowitz, B.P., & Graziano, A.M. (1976). Training parents as behavior therapists: A review. *Behavior Research and Therapy, 10*, 297–317.

Cianci, V. (1951). Home training for retarded children in New Jersey. *The Training School Bulletin, 48*, 131–139.

Evans, E.C. (1976). The grief reaction of parents of the retarded and the counselor's role. *Australian Journal of Mental Retardation, 4*, 8–12.

Hansen, C.C. (1968). An extended home visit with cojoint family therapy. *Family Process, 7*, 67–87.

Hawkins, R.P., Peterson, R.F., Schweid, E., & Bijou, S.W. (1966). Behavior therapy in the home: Amelioration of problem parent–child relations with the parent in a therapeutic role. *Journal of Exceptional Child Psychology, 4*, 99–107.

Heifetz, L.J. (1977). Behavioral training for parents of retarded children: Alternative formats based on instructional manuals. *American Journal of Mental Deficiency, 82*, 194–203.

Kinney, J.M., Madsen, B., Fleming, T., & Haapala, D. (1977). Homebuilders: Keeping families together. *Journal of Consulting and Clinical Psychology, 45*, 667–673.

O'Dell, S. (1974). Training parents in behavior modification: A review. *Psychology Bulletin, 81*, 418–433.

Tymchuck, A.J. (1975). Training parent therapists. *Mental Retardation, 13*, 19–22.

Tymchuck, A.J. (1979). *Parent and family therapy: An integrative approach to family interactions.* New York: Spectrum.

Tymchuck, A.J. (1983). Interventions with parents of the mentally retarded. In J. Matson & J. Mulick (Eds.), *Handbook of mental retardation* (pp. 369–380). New York: Pergamon Press.

Watson, L.S., & Bassinger, J.F. (1974). Parent training technology: A potential service delivery system. *Mental Retardation, 12*, 3–10.

Wolfensberger, W. (1967). Counseling the parents of retarded children. In A.A. Baumeister (Ed.), *Mental retardation: Appraisal, education, and rehabilitation.* Chicago, IL: Aldine.

# 25
# RIP: A Parent-Implemented Treatment Model for Families with Behaviorally Disordered and/or Developmentally Delayed Young Children

MATTHEW A. TIMM

The Regional Intervention Program for Preschoolers and Parents (RIP) represents a pioneering effort in the treatment of families with young handicapped children. The program model is characterized by the use of parents as primary therapists for their own children, as trainers of fellow parents, and as implementors of the service delivery system's daily operation. Founded in 1969 in Nashville, Tennessee, the current RIP network is composed of 21 certified programs in 15 communities in the United States, Canada, and Brazil.

This chapter describes four essential elements of the program model, including its unique management-by-objectives evaluation system based on principles and techniques derived from the industrial engineering sector. Data regarding documented program effectiveness are presented in summary form.

Parent implemented systems offer "built in consumer satisfaction" at a time of widespread discontent with all educational services as well as with other government services.... In a parent implemented system, the parents, especially the mothers can offer one another a tremendous amount of group support and enthusiasm.... Parent implemented systems or systems that involve parents are important because they pose a partial solution to the manpower problem in the helping professions.... All the service and maintenance systems in our society are strained. On every side we have various constituencies stating needs in terms that usually involve the phrase "if we only had . . ." to show what they could do with more resources. (Ora, 1972, p. 73)

The most frequently recommended solution to the problem of inadequate treatment resources for children and youth is to train more psychiatrists, clinical psychologists, psychiatric social workers, and psychiatric nurses. While we may indeed need more mental health experts, a few minutes with a sharp pencil will show the futility of trying to match numbers with numbers without altering the patterns of deployment of mental health specialists. (Hobbs, 1982, p. 7)

The Regional Intervention Program for Preschoolers and Parents (RIP), founded in 1969 at George Peabody College, Nashville, Tennessee, has been described as "a professionally administered, parent-operated therapeutic preschool for children who cut across a variety of diagnostic categories including the retarded, autistic, behavior-disordered, and multiply handicapped. Many of the children are delayed in language, motor, and/or cognitive development, with related behavior and emotional problems" (Fields, 1975, p. 3).

Examination of any program model in continuous operation for many years must include consideration of the extent to which the program's structure and approach have been adapted to meet changing demands. The original grant application proposal submitted to the U.S. Office of Education (Ora & Wiegerink, 1969) identified RIP's primary target population as "very young seriously disturbed children who are high risks for later, extended residential care." Particular emphasis was placed on autistic or autisticlike children below 36 months of age.

Within the first year of operation, requests from pediatricians, allied professionals, and parents produced the decision to expand the population to include children who were intact with regard to major developmental domains but who were characterized by disruptive, oppositional behavior in everyday life. Requests from these same sources in the second year produced the decision to expand the eligible population even further to include developmentally delayed children who were not necessarily presenting serious behavior management problems. While families containing severely behaviorally disordered young children remain majority participants in RIP programs, these early decisions established a policy regarding formal diagnostic requirements prior to enrollment, best described as *noncategorical*, which remains an important feature of the current program model.

A second major area in which significant alteration occurred relatively early in the program's history concerned redefinition of the parent implementation concept. From the outset, RIP was notable for its extensive reliance on parents as primary therapists and teachers for their own children. Additionally, RIP relied on parents to provide peer support via relatively informal contacts and to assist in the daily operation of the program by working in the preschool classrooms. However, the direct training of parents to prepare them for work with their children was conducted by the employed staff and graduate students.

By the end of the second year of operation, the convergence of three variables prompted extension of parent implementation into the case management sector (Ora, 1970). The demand for service had begun to exceed the ability of the program to respond, given existing staffing patterns. Graduated parents had begun to volunteer their time to the program even though their children were now in other educational or treatment settings; and many of these graduated parents demonstrated technical competence and support skills that equaled or surpassed skills possessed by staff members and assigned students. The decision to use parents as direct trainers and case managers for other parents was made. Decisions were also made to establish a formal "payback" system for all parents and to invite selected parents to become part-time, paid staff members. Parent implementation in this form remains an essential element of the program model.

The basic RIP program model, in which consumers of the service function simultaneously as key staff members, contains an intrinsic predisposition as well as capability to respond to changing needs. Since 1974, The RIP Expansion Project (the program's official training and replication component) has created a feedback loop within the larger system that encourages additions and refinements to the basic program model as well.

A comprehensive listing of methodological refinements and structural adaptations introduced over the years would exceed the scope of this presentation. Examples of methodological refinements include use of multiple settings for adult and child training to maximize generalization effects; reductions in the use of overcorrection, restitution, restraint, and seclusion time-out procedures with children; significant reductions in the use of edible reinforcers for consequation of child behavior; and introduction of various "incidental teaching" procedures in language and self-help skill training.

Examples of structural adaptations include development of evening programs to accommodate employed parents; development of supplementary "fathers' programs" for enrolled families; development of one day per week programs based on the RIP model for families with handicapped or at-risk infants; development of an Hispanic RIP in an American city as well as establishment of a certified program in Manaus, Brazil; modification of the "payback" component to permit a variety of fee structure arrangements; and placement of certified programs within a variety of sponsoring agencies including outpatient divisions of psychiatric hospitals, pediatric divisions of medical hospitals, community mental health centers, public education systems, universities, and Children's Aid Society systems in Canada.

The following description of the current edition of the RIP program model, based in Nashville, Tennessee, is offered within this context of change over time and variability of features across replication sites. Particular emphasis is placed on four, interlocking program model attributes, considered to be essential elements, which have remained relatively constant despite the passage of time and geographical diffusion (Timm, 1978).

*Parent implementation* is the fundamental element of the RIP model. Parents are responsible for clinical training and administrative functions that may be performed only by professionals in other service programs. Parents at RIP serve as primary therapists and teachers for their own children, as operators of the service delivery system on a daily basis, as trainers of newer parents learning to perform these same functions, and as ultimate evaluators of the program's strengths and deficits (Timm & Rule, 1981).

Because RIP is parent implemented, the program can provide a range of services not readily available in collective form in most other service delivery systems. One such service is the parent support system. A family's first direct contact with RIP, the intake interview, is conducted by another parent. As one mother described this initial experience, "When I first brought [my son] into the program, the first thing I learned was that I was not alone" (Smith, 1974, p. 2). New parents are assigned experienced parent case managers who work with them throughout treatment, ensuring continually available personal support.

Provision of parent support is not the only rationale for parent implementation. Since 1969, over 1,000 families have participated in the Nashville program. From July 1972 through June 1986, the program served an average of 73 families per year with a collective average of 3,868 treatment visits per year. Each treatment visit entailed one or more individual therapeutic sessions for each family plus a minimum of two hours of classroom activities for children and parents. It seems likely that provision of such services in a single professionally mediated program would result in prohibitive costs for many families (Gold Award, 1976).

Parent participation is organized into two phases—active treatment and payback. During treatment, parents work individually with their own children both at RIP and at home. When not engaged in individual sessions with their own children or in the training and feedback sessions with experienced parents that follow each session, the treatment parents are assisting in other program activities. They may teach in one of the classrooms, collect data, prepare instructional materials, or supervise the sibling nursery.

When a family's active treatment phase is completed, parents then participate in a system of payback of time and skills to the program. Payback in the Nashville program is based on a day-for-day formula with a ceiling on the maximum obligation incurred. The current average for families whose children are not developmentally delayed is 105 hours of treatment and 105 hours of payback; while families with developmentally delayed children average 180 hours of each phase. For families containing more severely delayed children, enrollment in the program may extend many months beyond the point at which the payback obligation is satisfied with no additional obligation incurred. Families may continue to bring their children during the payback phase.

During payback, parents concentrate on support and training of newer parents still in treatment. They observe individual therapeutic sessions, offer feedback, record and analyze data, supervise therapeutic sessions conducted in home and public facility settings, manage classrooms, and develop new training materials. Other activities might include assisting in intake interviews, serving as temporary support parents for newly enrolled families, or conducting visitors on tours of the program. The payback system and the policy of open enrollment throughout the calendar year result in an arrangement whereby, "RIP constantly replenishes its supply of parent/teachers and creates a key self-help group for parents of handicapped children" (Knitzer, 1982, p. 20). Or stated in somewhat different terms, "RIP always has a large number of enthusiastic well-trained parents who are able to give the program the support it needs for success" (Smith, 1974, p. 2).

Parent implementation is an integral part of the treatment approach for individual families as well as a fundamental component of program management. Since most young handicapped children spend a critical portion of their lives with their parents, it is imperative that parents have the skills to teach and live with the children on a daily basis, regardless of other services the children may receive.

During active treatment, parents acquire basic skills to address immediate presenting problems. They may learn to manage severe behavior problems or begin to teach specific developmental skills that the child lacks. This phase of treatment has been compared to boot camp, in concept, if not in atmosphere. It provides rehearsal of skills that must be applied in the community at large (The

Regional Intervention Program, 1979). During payback, generalized application of these basic skills through work with other families prepares parents for the inevitable emergence of new demands on family interactions that their own children will present.

Parent implementation in RIP programs does not exist in a vacuum bereft of professional expertise and guidance. The RIP program in Nashville includes a professional resource staff of five individuals (masters level in psychology, special education, child development, social work) who devote exclusive attention to the ongoing operation of the program. Two additional masters-level staff members devote exclusive attention to operation of The RIP Expansion Project. A doctoral-level staff member (developmental psychology and special education) serves as administrative and clinical director for both RIP and The RIP Expansion Project.

In addition, six professional consultants in the areas of pediatrics, child psychiatry, clinical psychology, speech and language development, pediatric motor development, and educational skills assessment are available to parents and staff members as needed. The RIP budget for fiscal year 1987–1988 provides for a collective total of 50 consultant hours per month at an annual cost of approximately $17,000.

It is helpful to examine relationships between professionals and parents associated with RIP programs by describing the three other essential elements of the model. One of these elements, *data-based clinical operation*, was present from the earliest stages of program development and has remained of crucial importance throughout the program's history. The behavioral orientation of the treatment methodology employed in RIP presupposes, to some extent, quantified measurement of treatment activities and outcomes. And while the use of such measurement systems in RIP programs is somewhat less novel (and controversial) in 1986 than it was in 1969, the extent of application remains significant.

Of greatest significance is the direct involvement of parents in virtually all aspects of the data-based system (Hester, 1977). Incorporation of ongoing measurement into treatment activities is not carried out by the professional staff behind closed doors. Each intervention program designed for use at RIP and across other settings includes specification of the task, the antecedent events (including parent behavior), and a criterion measure for desired change. Data for each program are recorded daily during interaction between a parent and child and are then portrayed in graphic form. Discussion and analysis of child and adult behavior change programs conducted at RIP, at home, and elsewhere are based on ongoing evaluation of clinical data collected by parents themselves. Thus, reliance on a data-based clinical operation in RIP emphasizes acquisition and use of data management skills by the enrolled clients of the program (Parrish & Hester, 1980).

Another of these interlocking essential elements, RIP's *modular system*, was also developed relatively early in the program's history (Timm & Rule, 1981). Services are divided by specific functions into modules: Generalization Training (GT), Individual Tutoring (IT), Preschool Classrooms, Administration, Referral and Intake, Liaison, and Media Services. Each module is supervised by a resource staff member and, with the exception of the Administration Module, is coordinated by parents.

The Referral and Intake Module is the initial point of contact between entering families and RIP. Families may enroll in the program with or without formal referrals from other agencies or professionals, but direct contact with the program must be made by a parent. During the past seven years, 38% of all referrals were made by the medical and psychological professionals, 23% by educational and human service agencies, 18% by evaluation centers, and 21% came from friends or family. The intake interview, which includes conversation with participating parents and observation of the program in operation, is conducted by a parent. The constantly available pool of trained parents and the size of the physical facility permits the Nashville RIP program to avoid a waiting list. During fiscal year 1986–1987, the average time between intake interview and first day of treatment was 3.7 working days. After intake, parents enter direct service modules appropriate to the needs of the family.

The Generalization Training (GT) Module is designed for families of children exhibiting behavior management problems (tantrums, aggression, opposition to parents, self-injurious behavior) so severe as to constitute a problem for themselves or family members. The GT Module teaches parents to use differential reinforcement techniques to manage their children's behavior in a variety of structured play sessions and simultaneously implemented home programs. As described in detail by Strain, Young, and Horowitz (1981), the training phases include Baseline, Differential Reinforcement I, Reversal, Differential Reinforcement II, and Follow-up. Data-based criteria are used to determine the movement across phases.

The Individual Tutoring (IT) Module is designed for families with children exhibiting delays in any of a wide variety of developmental areas including speech and language, cognition, motor functioning, and self-help skills. Training sessions, with the parents serving as primary teachers for their own children are conducted on a daily basis at RIP. Home programs are conducted simultaneously by parents and other family members. The operation of the IT Module has been described rather extensively by Eller, Jordan, Parish, and Elder (1979).

Dependent on need, individual families may participate in the GT Module only, the IT Module only, or both. All families, however, participate in the Preschool Classroom Module. The primary purposes of the classrooms are to teach appropriate skills necessary for children to function effectively in group instructional settings and to provide an important training setting for enrolled parents. Preschool siblings of target children serve as models in the classroom. Data-based observations of children's classroom behavior are made regularly. Movement from Intake Classroom (where social behavior is emphasized) to Toddler or Community Classroom (in which preacademic and language skills receive greater attention) is guided by specific behavioral criteria. Data-based observations of adult classroom behavior aid parents in generalizing basic instructional and management skills from individual treatment to group settings.

RIP classrooms have also served as research settings for investigators concerned with social behavior and language development of preschool children (Hester & Hendrickson, 1977; Shores, 1974; Shores, Hester, & Strain, 1976; Strain, Shores, & Kerr, 1976; Strain & Timm, 1974; Strain & Wiegerink, 1975, 1976; Timm, Strain, & Eller, 1979).

The fourth essential element, *management-by-objectives* (MBO), permits RIP to deliver the range of services described through parents rather than professionals. The parents bring commitment, compassion, skills, and a continual source of energy to the program. However, "channeling such energies and properly directing such vital assets is a chronic management problem particularly in a completely citizen implemented system in which information flows from parent to parent and in which there is a planned turnover among those responsible for information and transmission" (Ora, 1972, p. 74). This challenge is met through RIP's system of management by objectives, developed in 1972 in collaboration with the University of Tennessee Department of Industrial Engineering (Snider, Sullivan, & Manning, 1974).

Three major tiers of objectives comprise RIP's MBO system. The first tier contains all treatment programs, center-based and community-based, implemented by individual families or involving individual children in RIP classroom settings. Treatment objectives, treatment procedures, measurement methods, and behavioral criteria are specified on program sheets. Data collected on a per day or per session basis are displayed in graphic form to facilitate ongoing analysis. Review involving parents, parent case managers, and the resource staff occurs usually on a daily basis.

The second tier contains family objectives established and evaluated at six-week intervals throughout each family's treatment period in the program. The family objectives, including measurement methods and behavioral criteria, address child and parent performance in the program. Family objectives, initially and at each evaluation interval, are developed and revised by the parents, the parent case managers, and the appropriate resource person(s) in consensual fashion (see Table 25.1).

The third tier in RIP's MBO system contains modular objectives, evaluated on a semiannual and annual basis per module. Objectives for each direct service and support module are organized with regard to major functions and expected outcomes. Resource staff members are responsible for ongoing management of the various modules and are accountable for output to the RIP Evaluation Committees. The two committees, one for the AM Program and one for the PM Program, are composed of parents who have been served previously by RIP and may, at the parents' invitation, include representatives from the community at large. Each committee meets 10 times per calendar year to review objectives and outcome data from the respective modules. Although evaluation results are forwarded to appropriate state officials, the committees are not responsible for the state of Tennessee and operate independently to represent families served by RIP. As noted by Hester (1977), "Such evaluation by consumers is critical to any service system attempting to be responsive to the needs of its clients" (p. 267) (see Table 25.2).

TABLE 25.1. Six-week family objectives.

---

Objective 1

Ms. Smith to learn one-to-one IT teaching techniques.

*Measurement Method*: See activities

*Activity 1*: Ms. Smith to learn to take data on her own IT sessions (90% or above interobserver agreement).

*Activity 2*: Ms. Smith to begin running IT sessions at home, after demonstrating competency at the center, to record and report data.

Objective 2

Susan to do leg thrusts to build up her leg muscles.

*Measurement Method*: Within six weeks Susan will triple the number of independent leg thrusts during probes, as shown by pre–post training session data.

*Activity 1*: Ms. Smith to run four leg thrust sessions per week at RIP and collect and graph data.

*Activity 2*: Ms. Smith to run five leg thrust sessions per week at home and collect and graph data. (IT objectives 3 and 4 for Susan are omitted for the sake of brevity.)

Objective 3

Ms. Smith to assume a responsible position in the Center.

*Measurement Method*:
  (1) Ms. Smith to post and graph her own IT data daily.
  (2) Ms. Smith to begin rating at least two sessions per week.
  (3) Ms. Smith to conduct at least one classroom activity per day as scheduled with resource staff.

---

*Note*: From "RIP: A Cost-Effective Parent-Implemented Program for Young Handicapped Children" by M.A. Timm and S. Rule, 1981, *Early Child Development and Care*, 7, pp. 154–155. Copyright 1981 by Gordon and Beach Science Publishers, Inc., One Park Avenue, N.Y., N.Y. 10016. Reprinted by permission.

RIP's MBO system has served as the primary means of assessing ongoing program operations since 1972. This application of a system, more usually associated with industrial organizations, provides parents, staff, and administrative officials with a variety of sets of data regarding treatment effectiveness and managerial efficiency. It should be noted, however, that the MBO system is most directly applicable to the treatment process and related support functions that occur while families are enrolled in the program. Questions related to the generalization and maintenance of treatment effects across settings and over time have been addressed in five efforts conducted under the auspices of the Regional Intervention Program which are summarized below.

The first effort represents a seminal attempt in early intervention program evaluation to assess the relationships between program cost and program benefits. As reported in Snider et al. (1974), a team of investigators from the University of Tennessee Industrial Engineering Department examined actual program costs for the 1969–1972 period. From the 158 children admitted to the program during this time, 64 children were identified by a panel of professionals as probable candidates for institutional psychiatric care. Ten cases were selected from this group of 64 in which the evidence concerning the child's probable future commitment to institutional care was determined prior to treatment at RIP. Independent projections by a panel of professional experts were made regarding

TABLE 25.2. Individual tutoring module objectives.

Objective 2.1

Teach mother/father to relate to the child in a structured individual tutoring session so that the parent can train the child in language and basic skills development.

Criterion

Seventy-five percent of all families who run Individual Tutoring sessions and who meet their specified level of attendance during their first two evaluation periods meet their specified IT treatment objectives within those two evaluation periods.

Activity

2.1.1 Resource consultant to review data from assessment sessions.
2.1.2 Resource consultant, case manager, and parent to complete IT program sheet each program.
2.1.3 Resource consultant to oversee writing of treatment objectives, review with parent(s), and revise if necessary.
2.1.4 Resource consultant to arrange for instructions before and feedback after each session.
2.1.5 Resource consultant to provide consultation to discuss sessions, data, programming, and so forth, on an as-needed basis.
2.1.6 Resource consultant to arrange for services that exceed capabilities of progam when family requests such services.

*Note*: From "RIP: A Cost-Effective Parent-Implemented Program for Young Handicapped Children" by M.A. Timm and S. Rule, 1981, *Early Child Development and Care*, 7, p. 156. Copyright 1981 by Gordon and Beach Science Publishers, Inc., One Park Avenue, N.Y., N.Y. 10016. Reprinted by permission.

probable dates of admission and lengths of stay in institutional care, with and without involvement at RIP.

The investigators then imposed an economic analysis formula, which was based on assumptions termed "ultraconservative" (Snider et al., 1974). Given the anticipated dates of institutionalization for each child, assuming a 60-year life expectancy and an annual institutionalization cost of $4,000 coupled with 5% annual inflation, the projected costs of supporting each child with and without RIP were established. Differences between the two costs were interpreted as savings attributable directly to participation in the program. A basic benefit–cost ratio in dollars alone, not including human benefits to the child and family was calculated conservatively to be 7.79:1. That is, for every $1.00 expended by the state to operate the program, benefits of $7.79 would be realized.

A second effort, reported in Eller et al. (1979), verified current placements of children served previously by the RIP program based on the most recent Liaison Module contacts between 1969 and 1975. The 159 children included in the survey were divided into two major categories, based on diagnostic data available prior to and during enrollment at RIP. The "Handicapped" category contained 72 children with diagnostic labels including autistic, childhood schizophrenic, mentally retarded, brain-damaged, cerebral palsied, visually impaired, hearing impaired, and language disordered. The "Oppositional" category contained 87 children who were enrolled in the program because of significant behavior problems, but for whom no additional diagnostic label had been obtained.

Of the "handicapped" children, 58% were enrolled in self-contained special education classrooms and 29% were enrolled in regular classroom placements.

Another 7% were enrolled in regular classroom placements with tutoring or special services. Only 1% of the children were in residential care. The remaining children were at home (3%) or could not be located (2%). Of the "oppositional" children, 79% were enrolled in regular classroom placements, 1% in special education classrooms, 10% were still at home, and 10% could not be located.

A third effort, reported in Strain et al. (1981), examined demographic information and treatment outcome data for 109 families served within RIP's Generalization Training Module from 1969 to mid-1977. Of the 109 families, 85 had completed all phases of treatment and were referred to as the "follow-up" group. Families reaching the follow-up phase had produced reliable data supporting generalization and maintenance of positive behavior change for the child within the home setting after treatment activities had ceased. The remaining 29 families had failed to meet one or more specified criteria for completion of treatment and were referred to as the "no follow-up" group.

Examination of dichotomous and continuous variables across both groups included consideration of child characteristics such as age, sex, race, and birth order; and adult/family features such as number of siblings, mother's age, intactness of family, income, mother's formal educational level, and average attendance during treatment. Three significant trends were demonstrated, with clear implications for acquisition and maintenance of treatment effects. First, children who completed the entire treatment series were markedly younger than those who did not. Second, the percentage of scheduled session appointments honored by follow-up group families was significantly higher than the attendance percentage recorded for the no follow-up group. Third, significantly more children from intact families reached follow-up status than did those from nonintact families. Also of considerable interest was the lack of significant relationships between generalized treatment outcomes and variables often linked with poor treatment prognosis such as income, educational level, mother's age, race, and sex of child.

The fourth effort represents the most extensive attempt to date to assess the long-term effects of RIP treatment, reported in Strain, Steele, Ellis, and Timm (1982). This investigation involved 40 families served by RIP from 1969 to 1978 meeting the following criteria: (1) child currently in grades 1 through 6, (2) family currently residing within 20 miles of program, (3) family referred originally because of child oppositional behaviors, and (4) parents and children had met all behavioral criteria for Generalization Training. The 40 participating families represented 90% of all families on file meeting these criteria. In addition, four peers (matched by age, sex, and no previous history of behavioral difficulty) were selected randomly within each former RIP child's current classroom. Three class peers were lost owing to absenteeism, reducing the final number of 157 as reported in the study.

Direct observation measures of adult and child behaviors were obtained in group academic instruction (seven behavior categories) and unstructured recreation (four behavior categories) school settings for each former RIP child, his or her classroom peers, and teachers or aides without identifying the former RIP children's previous association with the program. A total of six 30-minute data collection sessions, three for each setting, were conducted for each child within a three-week interval. Direct observation measures of parent, child, and sibling behavior were obtained in the home setting for each participating RIP family (10 behavior categories) within a four-week interval. Blind screen use of the Walker Problem Behavior Checklist (Walker, 1970) was implemented with teachers in the school setting, and open use of the same instrument was implemented with parents of former RIP children.

Major findings in this investigation (which was designed to address several methodological problems presented by earlier examinations of parent training outcomes) include the following: (1) commands, demands, or requests made by parents were very likely to be followed by former clients' compliance; (2) former clients' social interactions in the home were overwhelmingly positive and their nonsocial behavior was by and large appropriate; (3) parent behavior in the home setting was consistent with the child management skills taught in RIP three to nine years earlier; (4) there were no differences between the compliant, on-task, social interaction, and nonsocial behaviors of former clients and randomly selected peers; (5) there were no differences in multiple categories of teacher behavior toward the two groups of children; (6) there was high correlation between teacher and parent ratings on the Checklist; (7) there were no differences in teacher ratings of former clients and class peers; and (8) of all the examined demographic variables, only age at which treatment began and family intactness were related to current levels of behavior. Of particular interest was the significant evidence that the younger the age of the child during treatment the more successful was the adjustment three to nine years later; no "wash out" effect was observed relative to length of time the children and families had been out of the program.

The fifth effort is a recent follow-up study initiated by the Preschool Intervention Program (PIP), Hartford, Connecticut, a certified replication site since 1976. As reported by Reisman (1985), the study involved a comparison of 20 program graduates who had completed the Generalization Training Module, with 20 families referred for similar presenting problems who chose not to participate in any early intervention service. Length of time elapsed since initial referral ranged from two to five years for PIP graduates, with a mean of 4.45 years; and a mean of just over four years for the nonparticipating families. All 40 families were asked to document various human services provided them with regard to the child's behavior difficulties from date of referral to time of the study. Included were such services as special education, family counseling for parenting issues and behavior management, and social service case management regarding inadequate parenting skills.

Aggregate data for the 20 former PIP families over the five-year period showed that approximately $122,842 was spent in human services. Aggregate data for the nontreatment group during the same period revealed total expenditures of $369,837. The comparative cost–benefit ratio indicates a $3.00 savings for every dollar spent. Of particular interest was the finding that the former PIP families incurred virtually all expenses during the initial treatment year in the five-year period, with virtually no further use of services in subsequent years. By contrast, the total expenses incurred by the nontreatment group were distributed relatively evenly over the five-year period.

The program model developed and refined by parents and staff associated with the Regional Intervention Program system, based in Nashville, Tennessee, provides one approach to the amelioration and prevention of significant problems faced by young children and their families that is of demonstrated effectiveness. Since 1974, The RIP Expansion Project has conducted training and consultation activities that have produced an additional 20 certified replication sites in 15 communities operating currently in the United States, Canada, and Brazil. Certified sites have served approximately 2,500 families to date. It is most encouraging to note that essential elements of the model appear to work effectively in these other communities as well (Innes, 1981). As the late Nicholas Hobbs (1978) observed:

RIP, of course, uses the mother primarily with younger children to address very specific problems, and teaches the mother how to handle these problems. Thus you magnify enormously the resources that are available to help the child. The fascinating thing is, of course, you get the intense motivation that parents tend to have and that professional people seldom can have.

## References

Eller, P., Jordan, H., Parish, A., & Elder, P. (1979). Professional qualification: Mother. In R.L. York & E. Edgar (Eds.), *Teaching the handicapped* (Vol. IV). Seattle, WA: American Association for the Education of the Severely/Profoundly Handicapped.

Fields, S. (1975). Parents as therapists. *Innovations, 2,* 3–8.

Gold Award. (1976). A parent implemented early intervention program for preschool children. *Hospital and Community Psychiatry, 27,* 728–731.

Hester, P. (1977). Evaluation and accountability in a parent-implemented early intervention service. *Community Mental Health Journal, 13,* 216–267.

Hester, P., & Hendrickson, J. (1977). Training functional expressive language: The acquisition and generalization of five-element syntactic responses. *Journal of Applied Behavior Analysis, 10,* 316.

Hobbs, N. (1978). In DMK Films, Inc. (Producer). *Parents helping parents helping children: A model for early intervention.* Nashville, TN: DMK Films. (Film)

Hobbs, N. (1982). *The troubled and troubling child.* San Francisco, CA: Jossey-Bass.

Innes, S. (1981). *An analytic description of the replication process of an early intervention program: A case study.* Unpublished doctoral dissertation, George Peabody College of Vanderbilt University, Nashville, TN.

Knitzer, J. (1982). *Unclaimed children.* Washington, DC: Children's Defense Fund.

Ora, J.P. (1970). *Final report: Regional Intervention Project for Preschoolers and Parents.* Unpublished manuscript, Regional Intervention Program, Nashville, TN.

Ora, J.P. (1972). The involvement and training of parent- and citizen-workers in early education for the handicapped and their implications. In *Not all little wagons are red.* Washington, DC: Council for Exceptional Children.

Ora, J.P., & Wiegerink, R. (1969). *The Regional Intervention Program for Preschoolers and Parents.* Unpublished grant application proposal, Regional Intervention Program, Nashville, TN.

Parrish, V., & Hester, P. (1980). Controlling behavior techniques in an early intervention program. *Community Mental Health Journal, 16,* 169–175.

Reisman, J. (1985). [Preschool Intervention Program]. Windsor, CT: Capitol Region Education Council. Unpublished raw data.

Shores, R. (1974). Research on development of social interactions in a preschool for handicapped children. In L. Bullock (Ed.), *Proceedings of the annual fall conference of teacher educators of children with behavior disorders.* Gainesville, FL: University of Florida Press.

Shores, R., Hester, P., & Strain, P. (1976). The effects of amount and type of teacher–child interaction on child–child interaction. *Psychology in the Schools, 13,* 171–175.

Smith, C. (1974). The preschool program that works. *Tennessee Mental Health Magazine, 2*(3), 1–5.

Snider, J., Sullivan, W., & Manning, D. (1974). Industrial engineering participation in a special education program. *Tennessee Engineer, 1,* 21–23.

Strain, P., Shores, R., & Kerr, M. (1976). An experimental analysis of "spillover" effects on social interaction among behaviorally handicapped preschool children. *Journal of Applied Behavior Analysis, 9,* 31–40.

Strain, P., Steele, P., Ellis, T., & Timm, M.A. (1982). Long term effects of oppositional child treatment with mothers as therapists and therapist trainers. *Journal of Applied Behavior Analysis, 15,* 163–169.

Strain, P., & Timm, M.A. (1974). An experimental analysis of social interaction between a behaviorally disordered preschool child and her classroom peers. *Journal of Applied Behavior Analysis, 7,* 583–590.

Strain, P., & Wiegerink, R. (1975). The social play of two behaviorally disordered children during four activities: A multiple baseline study. *Journal of Abnormal Child Psychology, 3,* 61–69.

Strain, P., & Wiegerink, R. (1976). The effects of sociodramatic activities on social interaction among behaviorally disordered preschool children. *Journal of Special Education, 10,* 71–75.

Strain, P., Young, C., & Horowitz, J. (1981). An examination of child and family demographic variables related to generalized behavior change during oppositional child training. *Behavior Modification, 5,* 15–26.

The Regional Intervention Program. (1979). In *Mental retardation: The leading edge.* 1978 Report, President's Committee on Mental Retardation. Washington, DC: U.S. Government Printing Office, DHEW (Publication No. [OHDS] 79-21018).

Timm, M.A. (1978). *A framework for analysis of the RIP replication process.* Nashville, TN: Regional Intervention Program. Unpublished manuscript.

Timm, M.A., & Rule, S. (1981). RIP: A cost-effective parent-implemented program for young handicapped children. *Early Child Development and Care, 7,* 147–163.

Timm, M.A., Strain, P., & Eller, P. (1979). The effects of systematic, response-dependent fading and thinning procedures on the maintenance of child–child interaction. *Journal of Applied Behavior Analysis, 12,* 142.

Walker, H.M. (1970). *The Walker Problem Behavior Identification Checklist: Test and Manual.* Los Angeles, CA: Western Psychological Service, Inc.

# 26
# The Education and Treatment of Behavior-Disordered Mentally Retarded Children

SIDNEY W. BIJOU

It is an accepted fact that public schools do not provide behavior-disordered mentally retarded children with the kind of attention they require to enhance their learning, cognitive functioning, and personal adjustment. This problem and recommendations for its solution are the focus of this chapter. First, a working functional basis for analyzing the conditions that bring about behavior-disordered mental retardation is discussed. Second, the kind of intervention that is essential for improving the learning, cognitive functioning, and adjustment levels of this group is presented. Third, four recommendations for actualizing such a program are given.

## Conceptualization of Behavior-Disordered Mentally Retarded Children

Like any child, the behavior-disordered mentally retarded child develops from a combination of (1) genetic factors, (2) his or her history of interactions with the environment (including interactions with the individual's own biological structure and functioning), and (3) current circumstances. Both the historical and current conditions are further divided into antecedent conditions (stimuli in actual interaction with the individual), the actions of the individual (what he or she says, does, and shows), and the context (the setting in which an interaction takes place). Research conducted from this perspective, which is referred to variously as learning theory, the natural science approach, behavior modification, behavior analysis, and applied behavior analysis, has yielded over the past 45 years a vast store of information on how an individual learns skills and knowledge; develops learned motivations, attitudes, and values; and acquires adjustment (personality patterns).

From this point of view, the behavior-disordered mentally retarded child is one who has a limited repertoire of behavior and an abnormal adjustment pattern generated by a history of restrictions in opportunities for learning and of abnormal stressful conditions. Let us consider each set of conditions.

## Restrictions in Opportunities for Learning

The retarded child, with or without personal adjustment problems, lacks a normal repertoire of skills, knowledge, learned motivations, and adjustment reactions because of restrictions in opportunities and support for their acquisition (Bijou & Dunitz-Johnson, 1981). These restraints fall into three categories: biomedical pathologies, biomedical pathologies in combination with regressive social practices, and sociocultural disadvantages.

### BIOMEDICAL PATHOLOGIES

Severe biomedical pathologies, which occur in 25 to 35% of the retarded population in the United States, originate in the genetic, prenatal, perinatal, or postnatal stage of development. A review and evaluation of the extensive literature on the biomedical pathologies that *contribute* to retarded development are beyond the scope of this chapter; however, we shall touch briefly on the nature of these conditions.

Note that we say "biomedical pathologies that *contribute* to retarded development." This serves to emphasize that no one condition can be considered *the* cause, or etiology, of retardation, as is strongly suggested in classification systems (see Menolascino, 1983). Multiple conditions — some biomedical and some sociocultural — interact in an individual's history to produce retardation, sometimes alone and sometimes in conjunction with personal maladjustment.

Research in genetics has revealed that biological pathologies may result from anomalies in chromosomal arrangements, relationships between dominant and recessive genes, and problems of sex-linkage. Pathologies originating in prenatal conditions include defects in the structural conditions of pregnancy, maternal factors, x-rays, and other forms of radiation. Perinatal conditions, which include severity of birth (as indicated by the length and difficulty of labor, presentation, forceps delivery, and complications of first births), may adversely affect the anatomy and the physiological functioning of the infant through injuries, deprivation of oxygen, and respiratory distress. Also operative at birth are certain infectious diseases of the mother, such as syphilis and gonorrhea. And finally, there are postnatal anomalies affecting physical growth and functioning, which include malnutrition, infections, illnesses, diseases, drug effects, and traumatic damage through accidents.

Regardless of the developmental stage in which a severe biomedical impairment occurs, its significance lies in the extent to which the damage impairs the individual's *reaction systems*. If the individual's response equipment is severely impaired, reactions to objects and events are reduced, and the potentiality for normal development is consequently reduced. Also significant is the extent to which the impairment affects *internal stimulation*. If stimulation from glands, muscles, viscera, and physiological connecting systems (e.g., the central nervous system) is impaired, the chances for normal development are also reduced because the individual's internal environment is incomplete or distorted.

In addition to the effects of biomedical pathologies on psychological development, one must take into account their regressive effects when they are combined with certain forms of social practices. We refer here to situations in which parents and other significant individuals (e.g., peers, teachers, and recreational workers) in a child's life treat a stigmatized child as being chronically ill, peculiar, disturbed, or undesirable. These practices shield the child from everyday experiences of childhood and thereby limit the opportunities to develop the usual social and motivational repertoires. Even a clinical label alone, attached to a particular child who has no visible impairment, tends to generate negative attitudes and actions toward that child.

## SOCIOCULTURAL DISADVANTAGES

Handicapping sociocultural conditions as dominant factors of retardation account for 65 to 75% of the retarded population in the United States. Among these conditions are combinations of (1) poverty socioeconomic-status families, which include marginal physical resources and lack of parental support for complying with cultural and educational practices; (2) abusive parental practices; and (3) childrearing practices with indifferent parent–child relationships. Like biomedical pathologies, these handicapping sociocultural conditions directly or indirectly restrict children's opportunities to develop normally.

## Abnormal Stressful Conditions

Many of the conditions that restrict opportunities for learning are also stressful and as such generate maladjusted forms of behavior. The principles described in any textbook on abnormal psychology apply here. For the purpose of this discussion, we mention that stressful conditions arise from frequent and/or strong aversive conditions, severe and prolonged deprivations, and damage from drugs, degenerative diseases, and traumas. The maladjustment patterns that emerge range from excessive aggressiveness, extremely shy and withdrawn behavior, and chronic delinquency, on the one hand, to disorganized, degenerative, dissociated, and traumatic reaction patterns, on the other.

## Summary

The behavior-disordered mentally retarded child is analyzed here as one who has a limited repertoire of behavior and persistent adjustment problems generated by a history of restrictions in opportunities for learning and frequent and/or strong stressful conditions.

We shall now examine the kind of educational and treatment programs that are appropriate for such children. Specifically, this group consists of children between 6 and 18 or 21 years, depending on local school practices, who are neither so severely retarded nor so severely maladjusted (prepsychotic or psychotic) as to preclude public school attendance.

# The Required Education and Treatment Strategy

Because of the complex history of the behavior-disordered mentally retarded child, he or she needs a special kind of individualized education and treatment program, one based on current knowledge from empirical research.

## Meaning of Terms

Educating a behavior-disordered mentally retarded child means applying empirical learning principles that facilitate not only the acquisition of new skills and knowledge, particularly in the academic tool subjects, but also those behaviors associated with learning (namely, academic work habits, pride in achievement, desire for learning, and the like). Treating such a behavior-disordered mentally retarded child means applying empirical behavior principles in an orderly and systematic manner so as to improve the child's adjustment by enhancing social skills and eliminating or reducing behaviors that are aversive to himself, herself, and others (Bijou & Redd, 1975).

Individualized education and treatment means tailoring material and task sequences and motivational and teaching techniques to fit the competencies, learning style, and personality of each child. It does not necessarily mean a one-to-one teacher–child relationship; educational and treatment goals can be achieved equally well in small groups. Here, each child works at his or her level of ability and pace on individualized assignments and receives meaningful positive assistance.

Teachers, aides, peers, parents, siblings, senior citizens, and high school students can all contribute to successful individualized instruction and treatment. But it is the responsibility of the teacher, who must him/herself be trained and experienced, to train and supervise those who participate in the instruction and treatment of the children.

## Characteristics of Empirically Oriented Education and Treatment Programs

Empirically oriented individualized education and treatment programs may be best described by listing their essential characteristics:

1. They involve individualized assessment, usually by criterion-referenced tests and the child's history, to establish reasonable instructional and treatment goals. This procedure is effective only when there is continuity between the assessment procedures and the programmed sequences that the child is to be taught.
2. The teaching techniques, which involve controlling attention, prompting corrected or desirable behaviors, and the judicious use of contingencies, are based on empirical learning principles.
3. Progress in academic achievement and adjustment is monitored on the basis of some objective system that includes daily or weekly recordings.

4. Evaluation of progress leads to modifications of programs and procedures and the resetting of educational and/or treatment goals. This aspect of the procedure functions like a servomechanism; the performance of the child dictates the corrections in the program that must be made to keep him or her on the course to the goal set.
5. Explicit procedures are established for helping each child make a transition to the next training or work assignment.

### Current Situation

Currently, behavior-disordered mentally retarded children are generally placed in special classes for mentally retarded or behavior-disordered children. Although the teacher typically works with small groups or individuals and has the assistance of an aide, instruction and treatment are not individualized according to the features mentioned above. One or more cardinal elements are omitted. Sometimes the materials or tasks are not appropriate for the child's competence or are not properly sequenced; sometimes records are too subjective to indicate actual performance in the programs; sometimes the contingencies for correct and desirable responses are not meaningful to the child; and sometimes contingencies are not applied in the most effective manner. Hence, the children tended to "mark time" rather than advance in learning, cognitive functioning, and adjustment.

In some schools, behavior-disordered mentally retarded children are placed in regular classes for mainstreaming purposes. Such placements rarely benefit the child and serve instead to create frustrations mainly because the teacher: (1) assigns work that is inappropriate for his or her level of competence, as a result of which he or she experiences boredom, failure, and sometimes punishment; (2) deals with problem behaviors on an emergency basis rather than devising a program aimed at enhancing the social adjustment of the child; and/or (3) involves the parents merely to alleviate problem behavior rather than to involve them in carrying out recommended programs.

## Recommendations

To provide behavior-disordered mentally retarded children with effective educational and treatment programs in our public schools, four far-reaching recommendations are indicated.

1. The U.S. Office of Education should make funds available to state departments of education for the purpose of encouraging local schools to provide in-service training courses on individualizing instruction and treatment for this population. Beneficiaries of such training would be special and general teachers, school psychologists, counselors, and administrators — all of whom are essential for instituting and maintaining the kind of program envisaged. Currently, in-service courses designed to improve teaching practices are a waste of time and money since the subjects selected for study are strongly influenced

by fads and fashions in education. The usual consequence of these courses is an initial acceptance and enthusiasm and some attempts to incorporate new ideas into classroom procedures, followed by a loss of interest and a reversion to one's previous way of thinking and teaching. To counteract this almost inevitable sequence, in-service training should cover a technique or method thoroughly and be followed by supervision of a visiting master teacher. The duration of supervision would depend on the time required for the teacher to become proficient in using the information and procedures that have been introduced.

2. The U.S. Office of Education should offer training and demonstration grants to colleges and universities to encourage experimenting with present-day curricula for the purpose of breaking down the almost impenetrable walls between general and special-degree teaching programs and open new vistas for meaningful refresher courses. Such revisions would benefit future and practicing elementary and secondary school teachers who would receive training in (a) mainstreaming through individualization of instruction of all children—normal, accelerated, retarded, and behavior-disordered; (b) the use of classroom management techniques to deal with discipline problems; (c) how to teach academic tool subjects to exceptional children (particularly behavior-disordered mentally retarded children); (d) how to enhance the social skills and personal adjustment of such children; (e) the use of methods and techniques for involving parents in the education of their exceptional children; and (f) how to use computers to facilitate individualization of instruction, particularly in the academic tool subjects.

3. The U.S. Office of Education and the National Institute of Mental Health should provide funds for identifying and disseminating to colleges of education, state departments of instruction, school districts, group homes, and mental health clinics current information on improving the learning, cognitive functioning, and personal adjustment of behavior-disordered mentally retarded children in an effort to close the gap, at least partially, between current knowledge and current practice.

4. These federal agencies, as well as the National Institute for Child Health and Human Development, should provide funds for research oriented toward the further advancement of knowledge on the learning, cognitive functioning, and personal adjustment of behavior-disordered mentally retarded school-age children.

## References

Bijou, S.W., & Dunitz-Johnson, E. (1981). Interbehavior analysis of developmental retardation. *Psychological Record, 31*, 305–329.

Bijou, S.W., & Redd, W.H. (1975). Child behavior therapy. In S. Arieti (Ed.), *American handbook of psychiatry* (2nd ed., Vol. 5, pp. 579–585). New York: Basic Books.

Menolascino, F.J. (1983). Bridging the gap between mental retardation and mental illness. In F.J. Menolascino & B.M. McCann (Eds.), *Mental health and mental retardation: Bridging the gap* (pp. 3–64). Baltimore, MD: University Park Press.

# 27
# Transitional Services in the Habilitation of Mentally Retarded Individuals with Mental Health Needs

JACK A. STARK, WILLIAM E. KIERNAN, and TAMMI GOLDSBURY

## Introduction

In the 1970s and first half of the 1980s, *mainstreaming* was the major new focus of our educational system in providing services to disabled children and adolescents. During the next 10 to 15 years, *transitional* services will be the primary new emphasis of our school programs. Evidence of this new emphasis is already apparent in funding allocations by the Directors of the Office of Special Education and Rehabilitation Services and Administration on Developmental Disabilities. Both of these directors have jointly pooled funds to encourage individual states, via financial incentives, to reevaluate their success at transitioning disabled individuals from school programs into residential and vocational service systems in cooperation with other state and local agencies.

The purpose of this chapter will be to build on the recommendations provided by Dr. Bijou (Chapter 26) on educational services to the mentally retarded individual with mental health needs via a bridge to the other service systems. While other chapters in this book cover issues ranging from the epidemiological aspects to treatment approaches, we hope to demonstrate the need for and provide a blueprint of an orderly transition from a school program to a residential/vocational program for this most difficult-to-serve population.

## Needs of the Adolescent and Young Adult

The needs of the adolescent and young adult transitioning from the school system to community programs are enormous. Since the landmark legislation in 1975 involving the Education of All Handicapped Children's Act (P.L. 94-142), unprecedented numbers of students with disabilities have been graduating from our school systems. It is estimated that approximately 250,000 to 300,000 students "graduate" from special education programs each year (Rehab Brief, April 1984). It is further estimated that 80 to 90% of these individuals, particularly those with the more severe disabilities, are not moving into an employment status. They are either unemployed or underemployed and living below the poverty line. This status of employment, and oftentimes inappropriate living conditions, leads to what the authors of this chapter consider the major problem of the mentally retarded individual with mental health needs in American today —that special education students are transitioning from school with no place to go in which to live or to work.

This terrible indictment of our system is analogous to what Dr. Bijou was involved in 20 years ago when he helped to establish the Head Start program for disadvantaged preschoolers. After conducting research and establishing a system based on successful outcome data, he and others found that when follow-up was not conducted the skills that these preschoolers gained were soon lost. As a result, the National Follow-Through Program was established to provide ongoing enriched programs for their early grades to these same individuals. In the same manner, we will also need to provide programmatic assistance to ensure successful transition and placement of these special education individuals leaving our school systems. Indeed, as we travel around the country, we find that much of the informal data reflect the fact that the median age of those individuals being placed in our institutions (or nursing homes and intermediate care facilities) today are from 18 to 25 years of age. The tendency has been for these men and women (who are no longer eligible for school programs), after sitting at home for six months to a year and a half with no programming, to begin to experience behavior deterioration resulting in placement in an institutional setting. And, indeed, they often remain there because there are no programs to send them to within the community. Unless this depressing phenomenon is reversed, those individuals who are responsible for cost–benefit analysis and the funding of such programs will soon be asking the question: "Why should we even spend money on these individuals since they eventually will wind up in institutional care anyway?"

The remaining portion of this chapter addresses these various needs. It presents a design on how to provide a transitional system with an emphasis on a new model and what our future challenges will be in accomplishing this task.

## Characteristics of This Population

There is a great deal of misunderstanding as to what constitutes mental illness in the mentally retarded individual. Numerous terms have been used synonomously with mental illness—behavioral impairment, emotional disturbance, or other specific diagnostic labels. For the purposes of this chapter, we are concerned primarily with those individuals whose abnormal or inappropriate behaviors, emotions, or interactions are sufficiently marked or prolonged that they have significant substantial functional limitations in three or more of the seven major life activities (i.e., self-care, receptive/expressive language, learning, mobility, self-direction, capacity for independent living, and economic self-sufficiency).

Our emphasis is therefore on *habilitation* as it applies to the integration and reintegration (socially, educationally, vocationally, and psychologically) of the mentally retarded individual with mental health needs into the least-restrictive environment. The following sections on programs and models emphasize these comprehensive areas of emphasis.

## Demographic Issues

Research on the frequency and types of emotional disorders in the mentally retarded individual has numerous major methodological problems. Studies conducted over the last 20 years indicate a prevalence rate of mental illness in the person with retardation at 10 to 40%. However, most of the studies were conducted on institutionalized individuals and it is therefore questionable as to whether this is a true cross section of the population. Additional research conducted by Menolascino (1972) indicates that the percentages are perhaps less among those mentally retarded individuals who live with their primary families or in their natural community. Of the 300,000 individuals that graduate each year from special education programs, some 10 to 20% (30,000 to 60,000 individuals) have severe behavioral disorders that prevent them from accomplishing successful transition (Stark, Kiernan, Goldsbury, & McGee, 1986).

## Transitional Placement

As we continue to add to these 30,000 to 60,000+ individuals each year, we also develop a backlog of individuals who have been graduating from programs for the last five to six years and who have not been able to receive adequate care and therefore may wind up back in institutional settings or quasi-institutional settings such as private ICF/MR facilities and nursing homes (see also Scheerenberger, Chapter 38).

It is a major concern of ours that this nationwide pool of some 60,000 people constitutes a group whose severe behavioral impairments make them a high priority to be served if for no other reason than because of the strong political, financial, and ethical implications. If we stop and think about it, these individuals with severe acting-out behaviors number approximately 1,000 individuals per state. It is this segment of the population that some feel are too difficult to be served in the community and therefore need to be placed in special settings (i.e., institutions). The authors of this chapter strongly believe in the need for preventing this regrettable phenomenon with early intervention during the junior-high and high-school years via interagency cooperation in order to provide for a smooth transition into the community.

# Transitional Models: Conceptual View

The role of work, for both the individual and society at large, is significant from both an economic and psychological perspective. This role of work is central to both the personal identity and achievement of economic self-sufficiency. The preparatory process aimed at providing an individual with the skills and maturity to enter the employment system is complex. The formal preparation in school must be directed at viable outcomes for the young adult. In essence, we need to create a model whereby people with mental retardation can be provided with a process by which they can enter more fully into the community—prepared with the skills that will at least give them a chance of being economically self-sufficient.

Currently, we have no specific model to follow in preparing those persons with severe mental health needs who are mentally retarded. And perhaps, such a specific model would be inappropriate. Indeed, the model presented in Figure 27.1 is one that all developmentally disabled individuals hopefully would find useful since it is a model that contains options and choices and provides for this process of leading to greater economic self-sufficiency.

This Pathways Model provides a visual illustration of how mentally retarded individuals with mental health needs can be presented with a decisionmaking process and its outcomes, which are available as an individual moves through these various stages. It is important to note that this model is significantly different from the traditional vocational rehabilitation model that emphasized the "flow-through" design where greater emphasis is placed on a sequential lock-step training or service mode (i.e., a person can move on to the next step when certain requisite criteria are met). This model is also different in that it primarily demonstrates options and choices available to individuals with a multitude of disabilities. This model reflects a system whereby an individual is able to choose from a number of options, all of which lead to an outcome directed at enhancing the degree of economic self-sufficiency. This particular outcome does not look at specific jobs, but rather at the effects of moving the individual into an employment status with a multitude of potential jobs from which he or she can choose.

Another key aspect of this particular Pathways Model is that it attempts to extend the variety of environments available to dually diagnosed individuals whereby they can obtain or maintain continuous employment and living support. While we do not have a sufficient data base or model program specifically aimed at this subpopulation, we do know from our past experiences as well as research by our colleagues that many '"severely disabled" individuals are capable of productive employment (Horner & Bellamy, 1979; Wehman, 1981). The underlying philosophy of this particular model recognizes that specific modifications (or what we refer to as "supports") are apt to be used for this particular group of workers. These supports (see also Reiss, Chapter 22, and Fletcher, Chapter 23) can be of an extended or even permanent nature, particularly for this difficult-to-serve subpopulation. This supported employment work model, however, may not

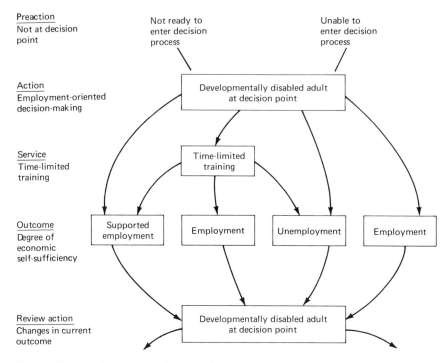

FIGURE 27.1. Pathways to employment for the developmentally disabled adult: a habilitation model. From *Pathways to Employment for Adults with Developmental Disabilities* by W.E. Kiernan and J.A. Stark (Eds.), 1986. Baltimore, MD: Paul H. Brookes Publishing Company. Copyright 1982 by the Paul H. Brookes Publishing Company. Reprinted by permission.

be realistic for an even smaller portion of this group who choose not to have employment as a goal; or because of medical, financial disincentives, or other personal reasons find that employment is not realistic at this particular time. It is our hope, however, based on progress of the past, that this group will become smaller and smaller as we continue to develop better technology, which can reduce the impairments that prevent them from fuller participation in the community.

This model contains four stages: (1) An action stage in which an employment-related decision should involve the decisionmaking process of the dually diagnosed individual. The purpose of this stage is to have sufficient information available as to what options can be achieved with specific assistance, support, and encouragement. Great care needs to be taken with these individuals before they graduate in order to explain the various options for both them and their family. (2) The second stage is service oriented. Training for this population, that is, specific training prior to placement or to simulating a placement, may be necessary in order that job requirements can be learned. In addition, supported assistance will vary according to the environmental demands in which the person works, resides, and socializes. The ultimate goal is to faze out the intensity of the support system (e.g., job coach, prosthetics) to a dually diagnosed individual in order to increase greater individual independence in our society. (3) An outcome stage—movement toward economic self-sufficiency through employment. (4) A review stage and opportunity to make a change in employment based on ongoing changes or crises in an individual's life that may also require a need to return back to a new decision point at any of the other stages.

## The Role of Secondary Schools in Transitional Services

The high unemployment and underemployment rates of developmentally disabled individuals, and more seriously those with a combination of mental illness and mental retardation, are largely due to a lack of systematic transitional planning and interagency cooperation. A number of studies have shown that between 40 and 75% of all disabled students are either unemployed or underemployed (Hasazi, Preskill, Gordon, & Collins, 1982; Mithaug & Horiuchi, 1983; Schalock, 1984).

Wehman and his associates (Wehman, Kregel, Barcus, & Schalock, 1986) have developed a three-stage model in the vocational transition of developmentally disabled youth. The model is particularly applicable to the dually diagnosed population. Facilitating this transition from a school setting into an employment and independent living environment involves three major stages:

*Stage I: School Instruction*
   Emphasis on functional curriculum
   Natural environment
   Integrated school environment
   Community-based service delivery
   Normalization principles
*Stage II: Transitional Process*
   The development of an individual transitional plan based on early planning and cooperation with parental and student input in conjunction with the school personnel, vocational habilitation staff, and community-based service providers in the development of a five-year transitional plan.
*Stage III: Employment and Living Placement*
   The placement into various employment settings that may require supportive assistance; two-year follow-up assistance and phase out.

These three stages address the issue that the major barrier to successful vocational employment and adjustment to demands of various living arrangements is often based on the inability of dually diagnosed individuals to generalize the training skills obtained in a school setting into a more complex community environment. This phenomenon can be minimized by focusing on the critical components and how each of these components can point toward the concept of generalization.

## Functional Curriculum

The major problem we see across the country is that many school systems try to use "canned" curriculum approaches. They try to fit students into their curriculum rather than vice versa. A functional curriculum needs to be based on those types of skills and abilities that will be critical to following an individual with these complex needs. This curriculum should begin five to six years before an individual is able to "graduate" from the school system, which will allow the individual to increase his or her skills gradually in a longitudinal and incremental manner. We need to focus on vocational skills, which will increase the stamina, production rates, ability to attend to task, and interactions with others in a socially appropriate manner while enhancing self-esteem and self-worth. There is a considerable amount of data that have been developed over the last 20 years on the necessity of training in the natural environment. This is often complicated by the limitations of the school system upon leaving the classroom premises. An emphasis needs to be made on natural environment simulation or using job sites within the school building as well as partial to full-day exposure to work experiences while still under the guidance of the school system. This natural-environment emphasis allows for less difficulty in adjusting to the community-based setting and essentially incorporates normalization principles. Integrated school programs are also going to be extremely important, particularly for those with severe emotional disorders who need to be with nonhandicapped peers who can provide modeling of age-appropriate behaviors.

Our ultimate desire for this individual is to be able to live as independently as possible in the community while being able to work in competitive employment settings, in structured specialized industrial training sites, or in sheltered enclaves in industry, with or without supported assistance.

## Individual Transition Plan

The school personnel may initially be somewhat hesitant to look at developing another plan requiring a great deal of paperwork and meeting time. Many complain that they do not have enough time to provide essential teaching because of all the planning and paperwork involved. However, the individualized education plan needs to be supplemented rather than replaced by the individual transition plan. Without this cooperation and understood emphasis, we have no direction and many individuals will wind up as they have been in the last few years—with no place to live and or work. The individual transition plan (as adapted from Wehman, et al., 1986, and originally conceived by Schalock) provides a good example of how such an excellent model can be used. Table 27.1 displays a five-year plan that begins with the development of specific goals, various procedures under which these goals can be accomplished, resources necessary to accomplish them, and the responsible persons involved in carrying out these activities. This sample case presentation demonstrates very clearly how planning over a five-year

TABLE 27.1. Individual transition plan.[a]

| Year | Goal(s)[b] | General procedure | Projected needed resources | Responsible persons | Completion date |
|------|-----------|-------------------|---------------------------|--------------------|-----------------|
| 1983 | Arrange orientation meeting with parent regarding ITP goal for job placement in five years | ITP team contacts parents | Community job training site and supervision | Vocational consultant<br><br>Resource teacher | |
| 1984 | Locate job training site for Chris (one–two days per week during last part of school year) | Advise superintendent of need<br><br>Contact community employers | Job site<br><br>Transportation | Home school superintendent<br><br>Vocational consultant | |
| 1985 | Have Chris in half-day job training | Orient employer<br><br>Place and do work adjustment<br><br>Conduct on-the-job assistance | Job site<br><br>Transportation | Facilitator/enabler<br><br>Employer | |
| 1986 | Coordinate job placement/training and transportation with community-based mental retardation program | Develop interagency agreement | Job site<br><br>Transportation | Vocational consultant<br><br>CBMR job supervisor and case manager | |
| 1987 | Have Chris participate in high-school graduation program | Place name on office list<br><br>Inform home district superintendent | | Parent<br><br>Resource teacher<br><br>School principal | |
| 1988 | Have Chris maintain full-time employment with occasional follow-along assistance | Provide assistance units by CBMR staff | 10 assistance units per month | CBMR job facilitator/assistance | |

[a] Attached to the student's regular individualized Education Plan.
[b] Begin at age 16.

*Note*: From "Vocational Transition for Developmentally Disabled Students" by P. H. Wehman, J. Krugel, J. Barcus, & R. L. Schalock, 1986. In W. E. Kiernan and J. A. Stark (Eds.), *Pathways to Employment for Adults with Developmental Disabilities*. Baltimore, MD: Paul H. Brookes Publishing Company. Copyright 1986 by Paul H. Brookes Publishing Company. Reprinted by permission.

period leads from initial orientation followed by partial-day job training to full-time employment with follow-along assistance. Critical to this plan is the cooperative efforts of the school personnel, community-based service staff, rehabilitation agency personnel, and the client with his or her family support.

## Transitional Services Applied to the Mentally Retarded Individual with Mental Health Needs: The Nebraska Psychiatric Institute Model

Now that we have discussed the conceptual model of transitional services along with specific recommendations for school and community personnel, we need to understand how such services can be applied to this population, particularly those with severe emotional disorders.

Our experience with schools and community-based service systems, as well as institutional programs working earnestly to deinstitutionalize this complex group, is that there exists a critical need for a *backup system*. When clients have a severe "acting out" problem, the school or community system frequently lacks staff expertise or the physical setting (particularly in rural settings) to bring these behaviors under control. Such a backup system has proved to be essential to prevent institutionalization or reinstitutionalization, particularly among the critical age group of 15 to 30 years (Menolascino & Stark, 1984).

The program at the Nebraska Psychiatric Institute (NPI) consists of a 12-bed inpatient unit designed to meet these backup needs via an interdisciplinary staff with extensive training and experience with this population. The average length of stay is 30 days and the individual is then returned to the home, community residential program, or ICF/MR with specific recommendations for maintaining appropriate behavior. Oftentimes, staff will accompany the client and receive individualized training (see also McGee, Chapter 20) in order to prevent additional adjustment problems.

Treatment consists of a team intake and assessment, individual and group therapy, vocational skill training, pharmacological management (if necessary), and other health care services needed for maximizing the client's abilities (i.e., physical and occupational therapy and medical treatment).

The data presented in Table 27.2 and also discussed by Menolascino in Chapter 10 illustrate information collected over the last six years at the NPI from our "dual diagnosis" program. A listing of the categories and the number of clients in each group reflect the complex psychiatric problems of this population, and in our opinion it is probably similar to what could be expected across the country. What this table does not reflect, however, is the age variance. Further analysis of these data demonstrates that over 40% of this large pool of dually diagnosed individuals cluster in the age range of 18 to 30 years. We think this is highly reflective of what is happening all over the country and once again demonstrates the critical need for backup services for this transitional age group, which owing to the lack of meaningful work and living options puts them at high risk to develop severe emotional problems.

Hopefully, each state or region can support such a backup center to provide the essential service and training needed. Perhaps the current system of University Affiliated Programs and other federal regional programs could take the lead in developing and maintaining this much needed component to assure ongoing success for this group of individuals.

## Future Directions

All of us need to be aware of the many major forces that will be achieved by society over the next one to two decades and that will have a dramatic impact on dually diagnosed individuals.

Economic and societal changes will have a direct and long-lasting impact on the provision of services to all developmentally disabled young adults and adults. Changes in employment at the marketplace will mandate a more sophisticated training at the high-school level as well as the postsecondary level if these individuals are going to be successful in entering the world of work. Allowing the continuation of fiscal disincentives for employment for these individuals, in such cases as Social Security, supplemental security income, and Medicaid, is being seriously questioned. The role of government is moving toward a more supportive partner. However, there are many dangers, which we must be aware of, that need additional amounts of our limited time and resources. We cannot ignore these factors that are going on around us, for they have great impact on our day-to-day concerns and services. The following is a list of those changes in our society that will greatly affect the success of working with this population.

1. *World economy.* Global economic problems in the next 10 years would seem to set a pattern for the following 30 years. We are entering a cycle now where a great deal of effort will be directed toward reducing the federal government, which will cause programs for all developmentally disabled individuals to come under great scrutiny, particularly at the state and local levels. As a result, a great understanding of the economic policies and the development of systematic advocacy skills will be essential in our efforts to secure funding. This expensive-to-serve population will require creative efforts in our administrative and fiscal operations during this period of time.

2. *Occupational changes.* The current restructuring of the U.S. economy is shifting from a manufacturing to information processing and telecommunications industry. The dominance of the United States in the field of production of goods and services is being challenged by foreign competition, particularly in technological fields. The majority of new jobs in the future will be in the service industry, which is an area that will be highly conducive for our planning of vocational success with this population. We will find that developmentally disabled individuals will be competing with a less-expensive labor force

TABLE 27.2. Mental illness in the mentally retarded.

| Psychiatric diagnosis | Total |
|---|---|
| Schizophrenic disorders | |
| Catatonic type | 10 |
| Paranoid type | 30 |
| Undifferentiated type | 53 |
| Residual type | 45 |
| | 138 |
| Organic brain disorders | |
| Behavioral reaction | 55 |
| Psychotic reaction | 43 |
| Presenile dementia | 7 |
| | 105 |
| Adjustment disorders | |
| Childhood and adolescence | 44 |
| Disturbance of conduct | 18 |
| Adulthood | 41 |
| | 103 |
| Personality disorders | |
| Schizoid | 6 |
| Paranoid | 3 |
| Narcissistic | 7 |
| Avoidant | 7 |
| Passive aggressive | 22 |
| Antisocial | 23 |
| | 68 |
| Affective disorders | |
| Unipolar manic disorder | 7 |
| Bipolar, affective | 5 |
| Major depression, recurrent | 32 |
| Cyclothymic disorder | 1 |
| | 45 |
| Psychosexual disorders | |
| Fetishism | 1 |
| Transvestism | 4 |
| Zoophilia | 1 |
| Pedophilia | 12 |
| Exhibitionism | 6 |
| Ego-dystonic homosexuality | 2 |
| Disorder not elsewhere classified | 8 |
| | 34 |
| Anxiety disorders | |
| Generalized anxiety | 9 |
| Posttraumatic stress | 10 |
| Obsessive compulsive | 1 |
| | 20 |

TABLE 27.2. *Continued.*

| Psychiatric diagnosis | Total |
|---|---|
| Other mental disorders | |
| Pervasive developmental | 16 |
| Anorexia nervosa | 6 |
| Oppositional | 2 |
| Substance use | 6 |
| | 30 |
| Total | 543 |

from foreign producers, which will require a sophisticated model as that described in the Pathways Model for supported employment.

3. *Population changes.* An increasing older population will significantly alter the social/economic landscape of America as well as resulting in a greater concentration of population in western and southern states. Because of increased costs in medical care and Social Security, we need to advocate for funding for the disabled population in planning for future needs and new programs, particularly in the southern and western areas of this country.

4. *Technological changes in education and training.* Computer and video technology will have a dramatic impact on our educational, occupational, and living environments in the future. This could be of great assistance to those individuals with moderate, severe, and profound retardation who could greatly benefit from these technological developments. The development of individually paced educational programs and training in more natural environments, as well as the home, which is specifically geared to the capability of the mentally retarded individual, could prove to be of great benefit in overcoming the complex barriers to jobs that preclude them from greater integration today.

5. *Demographic changes.* Changes in both the family and minority populations will also have a dramatic impact on services for the dually diagnosed population. Continued high divorce rates, minority family size increases, and 60% of the women in the work force all impact on how families are able to care for their sons and daughters. We will continue to see disproportionate growth in minority populations and also see increases in minority children living below the poverty index. One out of every four children will grow up below the poverty index and between 50 to 75% of minority children will grow up in a disadvantaged environment over the next 20 years.

6. *Changes in government decisionmaking.* The centralization of government control to transfer decisionmaking to state and local agencies will result in a return to the early 1960s when advocacy groups played a critical role in the development of services for this population. This new "federalism" will result in a shifting of financial burdens from the federal level to local and

state levels, where we will need to have better organization and advocacy if we are going to maintain what we have, let alone to improve services for this population.

## Conclusion

Hopefully, this chapter presentation of the needs and characteristics of this challenging population along with the review of model programs on how to transition them into the community will serve as a beginning to focus our future efforts on providing this critical link for successful programming of mentally retarded individuals with mental health needs.

## References

Hasazi, S., Preskill, H., Gordon, L., & Collins, C. (1982). *Factors associated with the employment status of handicapped youth*. Paper presented to the American Education Research Association, New York.

Horner, R., & Bellamy, G.T. (1979). Structured employment: Productivity and productive capacity. In G.T. Bellamy, G. O'Connor, & O. Karan (Eds.), *Vocational rehabilitation of severely handicapped persons*. Baltimore, MD: University Park Press.

Menolascino, F.J. (1972). Emotional disturbances in institutionalized retardates: Primitive, atypical and abnormal behavior. *Mental Retardation, 6*, 38.

Menolascino, F.J., & Stark, J.A. (1984). *Handbook of mental illness in the mentally retarded*. New York: Plenum Press.

Mithaug, D., & Horiuchi, C. (1983). *Colorado statewide follow-up survey of special education students*. Denver, CO: Colorado State Department of Education.

*Rehab Brief.* (1984). National Institute of Handicapped Research. Vol. III, No. 4.

Schalock, R.L. (1984). Comprehensive community services: A plea for interagency collaboration. In R. Bruininks & C.K. Lakin (Eds.), *Living and learning in the least restrictive environment*. Baltimore, MD: Paul H. Brookes Publishing Company.

Stark, J.A., Kiernan, W.E., Goldsbury, T.L., & McGee, J.J. (1986). Not entering employment: A system dilemma. In W.E. Kiernan & J.A. Stark (Eds.), *Pathways to employment for adults with developmental disabilities*. Baltimore, MD: Paul H. Brookes Publishing Company.

Wehman, P. (1981). *Competitive employment: Horizons for severely disabled individuals*. Baltimore, MD: Paul H. Brookes Publishing Company.

Wehman, P.H., Kregel, J., Barcus, J.M., & Schalock, R.L. (1986). Vocational transition for developmentally disabled students. In W.E. Kiernan & J.A. Stark (Eds.), *Pathways to employment for adults with developmental disabilities*. Baltimore, MD: Paul H. Brookes Publishing Company.

# Conclusion

PETER A. HOLMES

The model programs described in this section of the book all enthusiastically endorse common characteristics with their own unique components of their recommended models. Reiss, in chapter 23 in this section, describes his involvement with the Illinois–Chicago Mental Health Program along with its research, clinical, and educational components. This model program has developed a national reputation for providing outpatient services to this dually diagnosed population with specialized emphasis on those individuals' personality and conduct disorders. This highly effective model program should serve as an excellent example for those communities seeking to adapt and implement such a program for this specific subgroup in their community.

Robert Fletcher describes the array of Community Mental Health services in a rural setting in New York and refers to an individualization process based on the needs of each person in the program. The program array permits dually diagnosed persons to receive the most appropriate training possible, given the problems they have, and prevents dislocation to more restrictive treatment settings. This demand for individualized treatment recognizes that dually diagnosed persons have many different needs. Such an individualized approach is an effective way to meet these needs across many different situations.

In Bob Allin's Home Intervention Program (HIP), a male–female team works directly in a client's home with the parents or care providers. All phases of treatment including assessment, intervention design, intervention implementation, and follow-up are individualized to the conditions that occur while the therapists are in the home setting.

The HIP model provides "in vivo" training to care providers in the natural home setting. He reports that care providers sometimes ask for assistance even during times when they are successful at carrying out suggested interventions. Close supervision, modeling, and training by therapists during the critical periods when change occurs is an important implementation strategy.

The Regional Intervention Program (RIP), directed by Matthew Timm, is an excellent example of how early intervention (before age 5) can save states substantial amounts of money and human suffering. Children who graduate from the program are less likely to require mental health services as they grow older. The four evaluation methods used in the RIP program serve as excellent examples of how program outcome can be assessed.

Despite obvious advantages from implementing a RIP program, it is often difficult for state agencies to understand the wisdom of investing money now in preventive programs that promise future savings when more immediate problems exist. Incentive systems may be one way to move states to support preventive programs.

Bijou's chapter describes how in-service training is usually a waste of time for teachers, since this kind of short-term training seldom leads to any long-term changes in teacher behavior. His solution is a "Master Teacher" program. A Master Teacher would give in-service training to teachers and then engage in follow-up for several months with the teachers in their classrooms. This kind of intervention is more likely to change teacher behavior, which in turn would improve the kind of instruction special education students receive.

Bijou further indicates how schools can individualize their programs by attending to specific accomplishments of each student. When teaching is data-based, competency levels can be adjusted on a continuous ongoing basis according to student progress. Empirical behavioral analysis is the most successful way to individualized education via his model recommendations.

Stark, Kiernan, and Goldsbury outline a model program at the University of Nebraska Medical Center. The program uses the services of resident physicians, psychiatrists, psychologists, and social workers to help dually diagnosed persons develop more independent working and living skills. The professionals in training thus have the opportunity to work with dually diagnosed persons for an extended period of time. Both the clients and trainees benefit from this relationship.

When efforts to serve difficult dually diagnosed clients fail, more training in the form of workshops or seminars is frequently cited as an excellent approach. Unfortunately, in many programs today, training is not always given at the correct time, presented in a form that changes worker behavior, or aimed at methods that will modify problem behavior (Favell, Riddle, & Risley, 1984).

Recognition of dually diagnosed persons as a distinct population with special needs is a relatively new development. The chapters in this section show how model programs are beginning to address the problems raised in this book. This new recognition should bring awareness to what has been done and encourage others to develop even better program models.

## References

Favell, J.E., Riddle, J.I., & Risley, T.R. (1984). Promoting change in mental retardation facilities. In W.P. Christian, G.T. Hannah, & T.J. Glahn (Eds.), *Programming effective human services* (pp. 15–37). New York: Plenum Press.

# Section VI: Legal Issues
# Introduction

H. RUTHERFORD TURNBULL, III

It is clear from the chapters in Section VI that Boggs would not have advocates seek new federal laws, but instead, their more adequate administration; that Ellis would have advocates seek new state laws and improved administrative behaviors; that Luckasson would have advocates direct their attention to an underserved population, those people with mental retardation and/or mental illness who have been charged or convicted of crime; that Herr would have advocates litigate with vigor for the dually diagnosed person; and that Rosenberg also would pursue community-based litigation with vigor but not unbounded optimism. For myself, I applaud the integrated approach to law reform that these authors take, for they seek reform both at the federal and state level by way of legislation (and, presumably, accompanying appropriations and implementing regulations) and by way of litigation. But, as I suggested in my chapter, even after advocates solve the legal problems of how to get the dually diagnosed person into a suitable service system, the questions still remain: what do the professionals do with them, and why? It seems entirely appropriate that this book deals directly with those questions. It also may be that the rest of this book does so satisfactorily, but that is a matter that lawyers and other professionals will test over the years.

In a shift of emphasis, Mr. Rosenberg calls attention to the opportunities for using broad-based litigation strategies to establish new rights, or implement existing rights, for people with concurrent mental retardation and mental illness. He cautions against the overuse of litigation and insists that litigation must be used with caution and sensitivity, particularly in narrowly drawn litigation for residents of institutions, where the purpose is to obtain their discharge from the institutions. He also recommends the use of litigation to establish community-based services and a comprehensive service system within the community, arguing that litigation should be devised that would require the financing of services and that also would challenge zoning laws that exclude community-based services and residents. He then draws attention to the potential of using the "related services" provisions of the Education of the Handicapped Act as a means for obtaining psychological and psychiatric services for students who are mentally retarded and experience mental health problems.

Next, Mr. Rosenberg also discusses the potential for using the common law of tort as a means for obtaining compensation for the denial of services, having previously pointed out that the federal constitutional and statutory laws as well as state laws can be used to obtain services. Finally, he argues for the use of litigation in the federal entitlement programs, particularly supplemental security insurance, Medicaid, and early periodic screening and diagnosis and treatment. His point with respect to the federal entitlement programs is that litigation should ensure that eligible persons are placed on the rolls and receive their full benefits and should create an affirmative duty of state and local governments to offer services.

Professor Herr continues Mr. Rosenberg's theme of the use of litigation to advance the rights of dually diagnosed citizens. After reporting on several cases in which he has been involved in seeking rights within institutions and within the community, he discusses the limitations that face the organized bar in litigating on behalf of such citizens. Calling the limitations formidable, he recommends increased funding for P&As and shifts in priority setting to give greater emphasis to this subpopulation; establishment of developmental disabilities advocacy centers on a regional basis with universities and law schools taking a leadership role, developing courses, clinical offerings, training materials, workshops, and manuals.

In my chapter, I move the discussion away from the legal issues to 15 ethical issues that professionals, advocates, and parents need to confront in working with any citizen who has mental retardation, but particularly with those citizens who have both mental retardation and mental illness.

# 28
# The Role of Legislation

Elizabeth Monroe Boggs

## The Nature of Legislation

To the usual classification into "civil" and "criminal" laws detailing as they do the rights and responsibilities of individuals (or legal entities) toward each other, we should add, in the context of this chapter, laws that authorize or mandate programs. "Programmatic" legislation usually is explicit in authorizing both the appropriation of funds and the conduct of specified activities. The activities to be carried out may be designed to benefit the public generally or may be targeted by the language of the law toward a class of citizens deemed to need special attention. Whereas the judicial system has the primary responsibility for effectuating civil and criminal laws, a program is usually assigned to an agency in the executive branch of government at the appropriate level.

## Categorical Legislation

A program targeted on a particular class of people is often referred to as "categorical." Such categories may be broad or narrow. For example, "children of school age," "employees," "persons with incomes below the poverty level," or "farmers" are all broad categories. Examples of more narrowly defined categories actually covered under certain federal statutes include the elderly blind, veterans with service connected disabilities, employees of railroads engaged in interstate commerce, and owners of small businesses.

When legislation is directed to a category, the population to be benefitted must be defined in a way that is rationally related to a legitimate public purpose. It is unconstitutional to provide special benefits to any arbitrarily defined group. Likewise, when legislation places obligations on, or gives privileges to, individuals, the Constitution requires that persons "similarly situated" must be treated similarly. Compulsory school attendance, the internal revenue code, and election laws are all examples of broad class legislation that is intended to meet this test.

At the present time, there are no significant distinct pieces of federal legislation that apply uniquely to people with mental retardation to the exclusion of others, although mental retardation is present in a majority of the individuals encompassed under the functional definition used in the 1978 revisions of the Developmental Disabilities Assistance and Bill of Rights Act (P.L. 95-602). In many states, however, distinct legislation specific to people with mental retardation can be found; it may authorize programs, such as special residential services, or it may deal with civil commitment, or rights, or, less frequently, with other particulars (Sales, Powell, & Van Duizend, 1982).

The question to be addressed is whether there is a need to enact additional narrowly defined categorical legislation targeted on the population that we somewhat loosely encompass under the heading "dually diagnosed." That the needs of this group of people are not being adequately met is clear. That is not the issue. The question is: Is additional legislation over and above what is now in place (or should be in place in any case) needed to overcome the barriers to meeting the specific needs of mentally retarded individuals with mental health problems?

It is the thesis of this chapter that, by and large, the answer is no. If existing *programs* are implemented to the full extent of *authorizing* legislation, including the overarching mandates, it should be possible to do what has to be done to the extent that we now know how to do it.

In the areas of *civil* and *criminal* laws dealing with admission to service settings of those persons who are believed to lack capacity to appreciate their own needs or the consequences of their behavior, the law is currently in a state of flux, and it would appear that the changes that may be needed also apply more generally to persons with one or the other diagnosis as well as both. As such changes are further debated, it will be well to examine each proposed provision against the possible scenarios that might play out for dually diagnosed clients, patients, or offenders.

The reasons for this stance are several:

1. The knowledge base that undergirds renewed attention to these populations is in a state of rapid change and expansion; new laws based on whatever assumptions might muster sufficient political support at this time could become rapidly outdated and hence unduly restrictive.
2. The characteristics of this target group, small as it is, are nevertheless very heterogeneous. It would be difficult to fashion a meaningful common denominator that could meet the constitutional test of clarity as well as relevance in as much as (a) not all members of the class would meet the dangerousness test, (b) not all mental illness results in "acting out" behavior, although it is such behavior when exhibited in the community that is causing much of the heightened attention, and (c) not all acting out behavior is symptomatic of mental illness. Some of it may, in fact, be a manifestation of healthy efforts at self-assertion by nonverbal people opposing perceived oppression.
3. Dual eligibility can be an advantage.

# A Philosophical Foundation

It will be recalled that in the Kennedy era several pieces of relevant legislation were enacted by Congress at the request of the President. Public Laws 88-156 and 88-164 (Title I) were based on recommendations of the President's Panel on Mental Retardation (PPMR), appointed in 1961 and dissolved at the end of 1962. (This body is not to be confused with the present President's Committee on Mental Retardation, which was created by President Johnson in May 1966.) The work of PPMR was carried forward by five task forces, one of which, the Task Force on the Law, was chaired by U.S. District Court judge David Bazelon, who even at that time was already well known for his ground-breaking decisions pertaining to people with mental disorders. The following ideas excerpted from Section VII, the *Law and the Mentally Retarded*, in the Panel's report (PPMR, 1962) remain pertinent today.

Equality before the law is predicted on the assumption that everyone has roughly comparable capacities to invoke the law's protections and to abide by its proscriptions. This, "minimal set of personal characteristics in the population," which the law ordinarily takes for granted, may not be totally present in the mentally retarded person, but neither will it be totally absent. He will have, in some measure, the inadequate intellectual development and degree of impairment and ability to learn and adapt to the demands of society, which we discussed in the first section of the report. The law must take into account the pervading chronic character of mental retardation, along with the disparities and divergences and abilities and disabilities displayed by members of the group. . . .

With the development of new alternatives and treatment, our community and residential institutions are attempting to overcome certain rigidities of the law in the interests of giving the retarded individual the benefit of modern knowledge concerning his growth and development and his ability to learn and to modify his behavior in response to the various social structures and situations.

Responding to these trends and opportunities, we would minimize mandatory legal requirements wherever voluntary compliance can be obtained. The richer and better the services available to the retarded and those concerned with their welfare, the less need there is of coercive intervention to provide care. And, indeed, in dealing with the problems that arise with the retarded in the community, formal legal intervention should be regarded as a residual resource and should not occur where social or personal interests can be adequately served without it.

Where the law must intervene, the community should look first to see whether laws of general application would be adequate. If they are not, the community should turn to law which protects the disabled as a group. Only in the last resort should the community rely on *ad hoc* legislation for a specific handicapped group. (pp. 148–149)

These observations remain timely because they reflect the need for dynamic change, for continuous interaction between the law and the human sciences. They recognize that the law tends to be rigid and unresponsive to change and should therefore permit interpretation in the light of current circumstances and knowledge. Moreover, although these observations predated the invocation of the "principle of least restriction" in the field of mental retardation and mental illness by Bazelon in 1966 (Gutheil & Appelbaum, 1982, p. 84), they reflect this concept of least intrusion in personal and professional affairs.

The preference of the task force for using generic legislation or broad categorical legislation is also reinterpretable as circumstances change. In 1962, "ad hoc legislation for a specific handicapped group" was much more necessary than it is today. When what is now called the Association for Retarded Citizens of the United States was founded in 1950, discrimination against retarded children and adults with multiple handicaps was widespread. State schools for the deaf accepted only "normal" deaf children; in several states federal funds for "crippled children" would pay for braces for the child with cerebral palsy only if he were "of sound mind." The ARC early adopted as a principle that it would advocate for all persons who are retarded, regardless of their other handicaps, and that it would seek to assure that the services accorded for the second handicap must be equal in quality to those accorded to handicapped persons with single diagnoses other than retardation. Today this principle is well established.

This is not to say that categorical legislation is now out of style. On the contrary, it is more than ever necessary to fit the category to the public purpose. Some people with mental retardation and some people with mental illness share the needs associated with limited coping skills and capacity to protect their own interests. This need must be attended to in specific ways. Offenders who are retarded require special protections, as Ruth Luckasson documents elsewhere in this book (see Luckasson, Chapter 32). Because people who are retarded but not mentally ill seldom require emergency admissions based on alleged dangerousness, state legislation has in the past two decades moved toward a model in which the courts are used to permit an admission in the interests of the retarded individual, rather than to mandate detention for the protection of society. These nuances must be addressable, at least implicitly, in the legal frame of reference.

In the case of persons with mental illness, both state and federal laws are to be found that explicitly address this population. In some cases (e.g., typical laws—state or federal—dealing with criminal responsibility or capacity to stand trial), a law may be written in terms that are clearly inclusive of both categories. It is rare, however, to find a law pertaining to one category that expressly excepts or excludes persons because they have a second diagnosis.

To say that we do not need more narrowly targeted special-purpose legislation to grapple with the new or renewed concerns for persons of mixed diagnosis is not to say that existing laws are entirely adequate for the purposes to which they may now be applied. As Ellis and Luckasson point out in their respective chapters, existing laws may not be equitably applied or, especially in the case of state laws relative to commitment, may need revision in their own context. In view of the continuing tension between the law and psychiatry on these issues, however, as signaled by the debates now under way over the latest "model law" proposed by the American Psychiatric Association (Applebaum, 1985; Lamb, Sorkin, & Zusman, 1981; Stromberg & Stone, 1983; see also Barton & Sanborn, 1978), it would seem prudent to continue to use the advantages of duality available to us at present under both federal and state laws.

## Strategies at the Interface

This is not to ignore the "falling between the cracks" phenomenon. Such falls abound, not so much because of flaws in the law as because administrators faced with limited resources tend to draw their own boundaries more closely than they need to do by the terms of the laws under which they operate. Hard cases tend to get low priority in any system. Gaps between programmatic boundaries that are statutorily defined may require legislative remedy; overlaps usually can—and preferably should—be managed by negotiation among administrators at a policy or operational level.

In some instances, a dual authority may actually be useful. An example can be found in arrangements between the various institutes which make up the National Institutes of Health (NIH), and between them and the National Institute of Mental Health (NIMH). It has been mentioned that soon after the formation of the National Institute of Child Health and Human Development (NICHD), with a component mission to research the causes and treatment of mental retardation, a negotiation took place between NICHD and NIMH, which gave NIMH the lead in researching mental illness and emotional disorders (such as depression) in persons who are retarded. NIMH has, in fact, directed attention to these issues and may be encouraged to give even greater attention, now that the scope and urgency of these problems are being highlighted. There may, however, be some advantage in giving both institutes opportunities to venture into this domain, since each may have its own biases. The NIH internal rules even permit dual funding. Moreover, both have—and probably should retain—common ground with neurology, which has its own institute. (For an overview of the NICHD program in mental retardation, see Tjossem, 1985.)

In any such situation, the issue of allocation of resources will arise. If the leaders of the various institutes wish to retain their traditional professional discretion and academic freedom in selecting priorities for research, they must nevertheless consider the public interest. We may be sure that if the appropriate managers do not attend to the recommendations of this book, Congressional action is likely to settle the immediate question. Indeed, in November 1985, we saw the finale to a two-year struggle that raised, in broad terms, the issue of the extent to which the keepers of the public purse should influence or even control the selection of scientific priorities in federally funded health research (Culliton, 19 March 1985; 29 November 1985). H.R. 2409 was a reauthorization bill for NIH. It had enough bipartisan support to survive a veto in November 1985. Among other things, the law now directs increased NIH attention to spinal injury and mental retardation. These subjects are currently of interest to a large body of consumers and providers. Congress underlined them, even though there was already ample authority on the books to enable NIH to attend to these topics. Similarly, there is no need for an additional targeted authority for research on mental illness in people who are also mentally retarded. Managerial discretion is the better part of valor. In case this message is not heeded, the first and "least restrictive" step can be taken through the appropriations process. Each time such a step is provoked, however, some elements of autonomy for the scientific community are eroded.

A comparable situation is likely to pertain in the domain of service programs and their statutory bases. Authority already exists under which coordination among agencies is possible. In fact, it provides professional managers at the federal and state levels with greater flexibility than they will have if they wait to be told exactly what to do by a legislative body that acts under pressure from an exasperated public. Other chapters in this book offer examples of creative cooperation. Interagency and even interdepartmental contracting has proved possible and is now encouraged in the administration of both the Social Services Block Grant (Title XX of the Social Security Act) and Medicaid (Title XIX). In these cases, duality of diagnosis is not only no bar to eligibility but may, in fact, enhance it—especially under the recently rewritten rules defining "disability" for purposes of eligibility under various titles of the Social Security Act (20 Code of Federal Regulations part 404 Section 12.05, as amended August 28, 1985, Federal Register Part V, pp. 35068-9). These revisions retain the former presumptive disability of persons with "simple" mental retardation, evidenced by an IQ of 59 or less, and clarify the eligibility of those in the 60 to 69 range who have other work-relevant mental impairments (see specifically sections 12.05 C and D).

# The Application of Section 504 to Persons with Multiple Handicaps

One reason that we can, for some purposes, move with relatively greater security into more broadly defined groupings lies in the applicability of Section 504. This important piece of federal legislation applies with equal force to persons with physical, sensory, or mental disabilities. The designation refers to Section 504 of the Rehabilitation Act of 1973 (P.L. 93-112). As is well known by now, Section 504 declares that, "No otherwise qualified handicapped individual in the United States . . . shall solely by reason of his handicap, be excluded from the participation in, be denied the benefits of, or be subjected to discrimination under any program or activity receiving Federal financial assistance." The mandate applies explicitly not only to schools and transportation systems, but to health, mental health, welfare, and other human services and facilities.

The relevance of this statute to the subject of this book lies in the fact that it prohibits any federally aided agency or provider from denying treatment or accommodation to an individual for any disabling condition that the provider ordinarily treats or accommodates, solely because the individual also has another handicap. It now appears, therefore, that there is no basis for claiming a "legitimate public purpose" for discrimination by a provider against a person with a multiple diagnosis when the provider has competence to address even one aspect of the patient's or client's problem. This is true at least where federal funding can be tracked to the provide. Thus, Section 504 makes unnecessary most putative legislation that might be designed to assure that mental health agencies will provide mental health services to retarded individuals who also have a mental health problem, or vice versa.

This is not to say that persons with a dual or multiple diagnoses/disabilities can always be handled in a specialized provider agency without some accommodation. The 504 regulations recognize this by (for example) their explicit requirement that hospitals must be able to provide an interpreter for deaf patients. It should follow that community mental health centers should be prepared to treat psychiatric problems in people who are blind, deaf, or mentally retarded.

"Reasonable accommodation" may also require actual modification of the treatment modality. The physical therapist, for example, who is called on to treat an orthopedic impairment in a child or adult with mental retardation may not be able to count on the same motivation to persist as may be found in a child with the capacity to visualize the future and to forego present gratification for future benefit. Similarly, methods of psychiatric treatment must be used that can be accessed by the patient. Today's modalities provide a range of options, some of which are discussed by Menolascino and McGee, and others, elsewhere in this book.

During the period when psychoanalysis was the dominant style in psychiatry, the emotional disturbances and mental illnesses in persons with mental retardation tended to be set aside as untreatable. When George Stevenson became the medical director of the National Association for Mental Health on its foundation in 1950, he was one of the few psychiatrists with special concern for retarded children. In a plenary address to the American Association on Mental Deficiency in 1947, he spoke scathingly on how psychiatry had withdrawn from its earlier constructive role in treating mental retardation in community clinics as well as more traditional settings:

In the National Committee on Mental Hygiene the ground work for the child guidance clinic was laid by its Division on Mental Deficiency. . . . Today, however, child guidance clinics do not want to accept the mentally deficient "You can't do psychotherapy with them". Is that true? Maybe we would learn something about psychotherapy if we tried. . . . The concept of heredity has added to this rejection. . . . Then dynamic psychiatry came along to give the coup de grace to the field of mental deficiency. (Stevenson, 1947, p. 45)

In an era when verbalization by the patient seemed essential to treatment, perhaps it could have been argued that 504 did not apply because the person was "not otherwise qualified," but this scarcely holds water today. Other authors of chapters in this book attest to ways in which current methods of treatment can be adapted; perhaps even more importantly, the profession of psychiatry appears to be getting its act together in integrating new developments in neurobiology with current perspectives in psychoanalysis (Cooper, 1985; Pardes, 1986; Talbot, 1985a, 1985b).

In that connection, it may be noted that the diagnostic manuals of the American Association on Mental Deficiency (AAMD) and the American Psychiatric Association (APA) are now quite compatible. Mental retardation in its various degrees is a recognized diagnosis in DSM-III (APA, 1980, pp. 36–41). Psychosis is recognized as a possible cause and also as a notable concomitant of mental retardation in the 1983 edition of the AAMD manual (Grossman, 1983).

Finally, it is significant that programmatic integration across categories has progressed apace at the federal level during the last quarter century. The dominant funding sources for persons disabled by mental retardation, mental illness, or a combination of the two are to be found in the disability provisions contained in the income maintenance and health care programs of the Social Security Act, Titles, II, XVI, XVIII, and XIX. All of these use a common definition of disability. Thanks to yeoman efforts by advocates in recent years, adults with work disabilities based on mental impairment can count on assistance from these programs. As mentioned earlier, in the case of dually diagnosed patients, a combination of impairments neither of which would, by itself, be considered disabling may nevertheless offer the basis for entitlement.

Comparable generality characterizes many other pieces of federal legislation generated since 1960. A useful compendium of some 40 federal statutes, most of them applicable to a broad category of persons with disabilities, mental as well as physical, has been prepared by Turnbull and Barber (1986). Despite "Gramm–Rudman–Hollings," they continue to offer tools for creative advocates.

## References

American Psychiatric Association. (1980). *Diagnostic and statistical manual of mental disorders* (3rd ed.). Washington, DC: Author.

Appelbaum, P.S. (Ed.). (1985). Special section on APA's model commitment law. *Hospital and Community Psychiatry, 36*(6), 966–989.

Barton, W.E., & Sanborn, C.J. (Eds.). (1978). *Law and the mental health professions: Friction at the interface.* New York: International Universities Press.

Cooper, A.M. (1985). Will neurobiology influence psychoanalysis? *American Journal of Psychiatry, 142*(12), 1395–1401.

Culliton, B.J. (29 March 1985). Who runs NIH? *Science, 227,* 1562–1564.

Culliton, B.J. (29 November 1985). Reagan vetoes NIH bill: Override is likely. *Science, 230,* 1021.

Grossman, H.J. (Ed.). (1983). *Classification in mental retardation.* Washington, DC: American Association on Mental Deficiency.

Gutheil, T.G., & Appelbaum, P.S. (1982). *Clinical handbook of psychiatry and the law.* New York: McGraw Hill.

Lamb, H.R., Sorkin, M.A., & Zusman, J. (1981). Legislating social control of the mentally ill in California. *American Journal of Psychiatry, 138*(3), 334–339.

Pardes, H. (1986). Neuroscience and psychiatry: Marriage or coexistence? *American Journal of Psychiatry, 143,* 1205–1212.

President's Panel on Mental Retardation. (1962). *A proposed program for national action to combat mental retardation.* Washington, DC: U.S. Government Printing Office.

Sales, B.D., Powell, D.M., & Van Duizend, R. (1982). *Disabled persons and the law — State legislative issues.* New York: Plenum Press.

Stevenson, G.S. (1947). Where and whither in mental deficiency. *American Journal of Mental Deficiency, LII*(1), 43–47.

Stromberg, C.D., & Stone, A.A. (1983). A model state law on civil commitment of the mentally ill. *Harvard Journal on Legislation, 20*, 275–396.

Talbott, J.A. (1985a). Biological/psychological– Integration/separation. *Psychiatric News, XX*(2), 2,13.

Talbott, J.A. (1985b). Presidential address: Our patients' future in a changing world: The imperative for psychiatric involvement in public policy. *American Journal of Psychiatry, 142*(9), 1003–1008.

Tjossem, T.D. (1985). National Institute of Child Health and Human Development: Research program on mental retardation. *Mental Retardation, 23*(3), 101–104.

Turnbull, H.R., III, & Barber, P.A. (1986). Federal laws and adults with developmental disabilities. In J.A. Summers (Ed.), *The right to grow up* (pp. 255–265). Baltimore, MD: Paul H. Brookes Publishing Company.

# 29
# Residential Placement of "Dual Diagnosis" Clients: Emerging Legal Issues

JAMES W. ELLIS

## Introduction

Individuals who are "dually diagnosed"[1] as mentally retarded and mentally ill present difficult legal and administrative questions regarding the selection of appropriate residential placements. Residential placement is, of course, important in and of itself, just as decisions about where we live (and with whom) are important to all of us. The selection of an appropriate placement assumes even greater significance, however, because of its influence on other elements of a disabled person's life; it can dictate the availability of appropriate education, habilitation, employment, and mental health services. Therefore the procedures for determining where a disabled individual, who is both mentally ill and mentally retarded, will live are a matter of great importance, and it is startling that they have not received any attention in the professional or legal literature.[2]

The principal obstacles to appropriate placement of these clients may not be the difficulty of designing residential services appropriate to their needs,[3] but rather dysfunctional aspects of the commitment and admission system. These problems may result from the failure of legislators and other policymakers to recognize that mental illness and mental retardation, while distinct forms of mental disability, are not mutually exclusive. This misperception is particularly harmful for individuals with dual diagnoses because the commitment systems for mental illness and mental retardation are dissimilar in important respects.

## The Two Commitment Systems

The dissimilarities between the legal rules governing residential placement of mentally ill people and those governing people with mental retardation derive both from historical developments and from differences in the way the general public views the two groups and their role in society.

### Mental Health Commitment Laws

Commitment laws designed for people with mental illness have undergone a cyclical history in this country, with concerns about the need for expeditious confinement and treatment competing with worries that individuals who were not "insane" might be wrongfully committed. The development of mental institutions in the Jacksonian period was accompanied by an optimistic belief that they represented an opportunity for curing the ills that befell the insane, and thus by extension, the ills that befell society.[4] But admission procedures that reflected such attitudes were attacked in the period following the Civil War as tools for the unscrupulous who sought the permanent banishment of their sane but inconvenient relatives. This assault produced legal reforms that attempted to protect proposed patients from being "railroaded" into asylums.[5] Cycles of reforms and counter-reforms continued into this century.

The modern high water mark of unencumbered commitment laws accompanied the enhanced prestige of psychiatry in the decade after World War II. The view that commitment laws should be "streamlined" to place fewer obstacles between mentally ill people and the treatment they needed culminated in the promulgation of a model statute with few procedural protections for proposed patients.[6] Most states adopted this law in some form, and thus provided for involuntary commitment of those deemed "in need of treatment."[7]

These statutes, in turn, were attacked in the late 1960s and 1970s as insufficiently protective of civil liberties, both in regard to the broad scope of individuals subject to involuntary commitment and for providing too few procedural protections against unwarranted or inappropriate confinement. These proposed reforms, like their predecessors, found support in lingering popular suspicion of psychiatrists and the residential facilities they operated.[8] But with few exceptions,[9] the reforms of this era were either mandated or prodded by court rulings that declared existing statutes unconstitutional.[10] These judicial decisions held that patients were deprived of liberty without due process of law in two ways. First, the statutes were held unconstitutional to the extent that they permitted commitment merely upon a showing that the individual "needed" treatment without any proof that the person constituted a danger to self or to others. Second, the commitment laws were invalidated because they provided patients with inadequate procedural protection of their rights, such as the right to notice, counsel, confrontation and cross-examination of adverse witnesses, and access to their own expert witnesses.

In the wake of these court decisions, virtually all states have adopted new mental illness commitment statutes in the last 15 years, and these new laws are remarkably similar in the substantive and procedural protections they afford to persons whose commitment is sought.[11]

## Mental Retardation Commitment Laws

The origin and development of mental retardation laws was far different from those involving mental illness. In the late nineteenth and early twentieth centuries, mentally retarded people were viewed as a threat to society. Laws enacted to effect their institutional confinement sought segregation for its own sake, rather than as a means to effect individual improvement or cure.[12] As a result, the procedural provisions of these statutes were not designed to protect individuals from wrongful confinement or to facilitate release as soon as possible, but rather to guarantee that retarded individuals were subject to lifelong confinement. Similarly, the substantive criterion for commitment was not limited to those retarded persons who were demonstrated to constitute a danger to themselves or to others, because all retarded people (particularly if they had not been sterilized) were deemed a threat to society.

By the early decades of the twentieth century, this viewpoint became widespread among the general public as well as experts in the field of mental retardation. One leader of this alarmist movement summarized these beliefs:

The feebleminded . . . are by definition a burden rather than an asset, not only economically but still more because of their tendencies to become delinquent or criminal. To provide them with costly instruction for a few years, and then turn them loose upon society as soon as they are ripe for reproduction and crime, can hardly be accepted as an ultimate solution of the problem. The only effective way to deal with the hopelessly feebleminded is by permanent custodial care.[13]

Unfortunately, such misguided views were soon codified into state laws mandating sterilization and lifelong segregation of retarded people. These laws withstood constitutional challenge[14] and remained on the books, typically unexamined and unmodified, for decades.

The legal assault on mental health commitment statutes in the 1970s did not extend to mental retardation laws. Mentally retarded people won substantial victories in the courts and legislatures during this period, most notably in the area of education.[15] But despite substantial litigation on the issue of institutional conditions in mental retardation facilities and the right to habilitation for their residents,[16] far less attention was directed to the procedures under which those residents were admitted or committed.[17]

As a result, the current laws regarding placement of mentally retarded individuals are not as uniform as those in the area of mental health and within a particular state may differ substantially from the procedures for the commitment of mentally ill persons. In a few jurisdictions, the retardation statutes provide full due process hearings to all individuals who face residential placement.[18] The laws of some other states retain provisions inspired by the eugenics scare more than a half century ago.[19] A substantial number of states have enacted half-hearted reforms that give the appearance of due process without providing for a true adjudication of the need for an individual's commitment. And a few states have purported to repeal their mental retardation commitment laws altogether, relying exclusively on mental illness commitment laws and "voluntary" admission to provide for the residential placement of retarded individuals.[20]

Another key difference between mental illness commitment laws and those affecting people with mental retardation involves the substantive criteria for commitment. Virtually all mental health statues now require a showing of dangerousness to self or others.[21] Numerous courts have held this to be a constitutional requirement.[22] By contrast, typical mental retardation statutes have no comparable limitation. Only two jurisdictions limit commitment to those individuals whose mental retardation is in the moderate, severe, or profound ranges;[23] all the other statues permit the involuntary institutionalization of persons who fall within the category of mild mental retardation. Some statutes require a finding that the individual needs habilitation, but under many, the mere fact that the individual is mentally retarded is sufficient to justify commitment. State laws also vary substantially in the extent to which they require a finding that the proposed placement is consistent with the "least drastic means" principle of avoiding unnecessary restriction on individual liberty.[24]

But a more basic problem with mental retardation commitment statutes is that, even in those states that have them, they may not be used. There appear to be no published studies of national data on this topic, but anecdotal information from a substantial number of states indicates that statutes which appear on the books to offer some measure of due process are seldom or never enforced. The procedural protections described by these laws are illusory, since most or all residents are classified as "voluntary" clients.[25] This may be accomplished by either allowing the parent or guardian of a disabled adult to "volunteer" the individual into a placement or by accepting the purported "consent" of the disabled person, despite the fact that his or her apparent acquiescence may not meet the legal test for legally adequate consent.[26]

## Bridging the Gap Between Two Statutory Systems

There may be good and sufficient reasons for having different legal structures for the placement of people with different kinds of disabilities. For example, it may be useful as a means of directing the focus of the courts and other decisionmakers to the difference between mental health treatment and the habilitation of people with mental retardation. It may also be prudent to eliminate or reduce the emphasis on dangerousness in mental retardation laws, since its occurrence differs so substantially from the phenomenon among people with mental illness.

Nevertheless, the dissimilarities between the statutes for mental illness, on the one hand, and mental retardation, on the other, may create substantial anomalies in the service delivery system. For clients who are both mentally ill and mentally retarded, different legal procedures and standards in their state may skew the choices made by various professionals as to the services they should receive. If a particular facility (whether mental health or mental retardation) offers treatment and habilitation that a dual diagnosis client needs, the client may not find his way to it if he has been admitted or committed to the "wrong" system. And the choice of which legal procedures to pursue may be dictated by matters other than the nature of the individual's service needs.

# Transfer of Clients Between Systems

## Inadequacies in the Service System

The difficulties for dual diagnosis clients, created by the differences between the two legal systems for residential placement, are exacerbated in jurisdictions that lack sufficient facilities specializing in clients who are both mentally ill and mentally retarded. This may be a particular problem in smaller states that have only one or two principal public facilities for the treatment of mental illness and a similar number of mental retardation facilities. If substantial autonomy is held by each of these facilities, or if statewide planning authorities have made no provision for dual diagnosis clients, it may be that no facility has developed treatment and habilitation programs for clients who are both mentally ill and mentally retarded. Even if such programs have been established at one or more facilities in the state, they may not be able to accommodate all of the state's citizens with dual diagnoses who require residential services.

This problem stems, in part, from the fact that so few disability professionals have substantial training and experience both in treating mental illness and in providing habilitation services to persons with mental retardation. It is further complicated by concerns about the behavioral and management difficulties that dual diagnosis clients often pose. As a result, mental health facilities may conclude that they lack the expertise to provide habilitation services to persons who are mentally retarded, and mental retardation facilities may decline to accept clients whose mental illness is accompanied by behavioral problems.

These gaps in the service delivery system can have three possible consequences. The simplest and bleakest is that dual diagnosis clients may go completely unserved. Another possibility is that the client will be housed in a facility that addresses (or attempts to address) only one aspect of his or her disability. Since mentally retarded people who are mentally ill are likely to exhibit troublesome behaviors, they may be more likely to end up in a mental hospital than a mental retardation facility.[27] Such a mental hospital is likely to confront these behavioral symptoms with psychotropic drugs[28] or some other form of control, and to leave unattended the habilitation needs caused by the client's mental retardation.

A final possibility is that the client will be shuttled between mental health and mental retardation facilities, each of which repeatedly rejects him or her after perfunctory attempts to provide services. In New Mexico, such clients spend a disconcerting amount of time in transit on Interstate Highway 25, traveling between the state mental hospital at Las Vegas and the mental retardation institution at Los Lunas. The lives of these dually diagnosed citizens become reminiscent in some ways of "A Man Without A Country," and the absurd futility of this course of nontreatment becomes increasingly apparent as mental disability professionals take alternating turns at abdicating any responsibility for their care.

## Legal Issues Involved in Transfers Between Systems

The largest problem with these repeated transfers between the mental health and mental retardation systems is the inhumanity of failing to address the disabilities of these unfortunate individuals. But there may also be legal problems with such transfers.

Ordinarily, transfers between residential facilities, whether for mental retardation or mental illness, will not require any particular legal procedure unless there is such a requirement in state statutes.[29] There is no body of case law holding that, absent extraordinary circumstances, substantial federal constitutional rights are involved.[30] Nevertheless, a transfer from a mental retardation institution to one for mental illness (or vice versa) may trigger greater constitutional concern, even if it is permitted by state statute.

The reason an "intersystem" transfer may involve different constitutional rights is that such a placement may involve, explicitly or implicitly, an official designation that the individual has a "second" disability that is severe enough to require involuntary treatment or habilitation. This designation may constitute sufficient official stigmatization to implicate a constitutionally protected liberty interest.

The constitutional necessity of some procedural formality is suggested by a United States Supreme Court case involving the involuntary transfer of a convict from a prison to a mental health facility. In *Vitek v. Jones*,[31] the Court held that a prisoner would suffer an additional stigma by being labeled as mentally ill, and this additional stigmatization constituted a loss of liberty under the due process clause of the Fourteenth Amendment to the U.S. Constitution.[32] A noteworthy feature of the *Vitek* decision is that the Court identified a significant liberty interest even for an individual who would not suffer loss of physical freedom because of the placement (since he was already a prisoner). A persuasive argument can be made that similar considerations accompany an involuntary transfer between mental health and mental retardation facilities.

The nature of the hearing to which a "dual diagnosis transfer" client is entitled need not be excessively elaborate. The Court in *Vitek* held that due process required that the prisoner was entitled to notice, a hearing before an independent decisionmaker, the right to present his own witnesses and to cross-examine those presented by the state, and a written statement of the reasons for the decisionmaker's ultimate judgment.[33] The elements of the procedural due process balancing test[34] in *Vitek* are roughly equivalent for involuntary transfers between the two kinds of mental disability facilities, and therefore the same sort of hearing would probably suffice.

The provision of such a hearing could serve a number of useful purposes. At the most basic level, it would reduce the convenience (and thus lessen the incentive) of unwarranted reciprocal transfers between facilities when neither intends to provide the array of services that a dual diagnosis client needs. If there is a statutory requirement for an individualized treatment/habilitation plan, preparation for a hearing would also provide an appropriate occasion for service providers to evaluate carefully the treatment *and* habilitation needs of the client. Finally, the assistance of counsel or trained professional advocate and the requirement of an independent decisionmaker provide an opportunity and a forum for exploring whether the proposed transfer is well designed to serve the client's needs that arise from both aspects of his disability.

## Community-Based Services

The success of community-based services for mentally retarded people is well documented, even for clients whose disabilities were previously believed to require institutional care.[35] Despite the unquestionable success of these programs, the states have differed substantially in the extent to which they have implemented community-based residential programs.[36] In most (if not all) states, the number of retarded individuals who could be placed appropriately in community residential facilities exceeds the capacity of the facilities that are currently available. Some of these individuals are unserved by residential programs, continuing to live with their families or on their own without the assistance that a residential program would provide. Others remain institutionalized despite the fact that their disability does not require this additional restriction on their liberty.[37]

This shortage of community beds requires some system of allocation to determine which individuals will receive this scarce resource. Our society's typical means for allocating a scarce resource is rationing by price—allowing the system of supply and demand to set the price of the commodity and thereby to allocate it to those who are willing and able to pay the price. This system is inapplicable to the allocation of scarce opportunities for placement in the community, because few prospective consumers pay their own bills. The vast majority of community placements are subsidized, in whole or in part, by government. Therefore, government will have to decide who, among the "surplus" of eligible and willing consumers, will receive the opportunity to live in community residential facilities.

Another system, adopted in a number of states, is to delegate the rationing to private organizations. States choose this system when they contract with private companies or associations to operate community residential facilities and tell them they may select for admission whomever they prefer among those individuals who meet eligibility requirements. This system is attractive to the state because it lets others make the hard decisions of who will be served and who will not. It may also partially disguise government's role in creating the artificial scarcity in its decision to decline to fund the creation and operation of a sufficient number of community residential programs.

A major problem with the private delegation system is that it does not produce even-handed results. For example, where the private association that contracts with the state to provide the community services is a group of parents (such as a local ARC), it will not surprise anyone if the disabled people who receive the services include the sons and daughters of the parents active in that organization. Another bias built into the private delegation system is that the service provider has an incentive to select those disabled individuals who can be served most easily. This will seldom include dual diagnosis clients, particularly if those clients are believed likely to exhibit disruptive behaviors.

This bias is exacerbated if the contractual arrangement between the state and the service provider creates an incentive to select those clients who can be served at the lowest expense. If the service provider is reimbursed at a fixed rate, regardless of the nature of the client's disability or service needs, it is unlikely to choose clients who place additional burdens on its staff.

Therefore, a predictable consequence of a private delegation system is that mentally retarded people who also have a mental illness are likely to remain in institutions where they cannot receive the combination of treatment and habilitation that they need.

This result can be avoided if the government requires contractors to provide services on the basis of government-established priorities that include dual diagnosis clients or makes special contractual arrangements for the provision of services to individuals whose needs are likely to be unusually expensive to address.

But the principal reform that is needed is creation of a system that regularizes the process of admission to community facilities for all mentally retarded persons.[38] This provides a forum for implementation of priorities for admissions and ensures that admission decisions are based on individualized assessment of the habilitation needs of the proposed residents.

## Conclusion

Individuals who are both mentally ill and mentally retarded present unique challenges to the providers of residential services. They also raise significant legal issues. While it is essential that the service delivery system be adapted to accommodate the needs of this doubly disabled group of citizens, it would be advisable to create a separate legal mechanism for their placement. Rather, the existing procedures for admission of persons with mental illness or mental retardation can be adapted and employed, with special attention directed to ensuring that all the client's service needs are addressed.

## Footnotes

[1] I join my colleagues in this book in recognizing that the term "dual diagnosis" is at once awkward and imprecise. Nevertheless, since the term is commonly used and understood in the field of mental retardation, I will use it in this chapter as shorthand to describe mentally retarded individuals who have some form of mental illness.

[2] There is a wealth of literature on voluntary admission and involuntary commitment of persons who are mentally ill. *See. e.g.*, Developments in the Law – Civil Commitment of the Mentally Ill, 87 Harvard Law Review 1190 (1974); Legal Issues in State Mental Health Care: Proposals for Change – Civil Commitment, 2 Mental Disability Law Reporter 73-126 (1977); D. Wexler, Mental Health Law: Major Issues 1-113 (1981); Morse, A Preference for Liberty: The Case Against Involuntary Commitment of the Mentally Disordered, 70 California Law Review 54 (1982); R. Rock, M. Jacobson & R. Janopaul, Hospitalization and Discharge of the Mentally Ill (1968); C. Warren, Court of Last Resort: Mental Illness and the Law (1982). Substantially less research has been published on the processes by which mentally retarded people are placed in residential facilities. *See. e.g.*, Disabled Persons and the Law: State Legislative Issues 409-52 (B. Sales,

D. Powell & R. Van Duizend eds. 1982) (hereafter Disabled Persons and the Law); Dybwad & Herr, Unnecessary Coercion: An End to Involuntary Civil Commitment of Retarded Persons, 31 Stanford Law Review 753 (1979). There is no comparable analysis of clients who are both mentally ill and mentally retarded.

[3]Numerous communities have had success in providing services in the community to a wide range of clients, including those whose disabilities had previously been thought to be too severe for community placement. *See generally* K. Casey, J. McGee, J. Stark & F. Menolascino, A Community-Based System for the Mentally Retarded: The ENCOR Experience (1985); J. Conroy & V. Bradley, Pennhurst Longitudinal Study: A Report of Five Years of Research and Analysis (Temple University and Human Services Research Institute, 1985).

[4]*See* D. Rothman, The Discovery of the Asylum: Social Order and Disorder in the New Republic 130-54 (1971); N. Dain, Concepts of Insanity in the United States, 1789-1865 (1964).

[5]*See* Ellis, Volunteering Children: Parental Commitment of Minors to Mental Institutions, 62 California Law Review 840, 841-44 (1974). *See also* Dewey, The Jury Trial Law for Commitment of the Insane in Illinois (1867-1893), and Mrs. E.P.W. Packard, Its Author, 69 American Journal of Insanity 571 (1913).

[6]Draft Act Governing Hospitalization of the Mentally Ill (U.S. Public Health Service, 1951).

[7]For an example of such state statutes, *see* 1953 N.M. Laws ch. 182 § 5 ("in need of custody, care or treatment in a mental hospital and, because of his mental illness, lacks sufficient insight or capacity to make responsible decisions with respect to his hospitalization"), repealed 1977 N.M. Laws ch. 279 § 24.

[8]*See. e.g.*, T. Szasz, Law, Liberty and Psychiatry: An Inquiry into the Social Uses of Mental Health Practices (1963).

[9]*See* E. Bardach, The Skill Factor in Politics: Repealing the Mental Commitment Laws in California (1972) (describing the enactment of the Lanterman-Petris-Short commitment statute).

[10]*E.g.*, Bell v. Wayne County Gen. Hosp., 384 F. Supp. 1085 (E.D. Mich. 1974); Lynch v. Baxley, 386 F. Supp. 378 (M.D. Ala. 1974).

[11]*See* Van Duizend, McGraw & Keilitz, An Overview of State Involuntary Commitment Statutes, 8 Mental and Physical Disability Law Reporter 328 (1984).

[12]*See generally* P. Tyor & L. Bell, Caring for the Retarded in America: A History (1984); W. Wolfensberger, The Origin and Nature of Our Institutional Models (1975); R. Scheerenberger, A History of Mental Retardation (1983); The History of Mental Retardation: Collected Papers (M. Rosen, G. Clark & M. Kivitz eds. 2 vols. 1976).

[13]L. Terman, The Intelligence of School Children 132-33 (1919). *See generally* H. Goddard, The Criminal Imbecile: An Analysis of Three Remarkable Murder Cases (1915).

[14]*See. e.g.*, Buck v. Bell, 274 U.S. 200 (1927). It was in this case that Justice Oliver Wendell Holmes wrote the immortal (and infamous) line, "Three generations of imbeciles are enough." For a discussion of the factual context of the case (as well as proof that Holmes had his facts wrong), *see* Gould, Carrie Buck's Daughter, Natural History 14 (July 1984).

[15]*See, e.g.*, Education of the Handicapped Act, 20 U.S.C. § 1400 *et se.*; Mills v. Board of Education, 348 F. Supp. 866 (D.D.C. 1972). *See generally* S. Herr, Rights and Advocacy for Retarded People (1983).

[16]*See. e.g.*, Youngberg v. Romeo, 457 U.S. 307 (1982); Pennhurst State School & Hospital v. Halderman, 451 U.S. 1 (1981); Wyatt v. Aderholt, 503 F.2d 1305 (5th Cir.

1974). *See generally* Ellis, The Supreme Court and Institutions: A Comment on Young-berg v. Romeo, 20 Mental Retardation 197 (1982).

[17]This paradox is highlighted by the fact that the same federal judge who ruled that Pennhurst's very existence violated the Constitution stated in another case that providing hearings to children before placement in Pennhurst would constitute an "overdose of due process." *Compare* Halderman v. Pennhurst State School & Hospital, 446 F. Supp. 1295 (E.D.Pa. 1977), *reversed on other grounds*, 451 U.S. 1 (1981), *with* Bartley v. Kremens, 402 F. Supp. 1039, 1054 (1975) (Broderick J., dissenting), *remanded on other grounds*, 431 U.S. 119 (1977).

[18]*See. e.g.*, New Mexico Mental Health and Developmental Disabilities Code, N.M. Stat. Ann. § 43-1-13 (1984 repl.); District of Columbia Mentally Retarded Citizens Constitutional Rights and Dignity Act of 1978, D.C. Code § 6-1901 *et se.* The American Bar Association Commission on the Mentally Disabled proposed such a model statute. *See* Disabled Persons and the Law, *supra* note 2, at 409-52.

[19]For example, Alabama still places priority on committing mentally retarded women "of child-bearing age." Ala. Code § 22-52-51 (1984 repl.). Utah very recently provided as a substantive ground for commitment that the mentally retarded person constitutes a "social menace." 1929 Utah Laws ch. 75 § 29, repealed 1983 Utah Laws ch. 314 § 8.

[20]*See* Dybwad & Herr, *supra* note 2, at 760–61. The "voluntariness" of the voluntary admission of a residential client is often purely fictitious. *See generally* Gilboy, "Voluntary" Hospitalization of the Mentally Ill, 66 Northwestern University Law Review 429 (1971). This is particularly likely to be true when the client is seriously disabled, whether by mental retardation, mental illness, or both.

[21]*See* Van Duizend *et al.*, *supra* note 11. The statutes vary in their definitions of danger-ousness. Some states have a specific provision for those individuals whose mental illness renders them so "gravely disabled" that they cannot care for themselves. Others treat this as a form of dangerousness to self.

[22]*See e.g.*, note 10, *supra*. The United States Supreme Court has not directly ruled on this issue, but has observed that "A finding of 'mental illness' alone cannot justify a State's locking a person up against his will and keeping him indefinitely in simple custodial confinement. Assuming that that term can be given a reasonably precise content and that the 'mentally ill' can be identified with reasonable accuracy, there is still no constitutional basis for confining such persons involuntarily if they are dangerous to no one and can live safely in freedom." O'Connor v. Donaldson, 422 U.S. 563, 575 (1975).

[23]Ohio Rev. Code Ann. § 5123.01(L); District of Columbia Code Ann. § 6-1924 (1981).

[24]*See generally* American Association on Mental Deficiency, The Least Restrictive Alternative: Principles and Practices (H.R. Turnbull ed., 1981).

[25]*See* note 20, *supra*.

[26]*See generally* American Association on Mental Deficiency, Consent Handbook (H.R. Turnbull ed., 1977).

[27]This may be because the authorities or other persons who instigated the individual's commitment were able to identify the symptoms of mental disorder more readily than the subtler manifestation of mental retardation. *See generally* L. Teplin, Mental Health and Criminal Justice 157 (1984). Another possible explanation might be that many mental retardation facilities are particularly reluctant to accept clients who present behavioral problems and often such facilities are not prepared to manage such behavior or to provide habilitation which would address it.

[28]*See generally* Sprague & Baxley, Drugs for Behavior Management, with Comments on Some Legal Aspects, in 10 Mental Retardation and Developmental Disabilities: An

Annual Review 92 (J. Wortis ed., 1978); Plotkin & Gill, Invisible Manacles: Drugging Mentally Retarded People, 31 Stanford Law Review 637 (1979).

[29]Such a requirement may be implicit in those statutes that make an individualized treatment or habilitation plan a central part of the commitment proceedings. *See, e.g.*, N.M. Stat. Ann. § 43-1-13 (1984 repl.). Under these laws, the court is in the position of approving or disapproving a particular course of treatment or habilitation that is proposed for the client, and transfer from one type of facility to another would almost certainly require a new review by the court.

[30]If the original placement was by voluntary admission, any transfer would require legally adequate consent. If the person who consented to the original admission declines to approve the transfer, formal commitment proceedings would, of course, be required.

[31]445 U.S. 480 (1980).

[32]The Court also recognized a liberty interest in being free from "compelled treatment in the form of a mandatory behavior modification program" that Mr. Jones would face in the mental facility. 445 U.S. at 492. Similarly, a change in the character of "compelled treatment" would be likely to accompany any transfer between a mental hospital and a mental retardation facility.

[33]445 U.S. at 494–496. A plurality of the Court also declared that when such a prisoner was indigent he was also entitled to the appointment of counsel to represent him at the hearing. This did not become part of the majority opinion because Justice Powell believed that the prisoner could receive competent assistance from an advocate who was not an attorney. 445 U.S. at 499 (Powell, J., concurring). Since only five members of the Court reached the merits of the dispute (the other four believing that the case was moot), it is likely that if this issue were to reach all nine justices, a fifth vote would be cast in favor of the right to counsel in transfer hearings.

[34]In deciding how much process is due, the courts weigh four factors: (1) the nature of the interest of the individual in the outcome of the proceedings; (2) the risk that the hearing will produce an erroneous result if the additional requested procedure is not provided; (3) the likelihood that the requested procedure will reduce the risk of error; and (4) the government's interest in avoiding giving the individual the procedural protection he has requested. Mathews v. Eldridge, 424 U.S. 319, 335 (1976).

[35]*See* note 3, *supra*. There is now a substantial body of literature on community services. *See, e.g.*, Deinstitutionalization and Community Adjustment of Mentally Retarded People (R. Bruininks, C. Meyers, B. Sigford & K. Lakin eds. 1981); R. Scheerenberger, Deinstitutionalization and Institutional Reform (1976); B. Baker, G. Seltzer & M. Seltzer, As Close as Possible: Community Residences for Retarded Adults (1977); G. O'Connor, Home is a Good Place: A National Perspective of Community Residential Facilities for the Mentally Retarded (1976); D. Braddock, Opening Closed Doors: The Deinstitutionalization of Disabled Individuals (1977). The nature of life in the community for retarded people is illuminated by a recent collection of insightful anthropological studies. Lives in Process: Mildly Retarded Adults in a Large City (R. Edgerton ed., 1984).

[36]"Most states are stressing the development of community services as options to institutional services; but judging from their balance sheets, only a handful of states have made strong, relatively long-term financial commitments to a community-based system." D. Braddock, R. Hemp & R. Howes, Public Expenditures for Mental Retardation and Developmental Disabilities in the United States: Analytical Summary 84

(University of Illinois at Chicago Institute for the Study of Developmental Disabilities 1985).

[37]*See* note 24, *supra*.

[38]One model that could be adapted into a state statute or regulation is found at Disabled Persons and the Law, *supra* note 2, at 424–52.

# 30
## Clients in Limbo: Asserting the Rights of Persons with Dual Disabilities

STANLEY S. HERR

## Introduction

Protecting the rights of persons with dual disabilities[1] is a challenging enterprise. The mentally retarded population, as *City of Cleburne v. Cleburne Living Center* makes clear, continues to suffer from a legacy of degradation.[2] The mentally ill population fares little better and bears the additional burdens of exaggerated public fears of their "dangerousness."[3] It is therefore no surprise that individuals who bear the marks (or the labels) of both mental retardation and mental illness, are disadvantaged in their pursuit of services, liberty, and a dignified niche in society.

This chapter suggests that they are also disadvantaged in their access to advocates and legal services. As compared to other citizens and to other disabled persons, they are poor competitors for these scarce resources. There are many reasons why this is so, including (1) the problems of initiating client–attorney contacts; (2) the complexity of their potential cases; (3) the lack of adequate resources for advocacy in ethically sensitive, time-consuming cases; (4) the bifurcation of advocacy systems into developmental disability *or* mental health-focused systems; and (5) the reluctance of some advocates to take on clients who are poor and sometimes difficult to serve.

If any agency has a mandate to serve this multiply disabled population, it would be the protection and advocacy systems (P&As) created under the Developmental Disabilities and Bill of Rights Act.[4] Although this act does not expressly prohibit mentally ill persons from being served, and certainly includes dual diagnosed

---

[1]For the purposes of this chapter, persons with dual disabilities or dually diagnosed persons refers to persons classified as both mentally retarded and mentally ill. They may also have other disabilities, physical or sensory. This is obviously a heterogeneous population with diverse advocacy needs.

[2]473 U.S. 432 (1985).

[3]See Ennis & Litwack, Psychiatry and the presumption of expertise: Flipping coins in the courtroom, *California Law Review, 62*, 693 (1974).

[4]42 U.S.C. § 6042 (1987 Supp.).

persons within its ambit, very few such persons are served.[5] According to a recent U.S. Senate report, only 7% of the total number of persons served by P&As were mentally ill. No estimates are available as to the number of mentally retarded and mentally ill (hereinafter MR/MI) clients within P&A caseloads. But it is reasonable to assume that such clients constitute a minute proportion of the P&A's approximately 30,000 clients per year.[6] Congress has recently passed the Protection and Advocacy for Mentally Ill Individuals Act (P.L. 99-319), thereby clarifying P&A obligations to serve MR/MI clients and adding financial resources to do so. Because other legal services providers, such as Legal Services Corporation-funded programs, law school clinics, and private practitioners, do not gather statistics based on type of client disability, there are no data on which to generate reliable estimates of the number of MR/MI clients who seek or receive legal services.

There is, however, considerable evidence that this population will encounter substantial obstacles in gaining access to advocates and asserting their rights. They are in limbo because their place in service delivery systems, and hence advocacy systems, is so unclear, and because their multiple disabilities make them candidates for confinement and for being cast aside.

## Problems of Outreach

How does a severely retarded, physically aggressive, institutionalized man become the client of an attorney? How does a hallucinating, mildly retarded, homeless woman gain a defender of her legal and human rights? The traditional ways of initiating client–attorney contact simply will not work in such cases. If one relies on norms of lawyer passivity and client initiative, such individuals will remain outside the pale of justice systems.

The dually diagnosed face many impediments to bringing their problems to legal services providers. They lack awareness of these providers or the cognitive abilities to understand the legal process itself. They lack income to purchase services from the private bar or the assertiveness to demand service from the public bar. They may operate at the margins of basic subsistence, struggling for food, shelter, and safety, and have little energy or experience to cope with courts and bureaucrats. In short, it is unrealistic to expect many of these potential clients to walk into a lawyer's office, to call for an appointment, or to otherwise take the first step.

---

[5]See Staff Report on the Institutionalized Mentally Disabled, requested by Senator Lowell P. Weicker, Jr., p. 80. (Prepared for Joint Hearings Conducted by the Subcommittee on the Handicapped, Senate Committee on Labor and Human Resources and the Subcommittee on Labor, Health and Human Services, Education and Related Agencies, Senate Committee on Appropriations April 1-3, 1985.)

[6]See Staff Report on the Institutionalized Mentally Disabled, requested by Senator Lowell P. Weicker, Jr., p. 81 (data based on 40-state survey for P&A services in FY 1982.)

Homeless, dually diagnosed persons pose a particularly poignant illustration of clients who fall through the cracks of both social and legal services. Ella Wright, a 27-year-old Baltimore "street person," with a primary diagnosis of mental retardation, was first admitted to a state institution when she was 13 years old. Over the years, she had been released from mental hospitals six times, only to end up on the streets. After police found her eating scraps from a garbage can on a downtown street, she was committed to Spring Grove State Hospital. Through the commitment process and her involuntary patient status, a public defender was appointed to represent her. When her mental health problems stabilized and she refused to remain in the hospital as a voluntary patient, her lawyer pressed for her release. Under threat of litigation, the hospital administrators discharged her. After a fruitless search for alternative care (including calls to 10 agencies and the Rosewood Center—an institution for the mentally retarded), they brought Ella Wright to the Maryland Children's Society—an emergency shelter. Even that shelter was not prepared to keep her and provide her with the necessary supervision. She was ultimately placed in a foster home, but her physician was not optimistic about her prospects for staying there. As her doctor explained: "Yes, she could wander off again. Hopefully she can stay there, but she has a history of running away."[7]

Although her lawyer could win Ms. Wright's freedom from a large restrictive hospital, he could not secure for her a stable supportive home. And although social workers could identify the cycle of her exposure to physical and sexual abuse, they could not provide her with the services to break that cycle. More likely than not, Ella Wright will continue to drift in and out of institutions. Her contact with lawyers will, no doubt, be episodic and inconclusive—a result of her collision with police and coercive processes rather than the pursuit of some affirmative legal strategy.

Care providers can help bridge the gap between lawyers and such potential clients. One positive by-product of the publicity surrounding Ella Wright's plight was the formation of an Ad Hoc Committee to the Homeless Mentally Ill and Retarded. Their main task has been to develop and implement a proposal for emergency shelter and related services for such persons in central Maryland. The committee has recruited lawyers to advise them on lobbying strategies, to persuade state and local officials and to assess legal remedies for the affected class of dually diagnosed persons. To provide broader outreach and pro bono legal services, the Greater Baltimore Shelter Network has recently joined those lawyers to cosponsor the Homeless Persons Representation Project.

These are but two examples of how conscientious habilitation professionals can bring clients with serious needs together with reform-minded attorneys. Another illustration involved a lawsuit by a mildly handicapped individual detained in a mental retardation institution. There the staff contacted a Legal Aid lawyer to

---

[7]Robinson, Retarded woman falls through cracks of social service, *News American (Baltimore)*, November 25, 1983, p. 1A.

[8]*Clark v. Cohen*, 613 F. Supp. 684 (E.D. Pa. 1985), *aff'd* 794 F.2d 79 (3rd Cir. 1986), *cert.*

secure community placement for a woman who had experienced mental health problems.[8] Writing to law enforcement officials is another method of drawing attention to the systemic legal problems of the dually diagnosed population.[9] Before those problems can be resolved, individual clients must be identified and coalitions formed.

## Complexity of Cases

Although lawyers seldom encounter dually diagnosed clients, they know that the complexity of those clients' cases can be great. The client may be noncommunicative or noncompliant, or both. The factual issues may turn on the sciences of behavior modification, pharmacology, and other therapeutic technologies designed to control aggressive or disturbed conduct.[10] That conduct may have brought the client to the attention of the police, judges, advocates, community mental health centers, social services agencies, mental retardation program administrators, their mental health counterparts, shelter care providers, and others. In short, a dizzying array of private and public actors may touch on the client's life. But the providers' common refrain is likely to be, "We have no appropriate program/service/facility/treatment milieu for such a unique individual." If the service delivery system is incomplete, it is fair to say that the legal system has scarcely begun to frame the right questions to regulate that system or to respond to the needs of the dually diagnosed.

Two pioneering cases reveal the doctrinal and practical problems that lawyers confront when tackling those questions. These cases have received little discussion, in part, because they did not result in published opinions and because their implementation histories have not yet been studied. Analysis of these two federal cases, however, can offer an opportunity to understand the strengths and limitations of complex litigation in this field.

*Knott v. Hughes*[11] concerned a class of persons with a diagnosis of mental retardation who were confined to state institutions for the mentally ill. One event leading up to this suit was a letter by Maryland's Mental Health Association (MHA) to the state's attorney general. In April 1979, MHA complained of many failures by state mental hospitals "to comply with provisions of state law as conscientiously as we would hope," and the "relative unavailability" of legal guidance

---

*denied* 107 S.Ct. 459 (1986) (44-year-old mildly retarded woman, committed at age 15 when family life was tempestuous and disruptive to her development ordered transferred to community living arrangement).

[9]See, for example, letter from Jeff VanSickle, president of Mental Health Association of Maryland to Stephen H. Sachs, Maryland Attorney General, April 23, 1979 and the ensuing Sachs Report, discussed *infra* at text and notes, pp. 342–344.

[10]See Plotkin & Gill, "Invisible manacles: Drugging mentally retarded people, *Stanford Law Review, 31*, 637 (1979); J. Matson and J. Mulick (Eds.), *Handbook of mental retardation* (pp. 317–368) (1983).

[11]No. Y-80-2832 (D. Md. Jan. 18, 1982).

and counsel by the attorney general's office to state administrators.[12] The MHA was particularly troubled by the "inappropriate admission of persons who are mentally retarded rather than mentally ill to mental hygiene facilities."[13] In addition, MHA criticized court-ordered commitments of some retarded persons to mental hospitals in the absence of indications of need for psychiatric intervention, lack of discharge or aftercare planning for those ready for release, and delays in release that resulted in hospitals waiting for trial dates before releasing patients administratively. The attorney general's immediate response was to assign his chief general counsel to investigate these problems and to develop a funding proposal to provide administrators with more counseling and legal advice to implement patients' rights.[14] His longer-term response was to file the so-called Sachs Report, a 26-page evaluation of MHA's charges, with recommendations to deal with problems of noncompliance with state mental health laws. The Sachs Report acknowledged the accuracy of MHA's critique and the need for further change. Specifically, it concluded that hundreds of mentally retarded persons were improperly and illegally detained in mental hospitals. Despite a primary or sole diagnosis of mental retardation, they had been committed as suffering from a mental disorder, even though the term "mental disorder" had been defined to exclude mental retardation. Although they did not meet involuntary commitment tests (and had not been retained under voluntary admission standards), these individuals were stranded in state hospitals for want of more appropriate placements. While the Sachs Report dealt with broader issues, such as failures to create and implement aftercare plans, the concerned public viewed it as a means of rescuing what became known as the Sachs Population: mentally retarded citizens inappropriately placed in state psychiatric hospitals.

Sachs had not been the first official to publicize their plight. In 1975, the Maryland Humane Practices Commission had identified 382 such persons. For these "misplaced residents" they had urged interim programs "within existing institutions" until they could be transferred to "appropriate mental retardation facilities," preferably small and community based.[15] By 1978, the Department of Health and Mental Hygiene had reduced that estimate to 295 persons but had been stymied in its efforts to develop the interim program (which it proposed to locate in the Phillips Building on the grounds of the Crownsville State Hospital) or to expand community resources. The Sachs Report promised to end the improper detention of mentally retarded persons in mental hygiene facilities and to achieve their "proper care and treatment." Under this plan, 100 Sachs population clients would funnel through the Phillips Building as a way station to appro-

---

[12]Letter from Mrs. Max VanSickle, President of Mental Health Association of Maryland to Stephen H. Sachs, Attorney General of Maryland (April 23, 1979).

[13]See footnote 12, at p. 2.

[14]Letter from Stephen H. Sachs to Mrs. Max VanSickle, April 27, 1979.

[15]Maryland Humane Practices Commission, Second Report to the Governor and General Assembly (October 28, 1975).

priate community and institutional placements. The attorney general's office also advised DHMH officials of the unlawfulness of confining persons solely diagnosed as mentally retarded in state hospitals and the necessity of removing them "as soon as possible." For retarded persons who were also diagnosed as mentally ill, the lawyers urged that they should be notified of their due-process hearing rights, like any other mental patient, and be recertified.

But were they like other patients? By what processes would clinicians sort retarded clients destined to stay in mental health facilities from those bound for mental retardation institutions (SRCs) and group homes. And would the attorney general alone, or prodded by the Mental Health Association, be able to push through long-stalled reforms?

The Maryland P&A program believed that a federal lawsuit was needed to counter bureaucratic inaction. In their view, the attorney general's report had not gone far enough in terms of a remedy or a timetable. They criticized the lack of attention to placing dually diagnosed plaintiffs in their home communities or to providing them with interim treatment programs in the institutions in which they were then confined.[16] Skeptical of the state's implementation capabilities, the Maryland Advocacy Unit for the Developmentally Disabled (MAUDD) wanted third-party evaluations, independent monitors, and assurances that changes would result in something more than an interinstitutional shuffle of clients.

·On October 17, 1980, MAUDD filed a complaint in federal court on behalf of eight named plaintiffs and a class of similarly situated individuals.[17] The class was defined as all mentally retarded persons "now confined or in the future to be confined" in Maryland's state mental hospitals who did not have mental disorders of such nature as to require inpatient care under the state's mental health commitment statute.[18] The suit named 31 defendants, including the governor and ranking officials of the mental health, mental retardation, human resources, vocational rehabilitation, and public education bureaucracies.

The essence of *Knott v. Hughes* was that state officials had failed to provide the plaintiffs with appropriate and necessary habilitation and treatment in the least restrictive environment. The state had clearly identified this systemic problem as early as 1975. Yet, despite the attorney general's public statements that their rights were being violated, the plaintiffs remained in environments incapable of meeting their habilitation needs. As a result, they suffered social and intellectual regression and other harms, such as being subjected to seclusion in lieu of programs.

The *Knott* complaint called for a massive restructuring of services to the dually diagnosed population. Plaintiffs' attorneys sought declaratory and injunctive

---

[16]*Knott v. Hughes*, No. Y-80-2832, Complaint, para. 29 (October 4, 1980).

[17]The name plaintiffs sued by their "next friend" Anne Pecora, a University of Baltimore Law School clinical professor.

[18]Md. Ann. Code 1957, Art. 59, § 3 (f). Although that statute has now been recodified, mental disorder is still defined as not including mental retardation. Md. Health-Gen. Code Ann. § 10-101 (f) (3) (1982).

relief to protect them from harm in mental health (MH) institutions, such as the inappropriate use of drugs and seclusion. They wanted to enjoin transfers to large state mental retardation (MR) institutions or the use of the Phillips Building, a specialized treatment facility on the grounds of a mental hospital. They sought to prevent the admission to MH facilities of class members who did not meet the statutory criteria. The plaintiffs demanded an expansive, positive program: an interagency group to commit the defendants' services and resources; a multidisciplinary evaluation and planning team to determine the individual's interim, short-term, and long-term community placement and treatment; and a detailed plan for "the creation of an appropriate and adequately funded network of community-based residences and services" to provide class members with habilitation, training, education, and care. They also sought impartial outsider review: a monitor to oversee the implementation of court orders and to hear appeals from interdisciplinary team decisions, private physicians to review medication regimens, and private contractors to perform assessments and evaluations. Here was a demand for systemic changes on a dramatic scale.

The plaintiffs' legal theories relied on both federal and state law grounds. They raised constitutional claims for liberty and protection from harm. At a time when the U.S. Supreme Court had not yet blunted the promise of certain federal statutory claims,[19] they contended that Section 504, the Developmental Disabilities and Bill of Rights Act, and the Education for All Handicapped Children Act provided a basis for some relief. Lastly, the lawyers asked the federal court to base a remedy on state laws requiring education, training, and treatment for class members.

These legal issues were never fully adjudicated. The defendants acknowledged the illegality under state law of the continued confinement of the plaintiffs and their class in MH institutions and adopted their own plan of affirmative remedy.[20] Under the preventive law approach of Attorney General Sachs and his deputies, the defendants promised to fashion an appropriate placement for every class member.

Their plan had three main components. The state promised an infusion of new resources, a three-step evaluation and placement process, and the creation of new services and programs through initiatives with private community-based providers. The estimated cost of implementing their plan over four years was $23.5 million. The evaluation and placement process, already underway, was designed to identify all potential class members; assess the functional level and establish a diagnosis for each member; recommend a specific residential program and habilitation services based on an interdisciplinary review; and place each client in a community setting, an SRC, or the Phillips Building program.

Under the defendants' plan, "higher-functioning" individuals would move to community settings, while the more disabled individuals would transfer to SRCs.

---

[19]See, for example, *Pennhurst State School and Hospital v. Halderman*, 451 U.S. 1 (1981).

[20]*Knott v. Hughes*, No. Y-80-2832, Defendants' Proposed Placement Plan for Plaintiffs' Class (D. Md. March 16, 1981).

But even this line had its exceptions. Higher-functioning persons with MR and major MH needs would undergo an interim placement at Phillips. Lower-functioning persons, such as geriatric clients with 24-hour nursing care needs, might be placed in nursing homes. By classifying clients according to a matrix that correlated diagnosis and level of functioning, defendants could begin budgeting and aggregate planning for the *Knott* class.

Substantial obstacles stood in the way of carrying out this deinstitutionalization plan. The legislature would have to appropriate additional funds for a group that had little lobbying power in Annapolis. Even though more class clients could have been targeted for placement in the community, community services did not then exist in adequate quantity or quality. But community service providers needed inducements to create those alternative services. The defendants therefore proposed to create 76 community "equity" placements: new beds for clients living in their natural homes as a response to the charge that the state discriminated against those clients in favor of institutionalized clients.

Would this bargain work? Some private providers balked at accepting members of the heterogeneous *Knott* class, especially those who were elderly, had complex physical and mental health problems, or needed extensive support systems after decades of institutionalization. (The average class client had experienced 15 years of confinement, with the range extending from several months to 52 years.[21]) If the community providers chose not to grant trial visits to plaintiffs or accept their applications, the state had no public group homes or community living arrangements to offer. Despite these obstacles and uncertainties, the defendants expressed confidence that their plan could be implemented with dramatic gains in deinstitutionalization of mentally retarded persons. If they accomplished their goal of placing a total of 326 persons in the community in three years, this would represent a 50% increase in the number of community-based residences for retarded Marylanders.[22]

In an unpublished opinion, the court approved this plan, and ordered relief that would effectively dispose of most of the plaintiffs' claims. After plaintiffs' motion for a preliminary injunction, the parties attempted to settle their dispute concerning six areas of relief. They agreed to broaden the lists of persons entitled to priority access to appropriate habilitative programs and to increase educational and monitoring efforts to prevent inappropriate admissions of MR clients to MH institutions. But they were unable to agree that the state should not transfer class clients to MR institutions or that Phillips Building should not be certified as an ICF/MR facility. Although the parties agreed that seclusion and medication should not be used for other than therapeutic purposes, they disagreed on the need for independent outside reviews by qualified physicians and program

---

[21]See footnote 20, at 14.

[22]See footnote 20, at 15. This number of persons included SRC clients "displaced" by incoming *Knott* class members, clients living in the community going to the 76 "equity beds," and 22 borderline retarded individuals placed in foster homes under a Mental Hygiene Administration-sponsored program.

specialists.[23] On each of these disputed points, the court accepted the state's position as a sound and good faith attempt to "move the state significantly in the right direction." Thus, the court ratified the state's plan, but left the plaintiffs, or others, free to challenge the way in which it would be implemented. As Judge Joseph Young stated, the court's action in approving the plan "cannot be interpreted as a final endorsement of future efforts in this area on the part of the State . . . [m]uch remains to be done. This Plan represents one step, albeit a significant one, in the direction of fulfillment of the State's obligations under the Constitution and Federal and State statutory provisions."[24] In essence, if the state carried out its plan in good faith, the court would not disturb or burden those efforts.

The federal court maintained a continuing jurisdiction in this case until early 1985. It used this power, for example, to exempt elderly or other *Knott* class members from being transferred from state institutions for the mentally ill if they and their attorneys agreed that the individual should remain in such a facility.[25] Although the defendants' plan and the court's order had called for transfers for all class members, the parties realized that a more flexible policy was needed. The resulting policy articulated criteria for remaining, such as the individual's advanced age, length of stay, wishes, and risk of transfer trauma.[26] Because of the high degree of cooperation that marked this case, judicial intervention was relatively light. The parties chose to resolve their disputes amicably and to refer them to the state's MH/MR Coordinating Committee rather than to the judge. For practical purposes, the *Knott* case came to a close on January 10, 1985. On that date, the parties concluded that the systemic problem had been essentially resolved and approved a judicial order to deny supplemental relief to the plaintiff class. However, the *Knott* order can be construed as still having binding effect.

What had the *Knott* case accomplished? It had created a forum in which the systemic problems of certain dually diagnosed clients could be identified and addressed. Litigation had produced deadlines and a sense of emergency that allowed advocates—both inside and outside government—to mobilize new resources, refine plans, and keep the state on the right track. When the final statistics were tabulated, it appeared that significant movement and progress had taken place. Of the 398 persons identified as potential members of the *Knott* case, 291 (74%) were found to have a primary diagnosis of mental retardation. They therefore became the primary responsibility of the state's Mental Retardation and Developmental Disabilities Administration and gained access to more

---

[23]*Knott v. Hughes*, No. Y-80-2832 [hereinafter *Knott*], Plaintiffs' Report to the Court (Dec. 1980).

[24]*Knott*, Memorandum and Order, at 9 (D. Md. May 15, 1981).

[25]*Knott*, Consent Order (D. Md. Jan. 18, 1982).

[26]Department of Health and Mental Hygiene, Policy Concerning *Knott* Class Members Remaining in State Mental Health Facilities, October 19, 1981, incorporated in Consent Order (see footnote 25).

TABLE 30.1. Placement of Knott class.

| Placement | Number | Percentage |
|---|---|---|
| Supervised community settings | 131 | 34 |
| State residential center for the mentally retarded | 123 | 31 |
| State mental health facilities | 58 | 15 |
| Unsupervised community settings | 44 | 11 |
| Nursing homes | 20 | 5 |
| Deceased | 17 | 4 |

appropriate habilitation services. Nearly one-third now live in supervised community settings, another one-third are in state residential centers for the mentally retarded, and the remainder are in a variety of other settings or are deceased[27] (see Table 30.1).

What are the risks of even successful litigation of this type? Without detailed follow-up studies of the individuals who were transferred or were retained in MH facilities, it is difficult to assess precise gains and losses. Legal advocates can increase the pressure for action, but they may have difficulty ensuring that it is the right action at the right pace. Rapid expansion of services carries the dangers of experienced providers diluting their quality standards and inexperienced providers being unable to serve effectively individuals with complex clinical needs. As one observer of Maryland's process noted: "The 'most difficult' clients were not infrequently placed with those providers least able to cope."[28] This, in part, may have been due to their lack of sophistication in negotiating for resources and matching clients with services. It is difficult to provide the necessary monitoring of, and training for, service providers when numerical placement goals are a priority. Placements to the community may have taken place before support systems were available, such as behavior management and case management services from the MR system, and outpatient psychotherapy, crisis stabilization, and access to community mental health centers from the MH system. All these factors can lead to community resistance to bringing dually diagnosed clients into mainstreams. When a client "failed" in the community for want of those support systems, this experience reinforced the stigma that *Knott* clients already faced, owing to the untested assumption that they must have been severely disturbed to have been locked up in a mental health facility in the first place. In remedying past wrongs, good intentions may outrun systems capabilities. And if a state appears to be acting in a diligent and conscientious manner to meet placement objectives, courts may be reluctant to monitor or define what constitutes an effective systemic response.

---

[27]MAUDD, Statistical Survey of *Knott* Client Population (November 1, 1984).

[28]M. Smull, The deinstitutionalization of mentally retarded persons from mental health institutions (p. 7). University of Maryland School of Medicine, Mental Retardation Program, January 15, 1985.

If getting grossly misplaced MR/MH clients out of mental hospitals represented phase one litigation, obtaining appropriate services for MR/MH clients in developmental disabilities systems can be described as phase two litigation. *Grabau v. Hughes* posed precisely that issue.[29] Filed on June 22, 1981, by the Legal Aid Bureau, this class action suit sought adequate mental health services for dually diagnosed clients with maladaptive behavior or emotional disturbance. The federal court defined the class to include persons: confined in Maryland's State Residential Centers (SRCs) for the mentally retarded; who possessed levels of intellectual and personal skills to allow them to function outside the institution; and who were characterized by SRC staff as having maladaptive behavior or emotional disturbance of "sufficient severity as to require their continued confinement within the institution."[30] Although this class definition was somewhat convoluted, the thrust of the resulting consent agreement was clear. *Grabau* promised to provide adequate mental health services to MR class clients and thereby overcome the barriers to their successful placement in a community residential setting. For class clients subsequently placed in the community, it offered assurances that adequate mental health services would continue to be available to clients in alternative living arrangements.

Once again, Judge Young presided over a suit alleging that defendants inappropriately institutionalized dually diagnosed clients in violation of their rights to substantive due process and protection from harm. And once again, the State of Maryland averted legal judgment by consenting to an extensive plan of remediation. The settlement agreement reached by the parties called for a complex process of identifying class members, conducting comprehensive evaluations, and arranging special staffings to formulate individualized service plans. In addition, *Grabau* specified discharge planning that would detail aftercare services, recognize the importance of case management services to maintain clients in community-based programs, and create a dispute-resolution team to settle differences concerning enforcement, application, and interpretation of the settlement agreement.

The *Grabau* decree attempts to alter expectations and resources for clients the institution has too often failed in the past. Through a new round of comprehensive evaluations, and an infusion of finances, a sophisticated work force seeks to reformulate habilitation programs to decrease a client's aggressive and disruptive behaviors, and to replace them with acceptable skills and adaptive responses. The specific services to be implemented under the decree include therapy/counseling, behavior management, medication review, case management, a full-day-program, structured family interaction, intrainstitutional transfers to more appropriate areas, transfer to the IBMP (Intensive Behavior Management Pro-

---

[29]*Grabau v. Hughes*, No. Y-81-1582 (D. Md., filed June 22, 1981) [hereinafter *Grabau*].

[30]*Grabau*, Memorandum Opinion and Order (D. Md. December 22, 1981).

gram) at the University of Maryland's Carter Center, and community place-ment.[31] Through the Center's program, a special interdisciplinary unit, the Grabau Behavior Intervention Team (GBIT), performs evaluations and facilitates services. GBIT is composed of two psychologists, a psychiatrist, physician, social worker, activity therapist, speech pathologist, and three coordinators. A *Grabau* staffing consists of a 14-stage meeting in which GBIT recommendations are discussed by a group that includes the institution's senior social worker, SRC team members, a representative of the Mental Hygiene Administration, and a Legal Aid attorney.[32] In addition, the resident generally attends and his or her parents, guardian, or interested person are invited. The letter of notification strongly encourages them to attend and notes that if the client is found eligible for additional services under the *Grabau* criteria, one of three recommendations may occur:

Continued stay at the SRC with additional habilitative services for the emotional and/or behavior problem.
Transfer to the IBMP.
Transfer to an available community-based residential program.

In the two years since the court's approval of the *Grabau* agreement, there has been slow, but steady progress in bringing this blueprint to life. Much of this time has been spent in identifying class members and arranging their comprehensive evaluations and *Grabau* staffings. The typical report of such an evaluation is a detailed, carefully crafted, six- or seven-page document with recommendations and social, psychological, psychiatric, medical, nursing, speech-language and hearing, day program/activity therapy, and residential components.[33] To illustrate the recommendations that can result from this evaluation, A.D., a mildly retarded 34-year-old man, is to receive individual supportive counseling, a structured role-training group to improve socialization skills, adjustments in a behavioral contract to target running away and vomiting, psychiatric monitoring through a medication review program, and a neurological evaluation and EEG to rule out temporal lobe seizures. The team also recommended structured family interactions to promote consistency in client–family contact (especially during the transition period from institution to the community) and a community residential placement with "psychiatric consultation, behavioral consultation, 24-hour supervision, individual counseling in a community mental health setting

[31]Letter from Michael E. Schemm, *Grabau* Coordinator, to Eugene E. Kowalczuk, Chief Attorney, Mental Retardation Unit, Legal Aid Bureau (June 20, 1985).

[32]Letter from Michael E. Schemm to Eugene E. Kowalczuk, with attachment "Format for Conducting *Grabau* Staffings" (May 9, 1985).

[33]In preparing this paper, the author reviewed 16 comprehensive evaluations of Holly, Great Oaks, and Victor Cullen Centers clients, and 41 such evaluations of Rosewood clients.

and a location in an area removed from busy roads owing to client's periodic impulsive flight."[34]

Can existing service delivery systems, goaded by legal advocates, make all this happen? The jury is still out. At least in terms of evaluation services, *Grabau* is on track. As of October 30, 1985, 75 individuals have been determined to be *Grabau* class members. This process is still ongoing. At least 152 individuals have been identified by the parties as prospective class members; the membership of 43 individuals was in dispute, and the plaintiffs' counsel had proposed 65 additional individuals for consideration.[35] Well over $4 million in new funds has been spent or committed by the State of Maryland for *Grabau* and related purposes as of October 1985. Many more dollars will be needed to carry out the decisions and interventions proposed by *Grabau* staffings. Some conclusions are already clear. As a result of *Grabau*, vulnerable, neglected, and sometimes troublesome residents have received the individualized attention of an advocate and outside treatment specialists. They have had their priority claims for scarce services validated and enunciated.

The shortcomings in the process reflect the ambitiousness of this litigation and the limitations of consent decrees. Claims may pile up far faster than the resources to satisfy them. The energies of specialists may be absorbed in evaluations rather than direct services. The pace of implementation can also be discouraging. As one Legal Aid lawyer noted on April 9, 1985: "To date, as far as I know, no additional mental health services have been provided for any *Grabau* class members who reside at Rosewood, except for the evaluations themselves. The Settlement Agreement clearly contemplates provision of actual substantive services, not merely evaluations."[36] That criticism may have goaded officials into action, because by June 17, 1985, GBIT reported that by the end of the summer, 12 Rosewood clients would receive therapy or counseling, 28 would have behavior management problems, 20 would undergo medication reviews, and 11 would enter full-day programs.[37] Perhaps the most heartening news concerned the first three *Grabau* clients at Rosewood recommended for community placement: Two were scheduled to leave and, for the third, placement was "being actively pursued." This litigation, like similar complex, systemic lawsuits elsewhere,[38] is all about active pursuit of options for clients and the results that will free them from various forms of limbo.

---

[34]*Grabau* Behavior Intervention Team, Comprehensive Evaluation of A.D., July 15, 1985, at 6. A.D., one of the author's clients, has subsequently been ordered released by a Hearing Officer under Md. Health-Gen. Code Ann. § 7-505 (1982) and is now in a community placement.

[35]N. Nee, The *Grabau* settlement agreement: Illusory promise or material proposal for Maryland's dually diagnosed (December 7, 1984). (Unpublished paper).

[36]Eileen Franch, Report on *Grabau* Staffings Attended Through April 9, 1985 (in Legal Aid Bureau files).

[37]Letter from Michael E. Schemm, see footnote 31.

[38]See, for example, *Willie M. v. Hunt*, No. CC 79-0294, Consent Order (W.D.N.C. Feb. 20, 1981), 732 F.2d 383 (4th Cir. 1984); *Thomas S. v. Morrow*, 601 F. Supp. 1055

## Resources for Individual Representation

The toughest cases are not always complex class actions. The effective, ethically sensitive representation of dually diagnosed individuals can be intellectually demanding, time consuming, and expensive. *Romeo v. Youngberg*, which established a constitutional right to training for the institutionalized resident, creates a constitutional tort liability for certain injuries sustained by the dually disabled client.[39] Public Law 94-142 and its state law equivalents provide individualized remedies for the multiply handicapped child, remedies that include both specialized instruction and a variety of related services.[40] Individual representation of dually disabled clients in criminal, civil commitment, and guardianship matters can pose special difficulties.

Determining the clients' goals and coping with changes in those goals are threshold problems that can require patience and reflective analysis. For example, an elderly client, institutionalized for nearly three decades in a state mental hospital, asked her lawyers to obtain her release and placement in a group home. After intensive negotiation with three state and private agencies, the lawyers achieved that goal, only to encounter their client's adamant refusal to leave the hospital. The attorneys honored that change of desire, after attempting to present the choices to her, counsel her, and to arrange a trial weekend visit.

Increased public funding is needed to ensure effective representation of clients with multiple disabilities. Private attorneys may shun these clients for a host of reasons, including case complexity, lack of expertise, and the cost of multidisciplinary consultation.

The existing Protection and Advocacy systems and Legal Services Corporation program should therefore develop projects and materials to stimulate and provide effective representation in this field. Given the political climate marked by the Gramm-Rudman deficit-cutting measures,[41] this additional funding may have to come through shifts in priorities by advocacy programs or new revenues from state and local governments. In addition to civil legal assistance needs, the dually diagnosed population has unmet needs for competent aid in the criminal justice system, both as offenders and as victims. For the numerically small but morally significant problems of individuals with dual disabilities facing the imposition of

---

(W.D.N.C. 1984) *affd and remanded*, 781 F.2d 367 (4th Cir. 1986), *cert. denied, Kirk v. Thomas S.*, 106 S.Ct. 1992 (1986); *Nathan v. Levitt*, No. 74CH 4080 (Ill. Cir. Ct., Cook Cty., Oct. 23, 1985), 9 MPDLR 428 (1985) (consent decree on placing and treating dually diagnosed patients in the least-restrictive environment).

[39]457 U.S. 307 (1982).

[40]42 U.S.C. §§ 1400–1415 (1982); *Irving Independent School District v. Tatro*, 468 U.S. 883 (1984); *Abrahamson v. Hershman*, 701 F.2d 223 (1st Cir. 1983) (residential placement, such as a group home and 24-hour educational program can be ordered under P.L. 94-142 for a child with severe retardation and autistic behaviors).

[41]Gramm–Rudman Federal Deficit Reduction Amendment, H.J. Res. 372 (enacted December 12, 1985).

capital punishment, the provision of effective and well-supported legal representation is literally a matter of life and death.

The American Association on Mental Deficiency and the Association for Retarded Citizens of the United States have each recognized the gravity of this issue and called for legal reforms "that comport with the standards of civilized Common Law nations."[42]

A new federally funded P&A system for the mentally ill should improve access to advocacy for clients with dual diagnoses. In the past, the lack of a P&A system for the mentally ill, and the bifurcation in many states of advocacy programs for the mentally disabled along developmental disability and mental health lines, reduced the chance of such clients finding or being accepted for service. The Protection and Advocacy for Mentally Ill Individuals Act, signed into law on May 23, 1986, will help to remedy that problem.[43]

Under Public Law 99-319, Congress has authorized over $10 million a year to implement expanded advocacy programs. That money will go to developmental disabilities P&A systems for the purpose of advocating for the rights of persons in facilities for the mentally ill, including institutions, nursing homes, group homes, and board-and-care homes. These additional advocacy resources for the mentally disabled will ease, to some degree, allocation of resource pressures and make aid available to MR/MH clients in mental hospitals. Because the act defines an "eligible system" as the existing P&A program for the developmentally disabled, a unified system will minimize the problem of dually diagnosed clients being shunted between advocacy systems. This consolidation can also help third-parties to make appropriate referrals for advocacy services.

## Recruiting and Training Good Advocates for Hard-to-Serve Clients

Clients with dual disabilities, their families, and friends cannot rely on publicly funded advocacy programs to meet all their advocacy needs. Current and future practitioners will continue to avoid MR/MH clients unless they have supports, training, and incentives to undertake such representation. Universities, with law schools taking a leadership role, should develop regional advocacy and training centers that would provide training materials, workshops, and manuals. The missions of these centers would be sixfold:

1. To promote research on effective modes of advocacy for dually diagnosed clients.

---

[42]American Association on Mental Deficiency, Council Resolution (adopted January 11, 1986); Walton, Group assails executions of retarded inmates, *Kansas City Star*, January 12, 1986, p. 24A, col. 1.

[43]42 U.S.C. §§ 10801-10827 (1987 Pamphlet).

2. To train graduate and professional students, lawyers, providers, administrators, and officials on the rights of MR/MH clients.
3. To develop alternative dispute-resolution methods for settling interagency and intraagency conflicts over implementing these rights and providing clients with appropriate services.
4. To develop mediation assistance to gain community acceptance of community-based residences for dually diagnosed clients.
5. To provide interdisciplinary consultation and technical assistance in devising appropriate remedies for the individual and systemic legal problems of this minority.
6. To offer recognition and professional prestige for individuals who perform effective advocacy work for a hard-to-serve client population.

## Conclusion

The legal profession has only begun to map out the legal issues for clients saddled with multiple disabilities. It has done too little to entice pro bono practitioners in small and large firms or public lawyers in law enforcement offices to lend their talents to this cause. With the example of this conference, advocates should identify collaborators from many disciplines if our targets for reform and our remedies are to be selected wisely. We also need more applied research growing out of advocacy efforts, including studies on the costs and gains of particular advocacy initiatives to free clients from limbo. This freedom from limbo entails providing clients with relief from neglect, restraint, and confinement. For both the therapeutic and legal professions, it also requires replacing attitudes of rejection with patterns of acceptance. As the Maryland experience suggests, a start has been made in lifting clients with dual disabilities out of the cracks of institutions and service systems. With this national strategy conference, we can set our sights higher, mending these cracks on a national basis, and repatriating individuals with dual disabilities to their home communities so that they can live with the rest of us.

# 31
# The Dually Diagnosed Client in the Criminal Justice System

RUTH LUCKASSON

Persons with mental illness who come into contact with the criminal justice system have been and continue to be the subject of a great deal of attention. Both the popular media and scholars have long focused on the plight of mentally ill criminal defendants. In contrast, the legal problems of individuals with mental retardation who come into contact with the criminal justice system have, as a group, rarely attracted the attention of scholars.[1] Even criminal laws which on their face purport to address mental retardation often, upon examination, reveal considerations of mental illness but not of mental retardation. The individuals who are our focus here, those who have both mental retardation and mental illness, seem to have garnered even less reflection. They suffer the inattention accorded the defendants with mental retardation alone and engender none of the study for which people with mental illness are the focus. Consequently, this book is of vital importance in concentrating the efforts of leaders in the field and drawing the attention of policymakers to dually diagnosed individuals in the criminal justice system.

The reasons for the lack of attention accorded dually diagnosed defendants are varied. Primary among them must be that the individuals are not recognized and identified. It is clear that many defendants with mental retardation go undetected in the system.[2] Even the defendants who are identified as possibly having mental retardation rarely receive adequate evaluation services, and thus the complexity of their disabilities will not be explored.[3] Since the mental retardation may partially mask the mental disorder, it is not surprising that dually diagnosed individuals go unidentified. Other chapters in this book have ably documented the incidence and prevalence of dual diagnoses in several settings. From these

---

[1]But see, Ellis & Luckasson, Mentally Retarded Criminal Defendants, 53 *Geo. Washington Law Review* 414 (1985).

[2]See generally, Allen, The Retarded Offender: Unrecognized in Court and Untreated in Prison, 32 *Fed. Probation* 22 (Sept. 1968).

[3]See e.g., Ellis & Luckasson, supra n. 1, 484–90.

data, we can extrapolate that a substantial proportion of the people with mental retardation in the criminal justice system will have both diagnoses.

In this chapter, I address the historical understanding of the purported relationship between mental retardation and criminality and a modern analysis of the relationship. I then survey the legal issues for which individuals with mental retardation and mental illness may suffer special vulnerability and discuss some details of their predicament.

## Relationship Between Mental Retardation and Criminality

The original understanding of the relationship between mental retardation and criminality was that mental retardation caused criminality. Dr. Henry Goddard, a respected authority in the field of mental retardation, declared in 1915 that mentally retarded people constituted a "menace to society and civilization ... responsible in a large degree for many, if not all, of our social problems."[4] Dr. Goddard reported that 25 to 50% of *all* the people in prisons were mentally retarded.[5] This belief that mental retardation caused criminality led not only to "grotesque" discrimination[6] against individuals with mental retardation but also to their segregation and isolation in large institutions.

The revisionist view of criminality and mental retardation, popular by 1950, was that mental retardation had no relationship to crime.[7] And the extent to which mentally retarded people were involved in the criminal justice system was a function of the mental illness accompanying their mental retardation and not their mental retardation at all.

The modern analysis of the relationship of mental retardation to criminality admits of some complexity.[8] While mental retardation cannot be said to cause criminality, we may have previously both overemphasized (during the historical period) and underemphasized (during the revisionist period) some connections

---

[4]Goddard, The Possibilities of Research as Applied to the Prevention of Feeblemindedness, *Proc. of the Nat'l Conference of Charities and Corrections* 307 (1915).

[5]H. Goddard, *Feeble-Mindedness: Its Causes and Consequences* (1914). He ultimately renounced his alarmist and discriminatory views. See Goddard, Feeblemindedness: A Question of Definition, 33 *J. Psycho-Asthenics* 219, 223-27 (1928). For a review of Goddard's work and an evaluation of his influence, see S. Gould, *The Mismeasure of Man* 158-74 (1981).

[6]*City of Cleburne v. Cleburne Living Centers*, 105 S. Ct. 3249 (1985).

[7]See e.g., Biklen & Mlinarcik, Mental Retardation and Criminality: A Causal Link?, 10 *Mental Retardation and Developmental Disabilities: An Annual Review 172* (J. Wortis, ed. 1978).

[8]Edgerton, Crime, Deviance and Normalization: Reconsidered, in *Deinstitutionalization and Community Adjustment of Mentally Retarded People* 145 (R. Bruininks, C. Meyers, B. Sigford & K. Lakin eds. 1981).

between the two. One model of causation first employed in analyzing the relationship between mental illness and criminality may prove helpful on this issue. Monahan and Steadman suggest that there are three possible ways in which mental disorder may be related causally to criminality: mental disorder and criminal behavior may both be exhibited by an individual but coexist without causation; mental disorder may actually inhibit criminality in an individual, as in the case of an individual who is catatonic; and mental disorder may cause criminality, for example, in an individual whose paranoia, delusions, or irrationality lead directly to the commission of a crime.[9] This model can serve as a starting point in analyzing causation for people with mental retardation, although the irrational thinking that characterizes mental disorders is not an indicator of mental retardation.

Wilson and Herrnstein, in a recent review of the data, suggest that some of the frequently observed characteristics of people with mental retardation may be related to criminality.[10] Low intelligence, defective vocabularies, impaired ability to analyze, acquiescence in the face of perceived authority, susceptibility to individuals perceived as having high status, and attempts to avoid stigma often appear to contribute to criminal behavior. They also suggest that the average IQ of offenders is 92 and that verbal deficits seem to account for the depressed scores. It appears that criminals with lower intelligence commit different types of crimes. Forgery, embezzlement, and securities fraud are committed more frequently by criminals of higher intelligence; impulsive crimes more frequently by individuals with low intelligence; and property crimes and drug and alcohol offenses by individuals with average intelligence. Several possible explanations are offered including a suggestion that dimensions of mental retardation affect the types of crimes to which people have access, their ability to resist crime, and their ability to recognize crime. The relationship between mental retardation and criminality remains an important area for future study and analysis.

## Legal Issues

There are many issues in the criminal justice process to which dually diagnosed individuals are especially susceptible.[11] The most important issues in terms of the number of mentally disabled individuals affected are the competentence issues.

---

[9]Monahan & Steadman, Crime and Mental Disorder: An Epidemiological Approach, in 4 *Crime and Justice: An Annual Review of Research* 145 (M. Tonry & N. Morris eds. 1983).

[10]J. Wilson & R. Herrnstein, *Crime and Human Nature*, 148–172 (1985). See also, Hirschi & Hindelang, Intelligence and Delinquency: A Revisionist Review, 42 *Am. Sociological Rev.* 571 (1977).

[11]For detailed model state laws on mental health and mental retardation considerations in the criminal justice system, see American Bar Association Criminal Justice Mental Health Standards (1984) (Hereinafter ABA Mental Health Standards). The ABA Mental Health Standards were developed by task forces that included legal scholars and experts in mental retardation and mental illness. The author served as the mental retardation expert on competence issues.

These include competence to waive the Miranda right to remain silent, competence to confess to a crime,[12] competence to stand trial,[13] competence to plead guilty or agree to a plea bargain, competence to testify, and the like.

As in the case of competence issues outside the criminal area, the question of whether an individual is competent with regard to a criminal legal issue depends on several considerations. Questions concerning complexities of the task, the present ability and mental state of the individual, the information received by the individual, any outside pressures that might color voluntariness, and similar inquiries must be addressed. For each criminal legal issue, the law determining the precise specifications of the defendant's understanding must first be ascertained. Then the individual abilities and disabilities of the defendant must be measured against the requirements of the law. As in competence questions outside the criminal area, incompetence in one area or issue does not necessarily mean incompetence in another area or issue. Thus, a defendant's competence to stand trial should involve a different legal test than his competence to plead guilty.[14]

Competence to stand trial is the present ability to consult with one's lawyer with a reasonable degree of rational understanding and otherwise to assist in one's defense, and to have a rational and factual understanding of the proceedings.[15] Clearly, for many people with dual diagnoses, meeting this test will pose problems. However, the question often does not arise since many disabled individuals escape detection in the criminal justice system. The descriptions provided later will serve to illustrate this point.

The second major area involves the insanity defense or mental nonresponsibility. According to the American Bar Association, a person should not be held responsible for a crime if, at the time of the crime, and as a result of mental disease or defect, that person was "unable to appreciate the wrongfulness" of his conduct.[16] The ABA formulation makes it clear that individuals with mental

---

[12]In the mid-1800s, the Georgia Supreme Court suggested that the confessions of mentally retarded people ought to be exceptionally valuable since "experience teaches that, in point of fact, the cunning and crafty are much more likely to conceal and misrepresent the truth than those who are less gifted. It is the trite observation of all travelers that if you wish to learn the truth with respect to the health of a country, you must interrogate the children and servants about the matter." *Studstill v. State*, 7 Ga. 2, 12 (1849).

[13]Dr. Alan Stone has referred to competence to stand trial as "the most significant mental health inquiry pursued in the system of criminal law." A. Stone, *Mental Health and Law: A System in Transition* 200 (1975). Competence issues affect many more individuals than does the insanity defense but are often overlooked.

[14]See, e.g., *Sieling v. Eyman* 478 F. 2d 211, 214-15 (9th Cir. 1973) (mental illness); *United States v. Masthers*, 359 F. 2d 721, 726 n. 30 (D.C. Cir. 1976) (mental retardation).

[15]ABA Mental Health Standards 7-4.1.

[16]ABA Mental Health Standards 7-6.1. "Mental disease or defect" is defined as "impairments of mind" or "mental retardation" that substantially affected the mental or emotional processes of the defendant at the time of the alleged crime.

retardation are eligible to use the defense. However, the formulation omits the clause that would more accurately represent the effect of mental retardation. The "volitional prong," which added that as a result of the disability the defendant was unable to appreciate the wrongfulness of his conduct or *conform his conduct* to the requirements of the law, has been omitted. Thus, an individual who knows at a concrete or reflexive level that an action is "wrong" may, because of exceptional impulsivity (caused perhaps by prolonged institutionalization), exaggerated acquiescence, or other manifestations of his disability be unable to conform his conduct.

The third major issue is one that has been discussed at length by other panelists, albeit with regard to other problems of the dually diagnosed. Where can they go? What sort of habilitation and treatment can they get? Who can address their needs? How can the barriers of identification, service provision, and support be broken down?

## Individual Histories

To focus on the very human devastation that can, and often does, occur as people with mental retardation and mental illness come into contact with the criminal justice system, I summarize several cases that have come to my attention through various contacts.[17] These cases are typical in that, with individual variations, they represent what we know to be occurring and to have occurred across the country.

AA, very soon after he turned 18 and thus was legally an adult, acquiesced to the demands of his younger friends to come along while the friends participated in what was reported as a rape. He was charged with rape, while his friends were treated as delinquents. Even though AA has an IQ of about 65 and was in special education during his entire school career, he was never identified as mentally retarded at any point in the criminal justice process. AA expends a great deal of effort attempting to hide his disability through braggadocio and macho tatoos. His appointed lawyer appears to have spent very little time with him before his trial. AA was not evaluated for competence to stand trial or competence to plead guilty. On the advice of his lawyer, he pleaded guilty to rape and accepted a six-year sentence rather than take his case before a judge and jury or negotiate a more advantageous plea bargain.

AA understood little, if anything, of his entire ordeal. An alert prison teacher discovered the extent of his disability. Upon subsequent evalution, it was clear that AA had misunderstood the role of the district attorney ("he's your friend"), had misunderstood the role of his own lawyer, didn't understand whether 31 years

---

[17]The individuals will be identified by letters and certain details will be omitted or changed to protect confidentiality. The individuals do not all come from a single state nor are their cases all from the same time period. The contributions of the individuals themselves and their friends and advocates are gratefully acknowledged.

was longer or shorter than six years, and so on. AA also seriously misunderstood the concept of criminal guilt. Based at least in part on his early training and, of course, his limited ability to analyze difficult ideas, he understood the concept of guilt only in its most basic meaning—he felt terrible about what had happened the night of the alleged crime and readily "accepted" the guilt of being there. Upon more thorough probing, however, he made clear that he did not participate and never meant to suggest to the judge that he committed the actual offense. Unfortunately, the probing did not occur at any point before sentencing and incarceration.

AA never had a competency hearing. The judge routinely accepted the guilty plea and the entire issue was resolved in less than 30 minutes. AA spent a substantial period of time in prison, often in great physical danger, before the injustice was discovered and he received a new opportunity to explain his involvement in the incident. All parties eventually agreed that he had been incompetent to stand trial the first time. At the new hearing, he was offered a very advantageous plea bargain; but the new judge, having just heard about the extent of AA's disability, did not believe that AA was competent to plead guilty even to the lesser offense. Fortunately, the judge granted a week's extension for the purpose of teaching AA the skills he needed to make a competent decision. Because of his then tremendous motivation to learn and the application of special education teaching techniques, the week proved sufficient and his plea was accepted as competent.

BB is a man in his late 20s who has an IQ of about 64. He has never attended school, is bilingual, has a substantial hearing impairment that is readily apparent on visual observation, is brain damaged, has a speech defect, and was the victim of prolonged and serious child abuse. While driving his car (he had a valid driver's license), he accidentally drove into a child on a tricycle. This dreadful scene was witnessed by the child's parent who began screaming to stop the car. Being unable to hear the screams because of his hearing impairment, BB drove on. He was apprehended and charged with a long list of serious offenses including being a habitual offender. It appeared that he was grossly overcharged and that a person without disabilities would not have been charged at all. The habitual offender charge was based on previous traffic tickets to which BB had never responded because he could not read his mail. The prosecuting attorney offered a "deal," which was no bargain since the charges had already been inflated. BB pleaded guilty, not understanding what he was doing and is serving time in prison. He is physically very slight, which, combined with his limited intellectual ability, makes him devastatingly vulnerable to other inmates.

CC, an American Indian, has an apparent IQ in the 60s and has extensive psychiatric problems. He cannot read or write. His history of mental difficulties, combined with his mental retardation, cause communication with him to be fraught with obstacles. He was charged with a gruesome crime. Unlike many mentally disabled defendants, he did receive a competency hearing. However, the expert witnesses testified that he was competent without evaluating or testing him. Despite the inherent weakness of such testimony, he was found competent.

CC "signed" a document waiving his right to appeal even though he is not literate. He went to prison where he receives no psychiatric care or habilitation which might alleviate some of the effects of his disability or increase the likelihood he will succeed once he is released from prison.

Recently, DD came to my attention. He was found guilty of a serious offense after receiving no competency hearing. His mental disability is substantial. He is serving a very long prison sentence for a crime he did not commit. Fortunately, his case came to the attention of a persistent newspaper reporter who investigated the young man's plight and began to try to piece together the facts of the crime. One of the things that immediately became apparent was that DD could describe and identify the actual perpetrators. As a result of the reporter's ability to attract and focus the attention of the criminal justice system in a way that DD never could, a new grand jury indicted the real perpetrators. The prosecuting attorney then granted immunity to one of the perpetrators in exchange for testimony against the others, but refused to grant immunity to DD in exchange for his testimony. Even though it was DD's information that led to the arrest of the perpetrators, DD did not benefit because he was deemed to be an incompetent witness. The prosecuting attorney made the common mistake that incompetence for one issue necessarily means incompetence in all other issues.

These examples only begin to explore the complexities of the involvement of individuals with mental disabilities in the criminal justice system. But it is hoped that they will assist in focusing some of the discussion concerning dually diagnosed individuals on issues that are rarely addressed by mental retardation professionals. I would suggest two activities with which to begin efforts to help mentally disabled individuals who find themselves involved in the criminal justice system. Mental retardation professionals need to become more available to the criminal justice system as evaluators, expert witnesses, and program planners. We must be more assertive in accepting our proper role in helping the criminal justice system deal fairly with these individuals. Mental retardation and mental health professionals also need to focus more of their energies on those behaviors that cause individuals with mental disabilities to be susceptible to the criminal justice system. Of the possible futures for individuals with multiple mental disabilities, certainly unnecessary or unjustified imprisonment is one of the most horrible.

# 32
# Future Litigation Strategies

NORMAN S. ROSENBERG

It is gratifying that the task of meeting the needs of dually diagnosed people has at last reached the agendas of mental disability professionals, agencies, and the advocacy community. With research data suggesting that 25 to 50% of mentally retarded people have a coexisting mental illness, this population can no longer be ignored.

Nevertheless, in almost every state, dually diagnosed people remain unidentified, undiagnosed, and untreated. The reasons are clear: a lack of organizational or administrative focus on this group at the federal, state, or local levels; an absence of training and staff development among mental disability professionals; powerful systemic barriers—turf issues—between the mental retardation and mental health bureaucracies; and a dearth of sustained advocacy on behalf of this population.

Can litigation play a constructive role in protecting the rights of dually diagnosed people and securing services for them? It can. But it should be approached with caution, for several important reasons. Although court decrees have been extremely important in bringing about changes in the mental disability system in the last 15 years, serious questions have arisen recently about the continued usefulness of litigation as a reform strategy. System-changing cases have become exceedingly complex, protracted, and expensive. Implementation of decrees won in the landmark class actions of the 1970s has not been entirely successful. The Supreme Court has placed formidable procedural and substantive obstacles before litigants, restricting their access to the courts and limiting the scope of relief that may be granted. Finally, a wave of judicial and economic conservatism has reduced the opportunity to expand individual rights and generate major new programs, at least for the foreseeable future.

At the same time, experience has shown that when conventional advocacy channels fall short, litigation can be a valuable tool to focus attention on unserved or underserved populations, overcome bureaucratic and administrative barriers to service, and force reallocation of existing resources to meet the needs of a target population. With these considerations in mind, I discuss several litigation opportunities on behalf of both dually diagnosed people residing in institutions and those living in the community.

## Litigation on Behalf of Institutionalized People

In more than 25 states and the District of Columbia, mentally disabled people have won decrees ordering that institutions be improved, depopulated, or closed. Yet, the fact remains that many of the 400,000 residents of the nation's public psychiatric hospitals and mental retardation facilities continue to be subjected to physical harm, neglect, segregation, idleness, and regression. For as long as institutions exist, our society has a powerful moral and ethical imperative to make them as decent and humane as possible – to pry open the lid, permitting public scrutiny and forcing accountability. What I urge in this area is litigation with a narrow focus, aimed at achieving two distinct but related objectives: first, compelling the development of community placements for people who could readily leave the institution if such placements were available; and second, improving services for severely disabled inpatients who are not at the time considered candidates for outplacement.

One of only a few cases brought specifically on behalf of a dually diagnosed person is *Thomas S. v. Morrow*,[1] aimed at the first objective. *Thomas S.* was filed in July 1982, seeking declaratory and injunctive relief under federal and state law. The lawsuit claimed that the plaintiff, then an inpatient disabled by schizophrenia and borderline mental retardation, was entitled to more appropriate treatment in a less-restrictive, community-based setting. In ruling for the plaintiff on a motion for summary judgment, district court Judge James McMillan declared that the state had denied the plaintiff his substantive due process rights under the Fourteenth Amendment to the U.S. Constitution. Addressing the rationale frequently cited by states as justification for failing to serve dually diagnosed people – that it's difficult or impossible to treat them – Judge McMillan wrote:

[The court] fails to see how that fact can excuse defendants from providing the treatment to which plaintiff is entitled. People with problems are rarely easy to deal with. If plaintiff were "normal" then he would not need the treatment the professionals say he needs. The solution to whatever behavioral problems plaintiff may have is not to place him inappropriately . . . it is to provide him with appropriate treatment.[2]

The court then pointed out that the particular interventions required by such plaintiffs varied according to the professional making the assessment, but that the basic common elements of treatment appear to be: (1) a stable environment, that is a relatively permanent placement; (2) a noninstitutional adult foster care situation that would allow the plaintiff to function as a family member, with some supervision but relatively few restrictions; (3) basic educational and vocational training; and (4) therapy and counseling.[3] The court ordered the state to develop a treatment plan including each of these elements.

The relief ordered in *Thomas S.* is not feasible in all cases. For example, when professionals agree that the severity of a resident's disability makes release from

---

[1]601 F. Supp. 1055 (1984), 781 F.2d 367 (4th Cir.), *cert. den.*, 106 S.C. 1992 (1986).

[2]See footnote 1, at 1058.

[3]See footnote 1, at 1059.

an inpatient setting inappropriate, it may be very difficult to win an order for community-based care. But even so, it is reasonable to expect that litigation will at least highlight the needs of dually diagnosed patients and generate some services to meet these needs. A good illustration is *Armstead v. Pingree*,[4] filed in 1984 on behalf of patients at Northeast Florida State Hospital. During pretrial discovery, it was learned that at least 60 to 100 of the hospital's more than 800 inpatients had secondary diagnoses of mental retardation and that the institution had not been providing habilitation services for them. Under pressure from the plaintiffs, the state is evaluating each dually diagnosed resident and has established a 16-bed transitional group home and a specialized inpatient unit to serve patients who are not now candidates for outplacement. The plaintiffs are understandably concerned that the defendants are moving too slowly to meet the needs of this group and that improved inpatient services may unnecessarily prolong confinement. Nevertheless, the litigation has produced important outcomes, identifying serious gaps in services and generating programs to fill them.

Both the *Thomas S.* and *Armstead* cases relied on federal law. State statutes and common law remedies also have litigation potential. About two-thirds of the states have enacted legislation or promulgated regulations to protect institutionalized mentally disabled people. These laws vary in scope and detail, but they generally guarantee the right to appropriate treatment and habilitation, notwithstanding the nature or severity of the disability. Most also establish the right to a safe environment, the right to privacy, the right to freedom from abuse and restraint, and the right to live in the least-restrictive environment. Unfortunately, these statutes and regulations are often honored in the breach. But individual or class injunctive litigation may be a useful tool to achieve vigorous enforcement.

A final alternative is tort litigation. Anglo-American law has traditionally recognized that it is appropriate to compensate someone who has suffered harm through another's negligence. The twentieth century has brought awareness that disputes among individuals may also involve society's interests. As a result, tort remedies have been used as a form of social engineering—a means of regulating human behavior and promoting policy change.

The use of tort law on behalf of institutionalized people has uncertain implications. Comparatively few damage actions have been brought, and we have even fewer reports of their impact. But such cases can be extremely valuable levers for change, particularly in situations involving misuse of psychoactive medication on people whose primary diagnosis is mental retardation, or when a state has knowingly failed to provide services to dually diagnosed people.

## Access to Community-Based Services

With fanfare and eloquence, decisionmakers periodically announce plans for imaginative new programs and policies to serve mentally disabled people in the community. But even a cursory look at how services are funded, organized, and

---

[4]84-96-Civ-J-12.

delivered reveals a lack of commitment to this goal at the federal, state, and local levels.[5] The absence of such commitment has been a formidable barrier to meeting the needs of dually diagnosed people.

Federal dollars, always insufficient, are diminishing. Although the 1985 Alcohol, Drug Abuse and Mental Health Block Grant contains a set-aside of over $20 million for "underserved areas and underserved populations," it has no explicit requirement that dually diagnosed people be served at all. As a result, treatment of this population is uncertain, variable, and almost always inadequate, whether the client is rich or poor, rural or urban.

Sadly, this country has never fulfilled its promise to develop a system of community-based services to meet the needs of mentally disabled people. Accordingly, litigation aimed at establishing a comprehensive service system may be the only alternative. One recent and successful example is *Arnold v. Sarn*.[6] In *Arnold*, a class of indigent mentally ill residents of Maricopa County, Arizona, sought an order compelling state and local agencies to fulfill their state-law obligations to provide a unified and cohesive system of community mental health care, including a continuum of services and treatment plans for all class members, notwithstanding the nature or severity of their disabilities.

During the nearly month-long trial, plaintiffs introduced extensive evidence about the history of treatment of chronic mental illness, the requirements and benefits of an adequate community mental health system, and the deficiencies of Maricopa County's existing services. The state court ordered the defendants to fulfill their obligations, notwithstanding their claim of insufficient resources. A related case brought on behalf of dually diagnosed persons could reach a similar result.

While cases like *Arnold* compel local and state governments to finance much-needed community care, other litigation seeks to keep barriers unrelated to funding from inhibiting the development of community services. These generally involve challenges to local zoning laws and private restrictive covenants.

Expansion of independent apartment programs and community residential facilities (CRFs) is crucial to the integration of mentally disabled people into the mainstream of society. But discrimination against mentally disabled people as neighbors has been a formidable obstacle to such expansion. While in many communities it is difficult to establish a group home for mentally ill people, it has been nearly impossible to create community living opportunities for the so-called hard-to-place population, including those with multiple impairments.

Some relief may be at hand in the wake of the U.S. Supreme Court's decision in *City of Cleburne v. Cleburne Living Centers, Inc.*[7] In *Cleburne*, the court held

---

[5]See, e.g., Comptroller General of the United States Report to Congress. *Returning the Mentally Disabled to the Community Government Needs to Do More.* Washington, DC, 1977.

[6]No. C432355 (Arizona Superior Court, Maricopa County, June 25, 1985).

[7]53 U.S.L.W. 5022 (U.S. July 1, 1985).

that a community may not use zoning laws to discriminate against mentally retarded people. In declaring Cleburne's special-use permit unconstitutional as applied, the Court found that the city's ostensible justifications for denying it were either impermissible (neighbors' fears) or unworthy of belief (concern for residents' safety). The Court wrote that "mere negative attitudes, or fear, unsubstantiated by factors which are properly cognizable in a zoning proceeding, are not permissible bases for treating a home for the mentally retarded differently from apartment houses, multiple dwellings, and the like."[8] The Court's analysis in *Cleburne* may be helpful in litigation brought by providers who are ready, willing, and able to offer a community-based alternative for dually diagnosed people.

Recently, opponents have employed other strategies in attempts to block group homes, with results as yet unknown. For example, a group of taxpayers in Greenwich, Connecticut, convinced the local tax authority to reduce assessments on property surrounding a group home for mentally ill people. They argued that the proximity of the group home deflated property values. Suit was filed in state court to reinstate the original assessments.[9] If the taxpayers of Greenwich prevail in the case, they will have struck a serious blow to the community-living movement. To date, no court has agreed that fears of diminished property values are warranted. But clearly, advocates face an important challenge in defeating actions of this kind and increasing public understanding and eliminating prejudice about mentally disabled people.

Litigation under the Education for All Handicapped Children Act (P.L. 94-142)[10] may play an important role in expanding services for dually diagnosed children. After 10 years of litigation at all levels, P.L. 94-142 remains intact— indeed, enhanced benefits have actually been achieved in selected areas.[11] The basic right under the act to an appropriate program (defined by the Supreme Court as one "reasonably calculated" to enable the child to progress and receive minimal educational benefit) has been affirmed.[12] Procedural safeguards have also been upheld, including the right to a de novo hearing in federal court after administrative remedies have been exhausted.

One of the most promising opportunities for mentally retarded children who have a coexisting mental illness is in expanding related services, particularly in the area of psychotherapy. The requirement to provide psychotherapy as an element of a free appropriate education has been in a state of legal limbo for

---

[8]See footnote 7, at 5026.

[9]*Lieberman v. Board of Tax Review for the Town of Greenwich, Connecticut*, No. CV 85 0076085.

[10]20 U.S.C. S 1401 et seq.

[11]See, for example, N.W. Rosenberg & J.B. Yohalem. The future of children's litigation. *Mental & Physical Disability Law Reporter, 10*(1 & 2), January–February and March–April (1986).

[12]*Board of Education of the Hendrick-Hudson School District v. Rowley*, 458 U.S. 176 (1982).

years. Advocates have consistently urged that, unless administered by a psychiatrist, psychotherapy is a nonmedical related service. School officials have contended it is a medical service, therefore excluded by P.L. 94-142 no matter who provides it. "Counseling" is the school's obligation, they insist, but "treatment" is not. The plaintiffs' victory in 1984 in *Irving Independent School District v. Tatro*[13] (a case in which the Supreme Court rules that a school district was required to provide clean intermittent catheterization as an element of a free appropriate education), provides important support for the proposition that health services that can be administered by nonphysicians are nonmedical related services under P.L. 94-142. Although at least one court of appeals has since endorsed this view, in *T.G. v. Board of Education of Piscataway, New Jersey*,[14] the issue is far from resolved. But assuming it will be, for the dually diagnosed child, the provision of psychotherapy may make the difference between remaining in school and being forced to leave and/or be institutionalized. In the absence of other community-based resources, P.L. 94-142 may be the most important vehicle for assuring appropriate services for dually diagnosed people—at least, for those under the age of 22.

Finally, advocacy efforts on behalf of mentally disabled children have also begun to focus on federal entitlement programs under the Social Security Act. Many thousands of handicapped children have been deprived of needed benefits by substantial cuts in funds provided by these programs and by illegal application of their regulations and procedures. Two programs offer significant potential resources for poor handicapped children: Supplemental Security Income (SSI) and Medicaid. Of these, Medicaid may be especially susceptible to reform through litigation. Medicaid is a $40-billion health-care reimbursement program. Because reimbursement rates are usually low, finding providers of mental health services for disabled children can be difficult or, in rural areas, impossible. Early Periodic Screening, Diagnosis and Treatment (EPSDT), a special program for children within the Medicaid statute, offers promise.

Unlike the general Medicaid program, EPSDT places an affirmative obligation on state governments to ensure that eligible children actually receive the services they need. Since its enactment, efforts to implement EPSDT have largely been limited to the screening and diagnosis aspects, with little attention focused on treatment. In my view, EPSDT's affirmative obligation to assure that children receive services extends to treatment as well. If a child is diagnosed as having an emotional and developmental problem, relevant treatment covered by the state's Medicaid plan must be provided. Neither a state's lack of available providers nor providers' unwillingness to serve Medicaid patients is an acceptable excuse. A court could, I believe, require a state to find qualified providers or provide the necessary services itself. A test case might address the lack of psychi-

---

[13]82 L.Ed.2d 6764 (1984).
[14]576 F. Supp. 420 (D.N.J. 1983), affirmed 738 F.2d 420 (3rd Cir. 1984).

atric services for children who are also developmentally disabled and require the state to turn to community mental health centers or other resources to develop programs for such children.

This chapter has given an overview of some litigation possibilities on behalf of dually diagnosed people. But just as this group has taxed the energy, skill, and imagination of service providers, it presents a formidable challenge for lawyers and other advocates. Litigation can play an important role in this arena, but it will not succeed without consensus among treating professionals about the needs of dually diagnosed people, and without a willingness, both on the part of these professionals and of lawyers, to view each other as allies for reform.

# 33
# Fifteen Questions: Ethical Inquiries in Mental Retardation

## H. RUTHERFORD TURNBULL, III

## Introduction: Reluctance to Do Ethical Analyses

During the last several years, parents, professionals, self-advocates, physicians, ethicists, and others have engaged in a lively and sometimes heated debate concerning the moral dimensions of treating, or not treating, newborns who have serious birth disabilities. Whatever the other merits of that debate, there has been a clear sharpening of the field's ability to address the moral issues in mental retardation. Fortunately, some of that honing has found its way into debates about the moral dimensions of the educational placement of children with herpes,[1] the use of aversive procedures for behavioral control,[2] the limitations of choice in sterilization,[3] and the use of third-party consent.[4] Notwithstanding, we are generally reluctant as a field to be constructively self-critical by asking and analyzing ethical questions about ourselves and our work. Our hesitancy can impede our work by preventing us from seeing its shortcomings and attending to them and by leaving us open to charges that we do not seek self-improvement.

For example, in the area of aversive interventions, traditionally we have only barely come to grips with the moral issues involved in those interventions, largely by creating a presumption that compliance with the legal requirements for consent and approval by human subjects review committees suffice to pass

[1]P. Guess, M. Bronicki, K. Firmender, J. Mann, M. Merrill, S. Olin-Zimmerman, P. Wanat, E. Zamarripa, & H. Turnbull. Legal and moral considerations in educating children with herpes in public school settings. *Mental Retardation, 22*(5), 257–263(1984).

[2]H. Turnbull, P. Guess, L. Backus, P. Barber, C. Fiedler, E. Helmstetter, & J. Summers. A model for analyzing the moral aspects of education and behavioral interventions: The moral aspects of aversive procedures. In P. Dokecki & R. Zaner (Eds.), *Ethics and decision-making for persons with severe handicaps: Toward an ethically relevant research agenda.* Baltimore, MD: Paul H. Brookes Publishing Company, 1985.

[3]R. Maklin & W. Gaylin. *Mental retardation and sterilization.* New York: Plenum Press, 1981.

[4]W. Gaylin & R. Maklin. *Who speaks for the child.* New York: Plenum Press, 1982.

on the moral rightness or wrongness of an aversive intervention.[5] Recently, my colleagues and I have undertaken a critical review and analysis of the literature on aversive interventions.[6] Building on that work, we have published an analysis of the morality of aversive interventions that extends far beyond the previous comment on their moral dimensions.[7] Allow me to summarize that work and then to use the summary as a springboard for asking questions about morality and ethics in the field of mental retardation generally.

In our critical review, we concluded that the three major aversive interventions—punishment, overcorrection, and negative reinforcement—were only partially effective:

Published studies that used punishment or overcorrection show that these procedures can, either singly or as part of treatment packages, effectively reduce a wide range of behaviors. In addition, published studies using negative reinforcement demonstrated the effectiveness of this procedure for increasing adaptive behavior. Unfortunately, effectiveness cannot be assessed fully because research that shows weak or negative results is neither published nor submitted for review for publication.

Effects appear to be durable for short follow-up periods. Most researchers, however, fail to provide follow-up data or else do so for only 12 months or less. In addition, follow-up conditions are described poorly.

Most researchers failed to provide data on generalization of effects. Of those reporting on generalization, over half found some degree of transfer of effects. Typically, generalization was measured in these instances in only a subset of possible conditions to which effects must transfer in applied settings.

Side effects were reported for all three aversive procedures. These effects appeared to be balanced in terms of being negative or positive.

Adequate experimental designs were present in a relatively small number of studies. While understandable in cases treating self injury or severe stereotyped behavior, this situation was evident, nonetheless, across all target behaviors.

We also analyzed the literature on aversive interventions from a demographic perspective, trying to determine on whom the procedures were used and in what settings. We concluded:

A summary of 61 published articles using aversive procedures with persons who are disabled shows the following major findings.

1. Of the three aversive procedures, punishment has been used most extensively, followed closely by overcorrection. It should be noted, however, that the number of published articles reporting the use of punishers decreased following the appearance of over-

---

[5]See footnote 2.

[6]D. Guess, E. Helmstetter, H. Turnbull, & S. Knowlton. *Use of aversive procedures with persons who are disabled: An historical review and critical analysis.* The Association for Persons with Severe Handicaps. Seattle Washington, 1986.

[7]See footnote 2.

correction procedures in 1973. Negative reinforcement procedures have been reported infrequently in the published literature.

2. All three aversive procedures have been reported to be used most frequently with persons described as profoundly/severely mentally retarded. Persons identified as autistic/emotionally disturbed were the second most commonly identified subject population in the literature review.

3. Stereotyped/self-stimulation and self-injurious behaviors were targeted most frequently for punishment and overcorrection procedures. Punishers were used most often for self-injurious behavior, while overcorrection was used slightly more often with stereotyped/self-stimulation behavior. A variety of other behaviors, however, were targeted for aversive procedures.

4. By far, the most frequent age range for the use of aversive procedures is between 7 and 21 years. The remaining two age categories, 0 to 6 and over 21, were almost equally divided in relation to application of aversive procedures.

5. Institutions are the most commonly identified settings for the application of aversive procedures, especially punishers. Preschool settings ranked a close second in published studies using overcorrection procedures.

In our separate analysis of the moral dimensions of aversive interventions, we concluded that, by an large, the interventions must be judged to be not moral according to philosophical and ethical criteria.

What is especially relevant to this book on the mental health needs of people who are mentally retarded is the finding in our analysis that aversive interventions have been used most often with people who are mentally retarded, emotionally disturbed, or both; with people who are preschoolers or adults; and with people who are in public residential facilities — that is, with the most vulnerable of our citizens.

## The Relevance of a Moral Analysis of Aversive Procedures

As I reread these two analyses in writing this chapter, it seemed to me that it would be proper, although perhaps not popular, for me to state in a somewhat provocative way the questions that clearly emerge from these analyses. It also seemed to me that the questions are not confined solely to aversive procedures. Rather, they are germane to behavioral psychology as well as to other disciplines, such as law, medicine, and special education. As I reviewed the other chapters in this book written by my friends and colleagues, I was even more persuaded that these questions should be put to an audience of readers who are psychologists, lawyers, physicians, special educators, parent advocates, and other interested individuals in this field. (Parenthetically, let me say that I am a professor of law and of special education and a parent advocate because my son has mental retardation and has experienced mental health problems.)

In this chapter, I state the issues in the form of questions, expecting that any other formulation would be offensive and that the question-putting would at best engage the mental and moral imaginations of the reader. Here, again, I would like to state the questions, but not without characterizing them in a different way. Let me characterize them severally:

As untested assumptions, that is, as apparent verities that we have assumed to be true but that we have not sufficiently rigorously analyzed.
As arguable disguises, that is, as masks behind which we have taken protection so that our work may go forward without being subjected to an examination that we seem to dread.
As apparent fictions, that is, as ingenious creations that we accept as facts.
As tough questions, that is, as issues that we must grapple with and seek to answer.

Finally, let me say that all of us — psychologists, lawyers, physicians, educators, and parents — should address these questions thoughtfully and nondefensively. If we do, we will find that there are good but perhaps not perfect reasons for our practices. We will understand that, in many respects, we behave in reasonable and defensible, albeit in less than ideal, ways. There always will be a gap between the reasonable and defensible on the one hand and the ideal and perfect on the other. The point of these questions is to show the gap and prod us to close it, allowing us to see the shortcomings of our work and to attend to them by self-improvement.

# The Fifteen Questions

## Question 1

The legal doctrine of third-party consent allows a mentally competent person to give consent on behalf of a mentally incompetent person. In giving or withholding consent, the surrogate for the mentally incompetent person has the legal power to require the mentally incompetent person to do, or not do, something that he or she strongly desires to do or not do. Thus, there is an unavoidable element of coercion in third-party consent. More than that, there is an irretrievable fiction about third-party consent, which is that the mentally competent person acts for the mentally incompetent person. In fact, that cannot be, since by definition, the mentally incompetent person is incapable of acting; otherwise, the mentally competent surrogate is unnecessary, irrelevant, and undesirable. The question is not whether to abolish the fiction of third-party consent, since its abolition would paralyze and prevent any action. The question instead is: How can the fiction of a third-party consent, with its inherently coercive component, be sufficiently safeguarded by procedures so that a reasonable person can be satisfied that the coercion and fiction are minimized?

*Question 2*

One way that this question has been answered is found in *Superintendent v. Saikewicz*,[8] where the Massachusetts Supreme Judicial Court held that the proper test for third-party consent is the following:

> In short, the decision in cases such as this should be that which would be made by the incompetent person, if that person were competent, but taking into account the present and future incompetency of the individual as one of the factors which would necessarily enter into the decision-making process of the competent person.

In *Saikewicz*, the issue was whether chemotherapy should be ordered for a profoundly mentally retarded 67-year-old man who had an IQ of 10 and a mental age of two years and eight months, who had contracted leukemia that invariably would be fatal, and who would not understand and, in fact, would resist chemotherapy, which itself would be effective only in delaying death and which would cause significant side-effect discomforts. The court held that, given the substitute-decisionmaker test (set out above), the chemotherapy should not be ordered over the objections of Saikewicz's guardian. The court undoubtedly did its very best to put itself in Saikewicz's position—to adopt the "shoes" test and see the treatment/nontreatment decision from his perspective. But the court's version of the test is logically flawed: How can a mentally incompetent person be competent and simultaneously take into account his or her present and future mental incompetency? Moreover, the court's version can allow the substitute decisionmaker to substitute his or her own judgment for that of the person who is mentally incompetent on the basis (pretense?) that the incompetent would have made just that very decision and the shoes test (a sort of "agency" test, where the substitute consent giver is the "agent" of the incompetent "principal") justifies the decision. How are we to know that the substitute consent giver has not simply given the consent that justifies the outcome that he or she wants? Suppose that the surrogate decides that Saikewicz has lived long enough, that delaying his death is not justified from the perspective of the cost of care and treatment that the state would incur, and that no conceivable good can come from the delayed death, either for Saikewicz or anyone else. What is to assure that the surrogate simply does not substitute his or her preconceived notion of the "right" outcome and cloak it with the fiction of a "shoes"-tested consent?

*Question 3*

In substitute-consent giving, there often is a tendency for professionals to rely on the law's maxim that fair procedures produce fair results. Thus, a review of the surrogate's decision frequently is limited to an inquiry into whether the process of obtaining consent was satisfied: Was the person with a mental disability adjudicated to be incompetent; was the surrogate duly appointed; has the surrogate's

---

[8]*Superintendent of Belchertown State Hospital v. Saikewicz*, 370 N.E. 2d 417 (Mass. 1977).

consent been informed and voluntary; has judicial approval of the proposed action been obtained? Fixation on procedure can obfuscate substance, preventing an inquiry into whether the "shoes" ("agency") standard or some other test of surrogate consent (such as a "best interest" or "trustee" standard) has been satisfied. The question must be this: Does compliance with procedural process alone suffice for obtaining and acting on direct or substitute consent and on human rights committee approval of interventions? Are we truly willing to adopt the process approach and to believe that in all cases fair procedures produce fair (or acceptable) results?

## Question 4

Many surrogate decisions are reviewed by human rights committees charged with the duty of assuring the adequacy of the consent, the defensibility of the professional intervention that is proposed to be taken, and the acceptability of the intervention as a matter of morality and ethics. Human rights committees consist of members of the same profession as the person proposing an intervention; psychologists review psychology procedures, physicians review medical procedures. The committees also consist of laypersons, including lawyers, client advocates, and sometimes ethicists. (Query: What if the ethicist is not acceptable to the client? A Protestant might not want to have an intervention proposed for him or her judged by the moral standards of a Jew, Roman Catholic, Muslim, Hindu, or atheist.) The questions that must be asked, especially but not only when the proposed intervention is highly complex, experimental, research-oriented, or controversial, are these: Are the human rights committees sufficiently independent of the professions that they oversee? If not, how can they be made sufficiently independent and still capable of reaching informed judgements about the procedures? What is meant by "sufficiently independent"? Do we want independence, or are we content to have a basically self-judging professional review?

## Question 5

In our critical review of the literature on aversive interventions, my colleagues and I found many reasons to question whether aversive interventions ever should have been used on some behaviors. The behaviors were so nondangerous to the actor or others that there seemed to be good argument that any intervention, much less an aversive one, was not clearly justified. Yet there was intervention, and it was aversive. The question must be: Do the ends (habilitation or change of behavior) always justify all the means, especially where the means are aversive?

## Question 6

In our critical review of aversives, my colleagues and I examined the demographics of the use of aversive interventions. We found that the interventions are used most frequently with the people who are the most disabled, youngest, most institutionalized, and most vulnerable. We were compelled to ask a question that is essentially one of equal treatment and that goes to the heart of the status in society and in the professional–client relationship of people who are disabled: Are people who are mentally disabled treated to the maximum extent possible as nondichotomously (equally) with nondisabled people? If they are not, what does that say about how society and professionals view and value them?

## Question 7

Our analysis of the moral dimensions of aversives also pointed out the "conspiracy of success" that can plague professionals and parents. The conspiracy of success is the nearly irresistible impetus to apply any intervention that may work, simply because there is a seeming need to be successful in changing the behavior, whether or not the person who is mentally disabled wants to change that behavior. The questions that arise are these: Are all interventions truly directed by altruism and based on defensible client choices, or are they motivated by complex personal responses of professionals and parents that consist, in part, of a desire to change the behavior as well as by a need to prove that the intervention and the professional can change the behavior? Is there a "conspiracy of success"?

## Question 8

Related to and emerging from this question is another. Do professionals always act in the best interests of their clients or do they sometimes act to advance their own interests? One might well inquire whether the point of a lawsuit, the purpose of an intervention, the planning of a service, or the development of a service system always has the client's point of view and perspective as foremost in priority.

## Question 9

Particularly with respect to our analysis of the literature on aversive interventions but generally with respect to other interventions (whether medical or educational), it is germane to ask whether the theoretical construct underlying the intervention is sound. Behavioral interventions assume behavioral causes. But in the case of many behaviors, there may be other etiologies, particularly physiological ones. Likewise, neuropharmacological interventions (drug therapies) assume biological causes. Yet there may be behavioral etiologies. The question seems to be: Does the behavioral construct or the biological construct sufficiently explain all human behavior and therefore justify sole or primary reliance on behavioral or neuropharmacological interventions? Is human behavior so simply explained that human interventions can be simply prescribed?

## Question 10

Again, our analysis of the literature on aversive interventions found that the side effects of an intervention have been slighted in the research design and follow-up. Yet side effects of aversive interventions, as well as of other interventions, seem to be important in several respects. They can be determinants of the wisdom of the intervention (is the benefit–risk ratio favorable to the intervention?); measures of its efficacy (did the intervention result in a net benefit to the client, where it succeeded in its purpose but also did not create or exacerbate other pathologies?); and as indicators of the moral dilemmas arising from the power the therapist has over the client. The question must be: Do therapists (psychologists, physicians, or educators) give sufficient consideration to the side effects of an intervention, or is their attention too narrowly fixed on the direct and immediate effects of the intervention?

## Question 11

Again, our analysis of the literature on aversive interventions measured the interventions according to whether the interventions produced durable and generalizable learned responses/behaviors or simply temporary and situation-specific responses. Because we found that the interventions did not uniformly produce durable and generalizable behavior, we found their efficacy to be less than optimum. The question must be: Is an intervention justified, particularly one that is aversive, risky, irreversible, or intrusive, when the learning that it causes is not durable and generalizable? That question in particular must be asked not only about aversive interventions but also about special education training in non-natural environments.

## Question 12

It is unusual for professionals to seek to determine whether their interventions have any effects on themselves. They seek primarily to discover the effects of their interventions on their clients, service delivery system, or policy choices. Yet our analysis of the literature on aversive interventions raised an issue that only a few people have addressed: What effect does an intervention have on a professional? We have noted the tendency toward "procedural decay" in the use of aversive interventions: Professionals will use the procedures more and more often and for more people and behaviors, if there is some record of prior success. They seem to acquire a touch of fanaticism: They lose sight of their goals but redouble their efforts. Simply put, the questions are these: What effect, if any, does an intervention have on the intervenor? Is a behaviorist more inclined to use increasingly aversive interventions on more clients and for more behaviors if he or she has "succeeded" in using an aversive procedure with one client for one behavior? Is a physician more likely to use drug therapy? Is a lawyer more inclined to file lawsuits? Is an advocate more inclined to seek new and specialized law after achieving one legislative victory? If so, or if not, what is the effect of the "procedural decay" process on the professional and on the client?

## Question 13

With respect to aversive interventions, we found that the American Association on Mental Deficiency (now the American Association on Mental Retardation), the Association for Retarded Citizens–United States, and the American Psychological Association all had policy positions that allow for the use of aversive interventions, with limitation and after compliance with some procedural and substantive safeguards. (In 1985, ARC-US by its delegate body at the national convention adopted a resolution calling for a halt to the use of painful aversives.) The Association for Persons with Severe Handicaps (TASH) has called for an end to the use of aversives and the American Association on Mental Deficiency (now AAMR) in 1987 adopted similar resolutions. The questions must be these: Does the approval of an intervention by a professional or parent–advocacy organization suffice to condone the intervention? Do professionals and parents hide behind these policy statements? Do the organizations take professionals and parents off the hook, relieving them of responsibility to make a decision about the efficacy of the intervention and its moral and ethical rightness or wrongness? Have the organizations intended to do this? Have these resolutions been adopted? Is it time to reexamine the organizations' policies?

*Question 14*

Again, our analysis of the demographics of aversive interventions is instructive, as are our readings about the morality and ethics of any intervention. To restate, we found, with respect to aversive interventions, that they were used most often with preschoolers, persons in institutions, and persons with severe or multiple disabilities, that is, with persons who are the most vulnerable. And they were sought to be justified on moral and ethical grounds. Yet, as we applied a rigorous moral analysis to the aversive procedures and as we studied the policy positions taken with respect to them by various professional and parent–advocacy organizations, it seemed clear that a situation of moral and ethical ambiguity was developing. The questions are these: Is the morality or ethics of an intervention situationally specific, depending on the nature of the client and the setting in which he or she is found? Should the morality and ethics of any intervention be situationally specific, depending on the nature of the client and setting? If it is not right to use aversive procedures (or other interventions) with a school-aged moderately disabled person, is it right to use them with preschool or adult people who are more or even less disabled and who emit the same behavior? Are we willing to accept moral relativism in our work?

*Question 15*

Finally, our analysis of the moral dimensions of aversive intervention discovered a remarkable shallowness in the literature that purported to discuss those dimensions. Particularly absent were the types of analysis that have been brought to bear in the debate whether to treat (and, if so, how to treat) newborns who have serious birth disabilities. Even in the more recent discussion about the moral and ethical dimensions of including in public schools children and employees who have Acquired Immune Deficiency Syndrome or related conditions, there is a dearth of moral analysis. And the moral analysis that attends the issue of whether and how to prevent mental retardation clearly has not been brought into the disability field with any great success, although the analysis clearly is relevant to the questions whether it is an acceptable human condition to be disabled and, by extension, whether it is acceptable to be a human with a disability. The question seems to be this: Why is there an inability or unwillingness to bring rigorous moral analysis to bear on professional interventions? That question should be asked in the context of not just aversive interventions but others as well.

## Summary

As I said at the outset, the field of mental retardation seems to be reluctant to be constructively self-critical by asking questions about ourselves and our work. Here I have ventured to ask some of those questions, risking the judgment of my colleagues that I disapprove of their activities. I ask them to read carefully the work in which I have participated at The University of Kansas (the critical analysis and review of aversive interventions, and the moral analysis of aversive interventions) and then to pass judgment about whether I am critical of their activities, and if so, how and why? In the meantime, I ask only that we all approach our work with people who are mentally retarded with an openness to listen to questions that are meant to be constructive and that can be so if taken in the spirit in which offered, which is to improve the lives of people who are mentally retarded and their families. That, for me, always has been the bottom line and always will be.

# Conclusion

## H. RUTHERFORD TURNBULL, III

This section on the legal and ethical issues consists of contributions by Dr. Elizabeth M. Boggs, a member of the governmental affairs committee of the Association for Retarded Citizens–United States and a long-time specialist on federal policy in developmental disabilities; James W. Ellis, professor of law, The University of New Mexico, a specialist in disability legal matters, particularly involving civil commitment; Ruth A. Luckasson, professor of special education and practicing attorney, The University of New Mexico, a specialist in disability legal matters, particularly involving the criminal justice system and people with mental retardation; Norman Rosenberg, the chief attorney at the Mental Health Law Center, a disabilities litigation center; Stanley Herr, professor of law at The University of Maryland where he is a practicing attorney in the law school's clinical program and specializes in disabilities law; and H. Rutherford Turnbull, III, professor of special education and law, The University of Kansas, who has written extensively on legal and ethical matters in disabilities.

Dr. Boggs quotes extensively from the 1963 report of the Presidential's Panel on Mental Retardation, particularly from the remarks of Judge Bazelon. She concurs with Judge Bazelon that, essentially, people with disabilities should be dealt with under generic, generally applicable law. Accordingly, she argues that no new federal legislation is required to address the mental needs of people who are mentally retarded. She also recommends that no new law is required concerning the functions and activities of the National Institutes of Health, but instead she urges that there be "enlightened discretion" within the administration of the NIH with respect to the research priorities of persons who are mentally retarded and experience mental health needs. Dr. Boggs recommends the modification of administrative practices and clinical approaches to persons who are mentally retarded and who experience mental health problems.

While Dr. Boggs focuses on federal law and sees no need for changes in existing federal legislation, Professor Ellis concentrates on state law and concludes that there are pressing needs for substantial reform of state law involving people with concurrent mental retardation and mental illness. He discusses the reform of the statutes of the states dealing with the admission and discharge of persons who are mentally retarded and who live in, or seek to live in, community-based programs.

He argues that placement errors are made by clinicians and administrators and that the services provided by them should be increased. Errors occur when persons who are mentally retarded and have mental health needs are inappropriately or incorrectly admitted to or discharged from residential programs. Service augmentation is required to provide more and better services for such people. Specifically, Professor Ellis argues for the adoption of the procedural rights that persons who are mentally ill have; he notes that persons who are mentally retarded generally lack the panoply of rights of people who are mentally ill. In particular, they do not have the same amount of procedural due process in transfers from one institutional facility to another, or in the securing of community placements.

Professor Ellis argues that the obtaining of community placements for persons who are mentally retarded and also have mental health problems constitutes a system of rationing of scarce resources, where persons with mental retardation and mental health problems are generally excluded from community services. If more procedural rights can be furnished to them, where the results of these rights would be to reduce the errors in placement and to augment the services available to them, then the "rationing out" of the persons who have mental retardation and mental health problems can be reduced. Ultimately, the states should seek to obtain a "zero reject rule" for adult services, similar to the zero reject rule obtained under the Education for the Handicapped Act.

Continuing the focus on state law, Professor Luckasson concentrates on a different kind of commitment—criminal commitment. She addresses seven issues having to do with the mental competence of persons who are mentally retarded and mentally ill and who become involved in the criminal justice system. These are the issues of competence to confess and waive their rights to a police warning; to stand trial; to plead guilty or engage in plea bargaining; to testify; to be found guilty; to secure a proper disposition (sentencing); and to be executed. She recommends that mental retardation professionals become involved in the criminal justice system; insist on habilitation and treatment of persons who are mentally retarded and have mental health problems and are involved in the criminal justice system; develop their own expertise on habilitation and treatment of such persons who are mentally retarded and have mental health problems and become involved in the criminal justice system. She characterizes these persons as being in great need of help but being the most overlooked and underserved.

In a shift of emphasis, Mr. Rosenberg calls attention to the opportunities for using broad-based litigation strategies to establish new rights, or implement existing rights, for people with concurrent mental retardation and mental illness. He cautions against the overuse of litigation and insists that litigation must be used with caution and sensitivity, particularly in narrowly drawn litigation for residents of institutions, where the purpose is to obtain their discharge from the institutions. He also recommends the use of litigation to establish community-based services and a comprehensive service system within the community, arguing that litigation should be devised that would require the financing of services and that also would challenge zoning laws that exclude community-based services and residents. He then draws attention to the potential of using the "related services" provisions of the Education for the Handicapped Act as a means for obtaining psychological and psychiatric services for students who are mentally retarded and experience mental health problems. Next, he discusses the potential for using the common law of tort as a means for obtaining compensation for the denial of services, having previously pointed out that the federal constitutional and statutory laws as well as state laws can be used to obtain services. Finally, he argues for the use of litigation in the federal entitlement programs, particularly Supplemental Security Insurance, Medicaid, and early periodic screening and diagnosis and treatment. His point with respect to the federal entitlement programs is that litigation should ensure that eligible persons are placed on the rolls and receive their full benefits and that it create an affirmative duty of state and local governments to offer services.

Professor Herr continues Mr. Rosenberg's theme of the use of litigation to advance the rights of dually diagnosed citizens. After reporting on several cases in which he has been involved in seeking rights within institutions and within the community, he discusses the limitations that face the organized bar in litigating on behalf of such citizens. Calling the limitations formidable, he recommends increased funding for P&As and shifts in priority setting to give great emphasis to this subpopulation; establishment of developmental disabilities advocacy centers on a regional basis with universities and law schools taking a leadership role, developing courses, clinical offerings, training materials, workshops, and manuals.

I move the discussion away from the legal issues and to 15 ethical issues that professionals, advocates, and parents need to confront in working with any citizen who has mental retardation, but particularly with those citizens who have both mental retardation and mental illness.

It is clear from the chapters in this section that Boggs would not have advocates seek new state laws and improved administrative behaviors; that Luckasson would have advocates direct their attention to an underserved population, those people with mental retardation or mental illness who have been charged or convicted of crime; that Herr would have advocates litigate with vigor for the dually diagnosed person; and that Rosenberg also would pursue community-based litigation with vigor, but not unbounded optimism. For myself, I applaud the integrated approach to law reform that these panelists take, for they seek reform both at the federal and state level by way of legislation (and, presumably, the accompanying appropriations and implementing regulations) and by way of litigation. But, as I suggested in my chapter, even after advocates solve the legal problems of how to get the dually diagnosed person into a suitable service system, the questions still remain: what do the professionals do with them, and why? It seems entirely appropriate that this book deals directly with those questions. It also may be that the rest of this book does so satisfactorily, but that is a matter that lawyers and other professionals will test over the years.

# Section VII: Service Systems Introduction

Lenore Behar and Donald Taylor

In considering the problems of delivering services to people with the dual diagnosis of mental retardation and mental illness, the manner in which services are organized into a service system is critical. According to Gettings, the organization of human service programs has become primarily a state responsibility and in most states such organization theoretically could follow two general patterns. One approach would be to organize services based on the type of assistance needed, such as day services, residential services, or supervised work programs. The second approach would be to organize services based on the characteristics of the population to be served, such as services for retarded persons and services for mentally ill persons. Both approaches are beneficial for part of the population in need; but for persons with multiple problems and multiple service needs, neither service delivery approach provides the integration and coordination of services that are needed.

Furthermore, the delivery of services to people with dual diagnoses is complicated by the fact that there are at least five different patterns of administrative organization of state-level agencies across the country. In each of these configurations, the responsible agencies seem to have sufficient problems designing, funding, and implementing programs for their "own" single diagnosis populations; the dually diagnosed become no one's responsibility. This deficiency is addressed by Chanteau, who postulates a service-based model versus a facility-based approach to services for this population. In addition, the President's Commission on Mental Health (1978) identified these problems of providing mental health services to mentally retarded persons; now some ten years later the problem, for the most part, remains unaddressed.

To begin to remedy these problems in organizing systems of service and making them responsive to clients' needs for the client who is both mentally retarded and behaviorally disturbed, the traditional systems that separately serve mentally retarded clients and behaviorally disturbed clients must be broadened in scope. Both the mental retardation and mental health service systems are based on the continuum of care concept, adhering to principles of services in the least-restrictive, most-appropriate, and most-normalized environment. However, as these separate systems, formerly more theoretical than real, have developed, it has become clear that even for their own clients with single diagnoses, the continuum of care concept must be applied flexibly. The continuum of care concept is meaningful for broad-scale planning for aggregated needs of the target population; however, on an individual client basis, moving in the logical graduations assumed in the continuum of care concept may not apply. Within either system, planning for services to an individual usually is not on the basis of a single need, for example, education, but on the basis of multiple needs, such as education, socialization, and self-sufficiency. Human needs are far too complex to all be at the same level at the same time, or to change at equal rates.

The problem of applying a continuum of care concept to an individual client is ameliorated by using flexibility in planning, so that the client may be served at different levels for different needs at the same time. Smull reported that persons with mental retardation are a heterogeneous group and the presence of mental health needs increases the complexity of the issues to be considered. The need for a diverse set of approaches to meet the mental health needs of persons with mental retardation becomes easier to understand when seen within the context of the differing capabilities and disabilities that these persons present. Thus, the need for flexibility is magnified for the dually diagnosed or multiply diagnosed client who may be bridging several service systems concurrently. An example of this complexity is addressed by White and Wood in their chapter on the dually diagnosed offender.

This flexibility seems best achieved using the concept of needs-based planning for each individual, such as that found in the service system that the state of North Carolina has implemented in response to a lawsuit on behalf of multi-handicapped, assaultive children and adolescents (*Willie M. et al. v. James B. Hunt, Jr., et al.*), described by Taylor and Behar.

Needs-based planning requires broad assessment of clients' needs and skills. For clients with two or more diagnoses or disabilities, a multidisciplinary team is essential with professionals having a broad range of assessment skills. Additionally, the merging of the two traditional service systems to have components of each available to the client requires a method of linking the systems or accessing the systems' components. One method, exemplified by the services for seriously multiply impaired, assaultive children (Willie M. programs) in North Carolina, is the lead agency model where a designated agency oversees multi-agency planning and service delivery on a client-by-client basis. A vehicle for accomplishing such a task within the lead agency structure is broadly defined case management. This type of approach has proved very effective in the Willie M. programs and in other programs across the country in both the mental retardation and mental health systems, requiring a designated case manager to have day-to-day knowledge of the client's use of services, awareness of the effectiveness of the services, and an ongoing capacity to oversee the functioning of several agencies as they provide services to individual clients.

In addition to a lead agency concept, it is also essential to the linking of service agencies/systems that professionals in these systems modify their attitudes and commitments about the kinds of clients they can or should serve. It has not been a lack of awareness on the part of professionals that has prevented clients from accessing services across several systems. Rather, it has been a lack of willingness for the mental health system to serve retarded clients and a lack of willingness of the mental retardation system to serve clients with mental illness or behavioral problems. The issues of "primary diagnosis" have historically appeared to be a method of applying a label to a difficult client that clearly defines the client as someone else's responsibility. Changing such approaches to clients is difficult, particularly when both the mental retardation and the mental health systems are stressed by insufficient resources; to enhance the willingness to take responsibility for new populations requires cross training, improved understanding, and shared responsibilities.

As such sharing of programming across client populations will increase the populations and thus the responsibilities of both, new resources will be essential. The resources required are both programmatic and financial; that is, there is a need for more clearly defined treatment and rehabilitation strategies derived from research and exemplified through model programs or demonstration programs that are then effectively evaluated.

Scheerenberger in his chapter offers another alternative via the "new" role that institutions could play with this complex population, particularly among those individuals with significant cognitive impairment, and calls for the use of innovative approaches now available.

In addition to the need for new program models and their evaluation, there is a serious need to assess alternative administrative models to determine not only the most effective and different management structure but to clarify which models work best in which kinds of states or localities.

Gettings points out that, in addition to problems in organizing the delivery systems at the state level, there are problems in the organization of federal programs to the dually diagnosed within states. The federal problems stem from the fact that the two agencies with the programmatic missions and expertise regarding the mentally retarded and mentally ill populations— that is, the Administration on Developmental Disabilities and the National Institute of Mental Health—have little control or impact on the funding of services for these populations, which is controlled by Health Care and Financing Administration, an agency that has neither the statutory mandate to serve these populations nor the programmatic expertise to develop policies for services to these populations.

It is essential that Medicaid, Medicare, and other third-party coverage for services be reviewed, particularly to consider promulgating a definition of "conditions related to mental retardation" to recognize the dually diagnosed client for purposes of ICF/MR eligibility.

Furthermore, the responsible federal agencies should provide incentive grants to encourage crossover training, interagency case collaboration, and join planning and implementation of services for dually diagnosed, similar in concept to the Child and Adolescent System of Services Program (CASSP) funded by the National Institute of Mental Health.

Federal agencies could further encourage improvements in the delivery systems by developing a consistent data base across states, using common diagnosis criteria and terminology.

Last, Dokecki and Heflinger remind us of the critical role that families play in this prevention/remediation process and draw on the use of the biosocial model and family developmental (environmental) model in demonstrating this importance.

Clearly, to address this difficult-to-serve population, complex changes are needed in organization and delivery of services across the major agencies responsible for providing mental health, mental retardation, health, vocational rehabilitation, and welfare services. To effect such changes in systems, a special focus must be given to the dually diagnosed population of mentally retarded persons with serious mental health problems.

# 34
## Service Delivery Trends: A State–Federal Policy Perspective

ROBERT M. GETTINGS

Since human services programs were first organized, we have been faced with the fundamental choice of either arranging services according to the type of assistance provided or according to the characteristics of the population to be served. From one perspective, it makes eminent sense to organize services generically, by establishing agencies with broad mandates to deliver given types of services (e.g., health care, education, recreation, and housing) to all persons requiring such assistance. However, for persons with multiple service needs that cut across the boundaries of traditional generic health, education, and social service agencies, it also makes sense to organize the service delivery system in a manner that assures continuity of services to the entire spectrum of a particular subpopulation's needs, over time.

Regardless of which of these approaches is adopted, we run the risk of "fragmentation" and "lack of coordination." If agencies are organized by type of services, the danger exists that the needs of specific subpopulations – especially those requiring cross-disciplinary interventions – will not be dealt with in a wholistic manner. Conversely, if we choose to organize services around the needs of specific categories of clients, we may achieve improved integration of services on behalf of the particular target population, but at the risk of increased duplication, inequities, and service costs.

In reality, of course, we have (and no doubt will continue to have) a human services network in which generic and specialized agencies coexist, despite the fact that interaction between elements of this loosely knit network often leave much to be desired. Not surprisingly, identified groups of clients, whose needs span two or more existing generics or specialized service delivery systems, are the most susceptible to "getting lost in the shuffle" or "falling between the cracks."

Our aim in this chapter is to explore the intersection between the mental health and the mental retardation service systems as they deal with dually diagnosed persons. However, it is important to keep in mind that the service delivery problems posed by clients who need both mental health and mental retardation services are, in reality, a manifestation of a larger societal dilemma. Whether we are dealing with retarded persons with serious emotional disorders, the transition of handicapped adolescents from school to work, or the provision of mental health services to nursing home residents, our seeming inability to build reliable bridges between major service systems lies at the heart of the problem.

The principal aim of this chapter is to examine recent organizational trends in terms of their implications for the delivery of services to mentally retarded citizens in need of mental health services. In particular, the chapter reviews the general organizational structures of service systems at the federal, state, and local levels and asks how the responsiveness of service systems are influenced by their organizational structure.

## The Impact of Organization at the Federal Level

The decision to transfer mental retardation programs out of the National Institute of Mental Health in the early 1960s has led to the separate consideration of categorical mental health and mental retardation policies at the federal level, despite the fact that (as we discuss later) the two programs are still jointly administered in half the states. To examine the impact of federal legislative and administrative policy primarily in terms of categorical programs, however, makes very little sense in the current federal–state decisionmaking environment.

Traditional categorical programs administered by the National Institute of Mental Health (NIMH) and the Administration on Developmental Disabilities (ADD) now constitutes a minuscule proportion of total federal assistance on behalf of retarded and mentally ill clients. In FY 1985, ADD grants represented roughly 1% of total federal aid to the states on behalf of all developmentally disabled persons.[1] The pattern is similar in the area of mental health, where alcohol, drug abuse, and mental health block grant aid represented less than a quarter (22%) of all federal dollars allocated to state mental health agencies in FY 1983.[2]

The Medicaid program has emerged as the principal source of federal support for mental health and developmental disabilities services at the state and local levels. In FY 1984, Medicaid payments constituted almost nine out of every ten dollars of federal support (89%) for institutional and community-based services to developmentally disabled persons.[3] The same general pattern is evident in the field of mental health, where, in FY 1983, Medicaid payments made up over half (56.4%) of federal aid to the states on behalf of mentally ill clients.[4]

This dramatic shift in the sources of federal support for both mental health and mental retardation services poses a major dilemma, since the two federal agen-

---

[1]David Braddock, *Federal spending for mental retardation and developmental disabilities*, Institute for the Study of Developmental Disabilities, University of Illinois at Chicago, July 1985.

[2]Personal communication with the staff of the National Association of State Mental Health Program Directors, Inc., October, 1985.

[3]See footnote 1.

[4]See footnote 2.

cies with programmatic missions and staff expertise (NIMH and ADD) lack any control over the major funding sources and thus have very little influence with regard to the evolution of policies at the state and local levels. Conversely, the agency that controls the lion's share of federal service dollars (HCFA) lacks a clear statutory mandate to serve mentally retarded and mentally ill persons, as well as the staff expertise to design and implement differential policies addressing the particular needs of such clients.

One glaring consequence of this yawning gap between programmatic expertise and fiscal control is the oft-criticized institutional bias of current Medicaid policy. Given the grim fiscal outlook and the possible impact on the federal budget of severing the Gordian knot that ties Medicaid long-term care support to institutional eligibility, it is far from certain that the federal government will develop, in the foreseeable future, a rational set of fiscal and administrative policies that square with modern program principles and clinical practices.

Current federal policy also illustrates both the advantages and disadvantages of relying on major social entitlement programs, such as Social Security, SSI, Medicare, and Medicaid, as the primary mechanisms for supporting services to mentally ill and developmentally disabled individuals. On the one hand, it simply is inconceivable that federal support for MH and MR services could have reached more than a fraction of their current levels had we continued to rely almost exclusively on the categorical programs that constituted the main sources of funding through the late 1960s. On the other hand, there is little doubt that the need to conform to general policies governing major social entitlement programs has impeded the accomplishment of reasonable programmatic and systemic reforms at the state and local levels. For example, increases in Social Security and SSI benefits have provided millions of retarded and emotionally disturbed clients with the wherewithal to purchase adequate food and shelter that otherwise might not be available to them. But, it also has made it a good deal more risky for a client with marginal productive skills to enter or reenter the work force, knowing he or she could lose essential sustaining benefits as a consequence.

## The Impact of State Organizational Structures

Historically, federal policy has had relatively little influence on the way in which states organize services for mentally ill and mentally retarded persons, at least compared to other human services programs (e.g., vocational rehabilitation, education of the handicapped, and maternal and child health). Consequently, each state has evolved its own idiosyncratic organizational structure for furnishing such services.

While the particulars of each state's service system are unique, it is possible to group state organizational structures into several distinct categories. Let me suggest one such typology of organizational approaches:

1. *A COMBINED mental health/mental retardation (or developmental disabilities) agency within an umbrella human services department.* In roughly one-fifth of the states (10 of 51 jurisdictions) state-level administration of mental health and mental retardation programs are jointly administered by a subunit of a multipurpose human services department. Typically, this department is charged with managing a wide range of health, welfare, and social service functions in addition to mental health and mental retardation programs.
2. *SEPARATE, coequal divisions of mental health and mental retardation (or developmental disabilities) services within the framework of an umbrella human services department.* Approximately one-third of the states (15 out of 51 jurisdictions) maintain separate administrative units for mental health and mental retardation services within an umbrella human services department.
3. *A COMBINED cabinet-level department of mental health (or mental health and developmental disabilities) that has responsibility for mental retardation programs.* Roughly one-third of the states (14 out of 51) have a separate cabinet-level department of mental health (or mental health and mental retardation).
4. *SEPARATE, coequal cabinet-level departments of mental health and mental retardation (or developmental disabilities).* Six states have cabinet-level state departments of mental retardation and/or developmental disabilities, in addition to separate, parallel departments of mental health.
5. *SEPARATE, coequal mental health and mental retardation (or developmental disabilities) agencies within another, nonumbrella department.* Six states maintain separate mental health and mental retardation (or developmental disabilities) agencies within a department of institutions, health, or social services.

Although mental health and mental retardation services are jointly administered at the state level in half of the states, the general trend has been toward greater organizational differentiation between the two programs. This trend, which as George Tarjan suggested to us in his keynote address, is the by-product of the national schism that occurred in the early 1960s. It manifests itself in a number of ways. Certainly, the structural separation of the two programs in almost two dozen states over the past 20 years is the most visible and dramatic evidence of this trend. But, even in states that maintain a unified administrative structure, the management of MR/DD programs has become a much more identifiable and distinct part of the overall organization of the MH/MR agency.

In terms of our deliberations at this conference, the most significant, but as yet unanswered, question is: To what extent do alternative organizational approaches either facilitate or impede the delivery of mental health services to mentally retarded and other developmentally disabled persons? Or, to state the question somewhat differently: Does it make a difference which of the previously mentioned organizational models a state elects to adopt?

Unfortunately, there is no systematic research that helps us to understand the impact of organizational structures on the delivery of services to dually diagnosed clients. One might hypothesize that more and better services would be available to such clients in states with unified mental health/mental retardation agencies. But, observational data do not seem to support such a conclusion. It is this observer's view that the manner in which a state chooses to juxtapose mental health and mental retardation services organizationally has little, if any, bearing on the availability or quality of the mental health services provided to mentally retarded persons. Perhaps this is a reflection of the fact that the delivery of such services has rarely been a high priority goal of state administrators of either program.

## The Impact of Local Service Delivery Arrangements

As in the case of state-level organization, the structure of local or areawide service delivery networks for mentally retarded persons has been shaped largely by historical and geopolitical factors unique to the particular state. Unlike developments in the mental health field, where the enactment of the Community Mental Health Centers legislation in the early 1960s established a national paradigm for the organization of local service systems, each state has been free to adopt an organizational structure of mental retardation services that best suits its perceived needs. As a result, there are significant variations from state to state with respect to the way in which local or areawide services are organizationally configured. It is somewhat risky to try to identify common organizational models because of the subtle but often important differences in the modus operandi of local service networks in different states. However, any typology of local/area-wide MR/DD service systems would probably include at least some of the following approaches:

1. *Combined mental health/mental retardation (or developmental disabilities) catchment areas with administrative responsibility vested in a SINGLE community (usually a countywide or multicounty) agency or board.* Examples of states where this model is operational include Vermont, Virginia, Michigan, and Pennsylvania.
2. *Contiguous mental health and mental retardation (or developmental disabilities) catchment areas with separate, coequal community administering agencies.* New Hampshire and Wisconsin (at least in some counties) are examples of such states.
3. *Noncontiguous mental health and mental retardation (or developmental disabilities) catchment areas with separate, coequal community administrative agencies or boards.* Colorado and Missouri would be examples of states where this model exists.
4. *Integrated regional or area administrative offices of a unified state mental health (or mental health and mental retardation) agency, staffed by state employees, who are responsible for coordinating services to both target populations (i.e., MR and MH).* One basic difference between this model and the preceding approaches is that the regional or area office is an appendage of the state agency, rather than a unit of county/city government or a nonprofit

entity. Illinois and Massachusetts are illustrations of states that operate under this mode.

5. *Integrated human services catchment areas, staffed by state employees, where mental health and mental retardation (or developmental disabilities) are just two of a variety of program functions.* Florida probably has the most decentralized, integrated system of managing human services programs.

6. *Specialized regional or area administrative offices of the state mental retardation (or developmental disabilities) agency.* This type of arrangement has gained popularity in states where the number of vendorized community day and residential programs has grown rapidly and, consequently, the need for decentralized administration has become more apparent. Examples of this model can be found in Arizona, Maine, and New York.

7. *Categorical regional service centers, either operated by state employees or by nonprofit entities contracting with the state.* Idaho's regional child and adult development centers and Connecticut's regional mental retardation centers are two contrasting models of such state-operated entities. Certainly, the best known model of the nonprofit center approach is California's system of 21 regional centers.

8. *Direct contractual relationships between the state agency and individual MR or DD vendor agencies.* This type of arrangement is more prevalent in sparsely populated states such as Alaska, Arkansas, Delaware, New Mexico, and West Virginia.

9. *Coordination of local mental retardation (or developmental disabilities) functions through county welfare or social services agencies.* Minnesota and Utah are two states where day-to-day administrative control over community programs are delegated to the county welfare and social services agencies, respectively.

10. *Using existing state residential centers for the mentally retarded as the management hub of a network of regional day and residential services.* A number of southern states use this approach, including Alabama, Louisiana, South Carolina, Tennessee, and Texas (in certain areas of the state).

There are any number of variations of the basic models described above. For example, there are several states where, by law, local services are provided or managed through a county-based agency, but, in addition, the state MR/DD agency has delegated day-to-day management of state programs to a network of regional offices (e.g., Ohio and Pennsylvania). Moreover, alternative methods of classifying local service systems could be formulated with little difficulty. The important point to keep in mind is the rich diversity of approaches that currently characterizes local MR/DD delivery systems nationwide.

The general trend over the past 20 years has been toward the establishment of separate local and areawide mechanisms for delivering mental health and mental retardation services. Again, one can speculate that the growing separation between the two programs in local communities is a reflection of the increasing complexity of state and local service systems as well as the historic schism that has long characterized relations between the two fields. Currently, we have almost no evidence that sheds light on whether any one of the existing service delivery models is more or less efficacious with regard to the provision of mental health services to MR/DD clients. Yet clearly empirical evidence regarding the organizational factors that influence the responsiveness of service systems is vital if we are to evolve more effective and efficient systems for delivering services to dually diagnosed clients.

## Steps Toward Organizing a More Effective Service Delivery System

When a special advisory panel to the President's Committee on Mental Health examined the status of mental health services to mentally retarded persons several years ago, it concluded that, "traditionally these people [i.e., the dually diagnosed] have 'fallen through the cracks'. They have, unfortunately, been neglected by both the mental health and mental retardation systems."[5] Although nearly a decade has passed since the panel filed its report, there seems scant basis for reaching a different conclusion today.

The fundamental question remains: What steps can be taken to improve the responsiveness of existing service systems to the needs of mentally retarded clients who require mental health services? From this author's point of view, there are four basic strategies that must be pursued simultaneously. First, we must foster interagency collaboration and cooperation at the state and local levels. Second, we must assure that specialists in both mental health and mental retardation services are fully apprised of the importance of joint planning and service delivery on behalf of clients whose needs span the two service systems. Third, we must agree on common diagnostic terminology and functional responsibility for serving dually diagnosed clients, if we are to avoid having "mentally retarded clients . . . bouncing back and forth between mental health and mental retardation professionals, with neither agency offering an adequate service delivery plan to meet the client's needs."[6] And, finally, we must determine the efficacy of existing and newly formulated techniques of delivering mental health services to mentally retarded clients, in various diagnostic categories and age groupings.

Since the latter three areas will be the principal focus of other chapters in this book, let me suggest several basic considerations that should guide our efforts to improve collaboration between the two service systems at the state and local levels:

*First, while the ultimate aim is cooperation at the point of service delivery, it is essential that top management at the state and local levels is fully committed to*

---

[5]Report of the Liaison Task Panel on Mental Retardation, The President's Commission on Mental Health, February 15, 1978, p. 2007.

[6]See footnote 5.

*making interagency collaboration on behalf of dually diagnosed clients a reality.* Too often in the past, the goal of improving services to such clients has clearly been articulated, but it has not been backed up by firm commitments from state and local agency administrators.

As an initial step in this direction, state commissioners of mental health and mental retardation (or developmental disabilities) should be encouraged to establish inter (or intra) agency task forces that are broadly representative of parents and professionals who are interested and involved in serving dually diagnosed clients statewide.

The mission of such working groups should be (1) to identify specific steps that can be taken to facilitate the provision of mental health services to mentally retarded clients in need of such assistance, (2) to promote increased collaboration (e.g., joint training and problem solving) between mental health and mental retardation administrators and clinicians at the state and local levels, and (3) to develop joint strategies for assuring that dually diagnosed clients receive a comprehensive array of appropriate services in the least-restrictive setting compatible with their needs.

The National Institute of Mental Health, the Administration on Developmental Disabilities, and the Division of Maternal and Child Health could join hands to encourage such collaboration at the state and local levels by (1) supporting a national evaluation project aimed at determining the relative effectiveness of alternative administrative models for delivering mental health services to mentally retarded and other developmentally disabled clients and (2) funding a series of demonstration grants to stimulate statewide planning and implementation of service programs for dually diagnosed clients.

*Second, existing impediments to sharing financial and administrative responsibilities for serving dually diagnosed clients must be identified and removed.* Even where there is a willingness to cooperate, lack of funds and restrictions on the agencies' legal mandates often are significant roadblocks to interagency collaboration. Earmarked funding for programs serving dually diagnosed clients may be necessary in some instances; but, in many cases, a clear, unambiguous commitment to serving such clients, throughout the service system, will suffice.

One specific modification in federal policy that would be helpful is promulgation of a definition of "conditions related to mental retardation," for purposes of ICF/MR eligibility, which explicitly permits services to dually diagnosed clients, irrespective of the locus in which the client receives such habilitative service. Final regulations on this subject were recently published by the Health Care Financing Administration.[7]

---

[7]Subsequent to the presentation of this paper, HCFA issued final regulations (51 FR 19177) that permit eligible dually diagnosed clients to qualify for ICF/MR services, but deny such services to mentally ill persons without associated developmental disabilities.

# Conclusion

As the proceedings of this conference will no doubt demonstrate, the task of identifying the mental health needs of retarded citizens and organizing services to address these needs are mind boggling in scope and complexity. It is important, however, to keep in mind the human dimensions of the problems associated with serving dually diagnosed clients and proceed with all deliberate speed. We have spent too much time already ruminating about the problems. The time for concerted action is NOW.

Obviously, there is a great deal to be learned about proper methods of classifying the mental disorder of the retarded, as well as organizing effective prevention and treatment programs. But we cannot wait for our knowledge base to expand before taking steps to reform existing service delivery systems.

We are told by historians that the Wright brothers, in their initial experiments with powered flight, never flew their aircraft more than a quarter of a mile or exceeded a height of approximately 10 feet off the ground. Yet they demonstrated basic principles of aeronautics that are still used in the NASA space shuttle.

We, like the original pioneers of aviation, must be prepared to take chances if mental health services to mentally retarded clients are to be improved and expanded.

# 35
# System Issues in Meeting the Mental Health Needs of Persons with Mental Retardation

Michael W. Smull

"The mental health needs of mentally retarded persons are complex yet remain unmet" (President's Commission on Mental Health, 1978). Although this conclusion of the Liaison Task Panel on Mental Retardation of the President's Commission on Mental Health was articulated in its 1978 report, it is substantially valid today. In the intervening years, model service programs have been developed and the technology has grown substantially. Despite these strides in treatment and service delivery, anecdotal reports support a conclusion that most persons with mental retardation who have mental health needs do not receive adequate or appropriate treatment. The technology that has been developed is not being applied.

If the mental health needs of persons with mental retardation are to be met, diagnosis and treatment are not enough. The barriers to implementation of what has been learned must be identified and addressed. This chapter reviews those barriers that arise from the structure of the present service systems.

Persons with mental retardation who need mental health services are often trapped by the difference in orientation of the two service systems. Throughout much of the mental health service system, consumers are seen as persons who are responsible for their own lives with control over their own environments. The mental retardation service system perceives consumers as persons whose needs for services are lifelong in nature and whose ability to assume complete control over their environments is limited.

This can be seen as a reflection of the perception of mental health problems as illnesses and mental retardation as a condition. Historically, the psychiatric hospital, oriented toward acute care, has the expectation that it should be able to stabilize and then discharge persons. Placement after discharge is an issue for the person, not the mental health system. State psychiatric hospitals are under pressure to discharge persons who do not meet involuntary mental health admission criteria and to minimize long-term admissions in general. They rarely have the programs or personnel necessary to deal with the habilitative needs that persons with mental retardation present.

A result is great reluctance to admit persons with mental retardation unless there is an assurance of an available residential placement upon discharge. As many persons with mental retardation come to the attention of the mental health system only after the community mental retardation resources are "burned-out," the mental health system resists admission with all the clinical and administrative energy it can muster.

In the provision of outpatient psychotherapy, there is not only a lack of training but a lack of understanding of the effects of the orientation of the service systems. The mental health practitioner rarely understands the fundamental lack of control that a person with mental retardation has over his or her environment. The importance of the person–environment fit (Landesman-Dwyer, 1981; Schalock, 1985) and the possibility that the "problem" behavior or the depression may be a reflection of a lack of ability to change a poor person–environment fit is often not considered.

## Labels

The lack of desire by either the mental health or the mental retardation service system to serve persons with mental retardation who have mental health problems is reflected in the use of the label "primary diagnosis." When used with this group of persons, the issue of the primary diagnosis is typically an administrative issue masquerading as a clinical question. The intent is not to ensure the provision of appropriate services but to determine who gets "stuck" with responsibility for serving a person for whom appropriate services do not exist (Houston, 1984). The question of the "primary" diagnosis is often asked for persons with mild mental retardation who are aggressive, destructive of property, and/or engage in unacceptable sexual behavior. Neither the mental health nor the mental retardation service system feels that these are persons whom it wishes to serve (or that it has the programs to serve). The goal then becomes one of attributing the problem to a condition that is the responsibility of the other service system.

Labeling one condition as primary is useful only to the degree that it serves to focus treatment and habilitation. Where one condition (or sometimes both) is going to be ignored, the labeling serves no clinical purpose. It is a disservice to the individual when the efforts that should be devoted to treatment are devoted to demonstrating that each service system is not responsible. The real issue of a lack of appropriate services is lost in the process.

The complexities that the person and the environment present are obscured by the use of the label "dual diagnosis." Its convenience is alluring but its simplicity and lack of precise meaning (Szymanski & Grossman, 1984) obscure the diverse service needs presented by those who are given the label. When first used, the term dually-diagnosed was part of an effort to emphasize that persons with mental retardation could simultaneously experience severe mental illness. At a time when many professionals were denying that persons with mental retardation could experience any mental illness, the label had a utility. Today, it is as likely to be used for a person with mild mental retardation who has a history of antisocial behavior as for a person with moderate mental retardation who exhibits an active psychosis. While specific labels that specify the conditions present may be less convenient than the simple label of dually diagnosed, they help keep in focus the heterogeneous nature of both the services needed and the interventions required.

## The Service Continuum

As noted earlier, some of the mental health needs of persons with mental retardation are the result of a poor person–environment fit. In this context, the service continuum is often part of the problem. The concept of a continuum is appealing —a range of progressively less-restrictive services through which persons move as they develop. The reality is that most community service systems have few program models within their continuum and adults with mental retardation tend to stay at the level of service at which they entered (Bellamy, Rhodes, Bourbeau, & Mank, 1986). When a person exhibits behavior problems, the chances of movement toward a less-restrictive placement are further diminished. The irony is that it may be the restrictive environment that produces the behaviors to which the service system objects.

Movement within the service continuum is based on a developmental hierarchy that involves the expectation that skills are acquired in a particular order and that mastery of lower-level skills is a prerequisite for acquisition of higher-level skills. While this concept works well in reinforcing the understanding that persons with mental retardation continue to grow and develop, it is too often mistranslated into a "graduation" model. This model requires that specified skills be mastered or behaviors controlled before the person can move to the next level. "Level" is equated with environment within the continuum. Unfortunately, the "problem behaviors" that are seen as precluding movement may be manifestations of frustration with the environment or may reflect the behavioral norms of an isolated, devalued environment (e.g., episodic aggression in a sheltered workshop setting may not occur when the person is in a supported employment setting).

The continuum is actually a hierarchy organized by staff resources and the number of persons with disabilities who are congregated. Where individuals are served in the hierarchy depends on their perceived need for supervision and on performance in an isolated set of splinter skills. As the treatment resources are organized by the number of persons with disabilities who live together, the greater the perceived need for supervision, the greater the number of people who live together. For those persons with challenging behaviors, being with a large number of persons, especially other persons with challenging behaviors, may induce or sustain the behaviors.

Planning for a person with mental retardation often focuses on how to fit the person to the program rather than how to develop programs that match the person. Alternative conceptualizations have been developed. The service array concept (Hitzing, 1987) calls for individuals to be placed in the environment in which they can function optimally. The services necessary to support them in that environment are provided and as they master coping skills and behavioral norms, services are reduced. This perspective requires that the person be viewed from a more holistic framework than is typical of the service system. The person must be seen within a context. Behavior must be seen as a response to the environments in which the person spends time. The challenge for those who assist the individual is not to just develop programming to change behavior, but to determine the environment(s) in which the persons will be less likely to exhibit the behavior. This service system perspective on the criterion of ultimate functioning (Brown, Nietupski, & Hamre-Nietupski, 1977) provides a conceptual framework for the development of a service system that is responsive to individual need.

Planning on the individual level has been enhanced by personal futures planning (O'Brien, 1987). When used for persons with "problem behaviors," it elicits the environmental context in which the behavior occurs and focuses on how the person might like to live. As persons with mental retardation are placed in more valued environments, as their behavioral capabilities are met within the environment, and as they gain more control over their environments, the "problem behaviors" objected to may disappear rapidly.

A service system that is responsive to individual needs will not alleviate all the mental health problems that persons with mental retardation present. It will not prevent the occurrence of mental illness. It is reasonable to presume that it would substantially reduce the number of persons who exhibit behaviors that present problems for the mental health and the mental retardation service systems. It would allow the service systems to focus on meeting mental health needs rather than managing behavior.

## Conclusion

Meeting the mental health needs of persons with mental retardation requires aggressively addressing systems issues as much as it requires the application of appropriate therapies. Central to these service system issues is the lack of positive control that persons with mental retardation have over their environments.

Behaviors that have resulted in a perceived need for treatment should be examined to determine if they are expressions on the part of the individual that the environment is not meeting his or her needs. Unlike the general population, persons with mental retardation cannot change their jobs, move to a new location, or change the people with whom they live. The people with whom they spend their time, where they spend it, and how they spend it are typically matters over which persons with mental retardation have little or no choice. This lack of control over the basic aspects of life often results in passive compliance. Where the person objects to the decisions made, the only available recourse is aggression, destruction, or self-injury.

Where mental health problems exist, appropriate treatment is difficult to obtain. The technology that exists is often not applied. In part, the fault lies in a lack of training. But much of the problem lies in the orientation of the service systems and is reflected in the labels used in service provision. Members of each service system need to understand the orientation of the other. The issue of who will be "stuck" with the mentally ill/mentally retarded person needs to be changed to how can we develop services together. The heterogeneous service needs that this population presents must be recognized.

## References

Bellamy, G., Rhodes, L., Bourbeau, P., & Mank, D. (1986). Mental retardation services in sheltered workshops and day activity programs: Consumer outcomes and policy alternatives. In F. Rusch (Ed.), *Competitive employment: Service delivery models, methods, and issues.* Baltimore, MD: Paul H. Brookes Publishing Company.

Brown, L., Nietupski, J., & Hamre-Nietupski, S. (1977). The criterion of ultimate functioning and public school services for severely handicapped students. In B. Wilcox, F. Kohl, & T. Vogelsberg (Eds.), *The severely and profoundly handicapped child.* Springfield, IL: State Board of Education.

Hitzing, W. (1987). Living options for persons with severe behavior problems. In A. Donnellan & R. Raul (Eds.), *The handbook on autism.* New York: Wiley.

Houston, H. (1984). A plan designed to deliver services to the multiply mentally handicapped. In F.J. Menolascino & J.A. Stark (Eds.), *Handbook of mental illness in the mentally retarded.* New York: Plenum Press.

Landesman-Dwyer, S. (1981). Living in the community. *American Journal of Mental Deficiency, 86*(3), 223–234.

O'Brien, J. (1987). A guide to personal futures planning. In B. Wilcox and G. Thomas Bellamy (Eds.), *A comprehensive guide to the the activities catalogue: An alternative curriculum for youth and adults with severe disabilities.* Baltimore, MD: Paul H. Brookes Publishing Company.

President's Commission on Mental Health. (1978). Liaison Task Panel on Mental Retardation, Volume 4, 2001–2016. Washington, DC.

Schalock, R.L. (1985). Comprehensive community services: A plea for interagency collaboration. In R.H. Bruininks & K.C. Lakin (Eds.), *Living and learning in the least restrictive environment.* Baltimore, MD: Paul H. Brookes Publishing Company.

Szymanski, L., & Grossman, H. (1984). Dual implications of "dual diagnosis." *Mental Retardation, 22*, 55–56.

# 36
# Abandoning Facility-Based Programs: Evolving Toward a Service-Based Model (The Rock Creek Foundation)

FREDERIC B. CHANTEAU

The Rock Creek Foundation has served the needs of the dually diagnosed since 1973, offering comprehensive services that include psychiatric day treatment, psychosocial vocational rehabilitation, residential services, and a full outpatient psychiatric clinic. The focus of this chapter is not these particular services but instead the evolution of our system. In terms of the process by which we are now attempting the delivery of our services, I would like to propose that given the opportunity to develop mental health services for mentally retarded individuals, we move toward what I am referring to as a "service model," and away from "facility-based programs." This is akin to an employee assistance program for mentally retarded individuals — one that would extend beyond the workplace into the home and other generic environments for the mentally retarded.

It is clear that there are some common denominators for any potentially successful model serving the dually diagnosed. First, mental health services must be integrated with ongoing rehabilitative activities; and second, they must interface with and closely consider all aspects of the mentally retarded person's life.

Fifteen years ago, Rock Creek embarked on the evolution of a community support system for dually diagnosed individuals. We developed what seemed to work with almost any resource that was available. I realize now how much this pragmatic approach continues to drive my thinking in program development. Today, we must deal with a dearth of mental health services for the mentally retarded within an environment of diminishing resources for program development, while faced with a rapidly expanding need. Any model one considers should therefore have the potential for immediate impact while maximizing the conservation of resources. It should be value- and community-based, promote normalization, have community-based vocational opportunities, and have the capacity to serve those in need of acute services as well as those in need of support services. In short, the model must be accessible, flexible, and community-based, provide an array of services, and be cost-effective. Particular resources were available in the initial stages of Rock Creek's development, which made the system possible. Unlike that time 15 years ago, the diminishing availability of financial and staff resources necessitates our exploring the integration and infiltration of mental health services into generic programs for the mentally retarded, rather than the development of specific facility-based programs for the dually diagnosed. A "service-based" model would mean that services would be individualized for clients within their existing environments, such as their home, a sheltered workshop, their job, or a developmental center. This is in contrast to a program facility defining the array of needs that it has the capacity to address. This "'service model" would necessitate the availability of the treatment resources of a community support system network. Aggressive outreach and integrating these services within available programs would avoid many of the accessibility and coordination difficulties that we have traditionally experienced with the chronically mentally ill population.

The "service model" would also address some of the basic shortcomings of facility-based programming, such as high costs, limited accessibility, and lack of flexibility. Expenditure of resources, as well as the extended time lines required for facility-based program development, could be avoided, thus providing dually diagnosed individuals with a more immediate opportunity for treatment.

Successful community-based programs for the dually diagnosed have integrated, at a minimum, psychiatric, behavioral, and rehabilitative services within a structured environment. A "service model" would make accessible psychiatric interventions such as individual, group, family, dance and movement, art, and chemotherapies in existing rehabilitative facilities. This would liberate limited resources for the development of acute care community-based services to mentally retarded people.

This approach would also avoid the potential fragmentation that can occur if a typical clinic model were employed for the delivery of the same mental health services. On-site services would also accelerate cross-training and the assimilation of mental health and mental retardation technologies by all team members involved. Flexibility of facility-based services would also be enhanced, given that it would increase the number of dually diagnosed individuals being treated in the community. A good example of a facility-based program's inflexibility is when a moderately retarded individual applies to a developmental center for admission, but because of a mild to moderate emotional overlay is excluded from that facility's program services because of its admission criteria. The availability of integrated mental health services within these environments might preclude that individual being served in a more-restrictive setting.

This "service model" is also cost effective in that it avoids the expenditure of resources, especially capital expenditures, for the development of a continuum of facility-based programs. Resources no longer exist that will allow us the luxury of a parallel-track service system for this population. The "service model" allows for the reallocation of resources toward the development of a limited number of community-based acute care facilities that would be required to address the needs of those clients whom we are not able to maintain in community-based programs.

A primary ingredient to the success of this type of model is the availability of mental health professionals trained in working with the developmentally disabled. The availability of trained professionals is the major obstacle to the successful delivery of any mental health services to this population and must be addressed quickly. The foundation's experience has shown though that if clinical skills levels are equal, a willingness to work with the population may be paramount to having knowledge of very specific techniques.

Funding is always an issue. Current funding streams exist, such as Medicaid, to support the operation of a "services model." Finally, this service system may also allow for clearer lines of fiscal, as well as programmatic, responsibilities between mental retardation and mental health administrations. Each could fund discrete activities within an integrated program environment.

In conclusion, let us keep in mind that there are no perfect solutions or models in human services; there are only working ones. It is time to begin to place our collective working knowledge increasingly into the world of those whom we are attempting to serve.

# 37
# The Lancaster County Mentally Retarded Offenders Program

DAVID L. WHITE and HUBERT WOOD

The Lancaster County Mentally Retarded Offenders (MRO) Program is the only program in the United States that has combined the services of an adult probation department and MH/MR unit to deal with the special needs of mentally retarded offenders. Since its beginning in 1980, Lancaster County MRO Program has won awards from the National Association of Counties and Pennsylvania MH/MR Service Providers Association.

Other states across the country have adopted the Lancaster County model as an ideal way to work with mentally retarded offenders. The state of Pennsylvania has recently provided funding to replicate this program in other counties. Issues to be examined include whether or not MRO programs can be effective in a large metropolitan area and whether the MRO program model, or the people operating the model, makes the difference for mentally retarded offenders. Lancaster County has recently expanded its program to begin serving juvenile offenders.

It is common for convicted persons leaving a courtroom to feel that they have met their obligation to the court. This attitude among the mentally retarded offender population allows them to fail while under probation or parole supervision. (This phenomenon is eloquently addressed also by Luckasson, Chapter 31.) It is this attitude that Lancaster County MRO Program changes for its clients.

In addition to the individual not feeling punished, he or she enters a probation/parole system where caseload numbers are high and professionals are not trained to work with clients having special disabilities. Complicating these problems is the common view that a mentally retarded offender is a nonachiever and is very difficult to manage in traditional probation and parole settings. These factors create lower expectations, which enable the retarded offenders to become irresponsible and unaccountable for their actions. Irresponsibility and a lack of accountability for mentally retarded offenders directly contribute to a recidivism rate among this population estimated at 60% nationally.

Not without blame, the community MH/MR system has often been unaware of, or uninterested in, the special needs of mentally retarded offenders. Once a retarded citizen becomes an offender, the advocate system tends to look for the criminal justice system to assume responsibility for the client and his actions. Conversely, the criminal justice system expects MR "experts" to provide more services or intervention for the offender. Workers in both the criminal justice system and the community mental health and mental retardation system often do not know how to deal effectively with the reciprocal systems or do not have time to deal with each others' systems. This results in the mentally retarded offender falling through cracks in each system and eventually receiving less than adequate services from either.

The uniqueness of the Lancaster County model is that two systems (MH/MR and criminal justice) have combined resources and professionals in order to habilitate the mentally retarded offender. The Lancaster County MRO Program began operation believing that traditional probation officer and case manager roles could be maintained. After a brief period of shuffling clients between two buildings, program staff realized that a systems gap continued to exist and that offenders were quick to use their manipulative skills to sabotage programming. By using an off-site location, somewhat separated from each parent organization, a team approach to the habilitation of the mentally retarded offender was developed. Community-based mentally retarded clients maintain a right to refuse treatment. However, because of probation or parole rules and regulations, compliance with the demands of the probation officer and case manager can be enforced. When necessary, the probation officer will approach the court for the imposition of special probation/parole conditions. Because of training offered county judges, these special conditions are usually granted, since they are recognized as a necessary step toward successful completion of probation or parole.

The Lancaster County MRO Program does little that probation officers and case managers could not do if they had a cooperative relationship and the time necessary to work together. Again, the Lancaster County MRO Program is a team of both the MH/MR and criminal justice systems. The Lancaster caseload has averaged 45 clients instead of the normal 100 to 125 client caseloads. A small caseload allows time to design and implement specific behavior plans for each client. It also allows the opportunity to see clients on a daily basis and the ability to respond immediately to crisis situations. Since all clients are seen by both team members, a crisis can be dealt with by either member of the team. This cooperative relationship and ability to discuss clients' day-to-day activities allow the project team to formulate mutually agreeable expectations of the client and continuity of response to client needs and problems. Daily client visitation allows the project team the opportunity to review the previous day's difficulties experienced by the offender. By allowing the client to discuss a variety of alternatives to his difficulties, the individual has the opportunity to eliminate the frustrations of daily living that are enhanced because of his or her mental retardation. This continuous intervention builds improved problem-solving skills for the client and improves the client's ability to make responsible decisions. Successful problem solving and decisionmaking lead to a more positive self-image.

The program emphasizes as its first priority for all clients the successful completion of probation and parole supervision. Once penetrating the criminal justice system, most mentally retarded offenders become victims within the system. This usually occurs because of the offenders' inability to meet the minimal demands of probation/parole rules and regulations. Because of his disability, the mentally retarded offender is not held accountable for his behavior by family and friends. This lack of responsibility tends to reinforce for the retarded that criminal behavior will be tolerated or overlooked. Therefore, the recommitment of crime is the usual. Additional court sentences are imposed and the client is drawn deeper into the criminal justice system. This phenomenon was not uncommon in Lancaster prior to the Lancaster County program. Numerous clients, having successfully completed their probation/parole obligation under the MRO program, are now free of involvement with the criminal justice system for the first time in 20 years of their lives. As cited previously, recidivism nationally for mentally retarded offenders is estimated at 60%. During the five years of operation of the MRO program, recidivism in Lancaster County has ranged from 3 to 5%.

The majority of offenders in the Lancaster County program are diagnosed as mildly mentally retarded and are extremely streetwise. When the program was developed, it was assumed that deinstitutionalized retarded adults would be the population served. However, most have been lifelong Lancaster County residents, protected by their parents and sheltered from many responsibilities normally handled by adults. Most of the mentally retarded offender clients have a very minimal or sporadic work history. Social services have not been used, either because of ignorance of what the services offer or inability to deal with agency demands. Also this population does not see itself as mentally retarded, but rather as a "slow learner." Data related to criminal history indicate that the Lancaster County mentally retarded offender is arrested with another individual and charged with a felony offense. The majority of offenses are property related. Most clients have spent some time in jail, usually because of lack of bail. The Lancaster County mentally retarded offender is less likely to retain private counsel and usually pleads guilty to the original offense without benefit of a plea bargain or presentence investigation.

Caseload size at any one time has averaged 40 to 50 clients. Approximately 60 clients are served per year. The treatment philosophy is a form of "reality orientation," which includes prevention, education, and supportive therapy. Mentally retarded offender clients are seen on a daily or weekly basis, depending on the stability and specific need of the client. Staff attempt to involve the family of clients in the treatment plan as much as possible. However, the finding has been that, for some clients, moving away from home and becoming independent increase the possibility of successfully completing probation and parole supervision. Responsibility is placed on the retarded offender to report for scheduled appointments and obey the rules of his or her probation and parole. Daily sessions include work orientation, social skills training, time management, budgeting and banking skills, supportive counseling, and attention to good citizenship. When improvement in these areas or other appropriate behaviors are attained, behavioral rewards, such as time off from reporting, are offered. Failure to comply with these rules results in a return to the county prison.

Clients are assisted in securing employment that is best suited for their skill level and personal interest. This is achieved through vocational testing and personal job interest evaluation. Often, disabled citizens and offenders are expected to accept any employment regardless of ability or interest in that position, which often leads to job dissatisfaction or termination. Employment leads to payment of state, federal, and local taxes, as well as fines, court costs, and restitution. Instead of being a community burden, mentally retarded offenders become assets to their community.

Many probation officers and case managers measure their personal success by the number of referrals they make for their clients. The MRO program established a different philosophy. Instead of making an immediate referral, the client needs to indicate behaviorally that he or she is interested in the service. For example, a client who is immediately referred to a vocational evaluation is less likely to succeed than a client who has learned the value of being on time, dressing appropriately, what the benefit of the evaluation will be, and that there are consequences for not completing the evaluation. The MRO program staff are knowledgeable about community services; this allows appropriate referrals to be made and leads to a high degree of success and a positive experience for the client.

Many police officers, district justices, judges, and attorneys recognize the special problems created within the criminal justice system by mentally retarded offenders, but they have no specific knowledge about how to deal with these problems. By providing continued training to members of the criminal justice system and becoming a resource to these individuals, this problem has been eliminated. Training focuses on issues such as:

Defining mental retardation
How mental illness differs from mental retardation
How Miranda advice should be read to a potential mentally retarded suspect
How a police officer can determine the possibility of mental retardation
What behaviors to expect from a mentally retarded suspect
How attorneys can serve mentally retarded clients
Should the mentally retarded offender be arrested
What behaviors a judge should expect in court from a mentally retarded defendant
How a judge can explain the mentally retarded individual's rights so that it is understood by the defendant

Because the case manager is not a member of the criminal justice system, he or she is able to consult with police prior to charges being filed against mentally retarded suspects. The case manager is able to sit with the police officer and mentally retarded suspect to see that the rights of the suspect are understood and protected. In this situation, the case manager acts as an advocate for the suspect.

The Lancaster County MRO Program has provided judges with an alternative to incarceration for mentally retarded offenders. The information provided to judges by the MRO program staff about the offender allows the judge to explain the legal system so that the offender understands what his or her involvement in the legal system means. Judges, without background information, often misinterpret a lack of understanding as a display of arrogance. Upon adjudication, offenders are placed on probation or parole not directly to the Lancaster County MRO Program, thereby avoiding the stigma associated with being mentally retarded.

The Lancaster County model has proved that with special intervention, probation and parole are effective means of providing habilitation to mentally retarded offenders. On this caseload, clients are taught that probation/parole is a privilege and that their responsibility to the court is continuous. The client does not initially view the program as pleasant or therapeutic, but comes to accept his or her status as better than incarceration. Smaller caseload size leads to extensive contact with the client and enables staff the opportunity to confront and deal with issues in an immediate fashion.

As stated previously, the recidivism rate for mentally retarded offenders in Lancaster County has ranged from 3 to 5% when compared to a national estimate of 60%. This reduction in recidivism indicates a reduction in the number of crimes this population would have committed. If fewer crimes are committed, less money needs to be spent to solve crimes and more attention can be focused on other areas. Clients who complete supervision under the Lancaster County MRO Program have learned that they will be held accountable for their actions in the future and that there are consequences for making mistakes. Probation and parole give them the opportunity to make amends to society and to change their lives so that the need to return to illegal activities is diminished. Ideally, a client leaving the MRO program is more self-confident, is employed in a job at his or her level of ability, is living independently, handles finances independently, and is more aware of his or her limitations.

To the criminal justice system, the MRO program is a cost-effective program that is successful. The cost of keeping an inmate in the Lancaster County prison is estimated to be $13,000 per year. However, the cost of a client participating in this specialized service is approximately $1,000 per year. In addition to the cost saving to the prison system, overcrowding is reduced and the prison avoids the problems often associated with the retarded offender in a prison setting.

Debate continues among criminal justice, MH/MR, and community advocates as to whether or not the mentally retarded should be arrested. The philosophy of the Lancaster County Program is that mentally retarded individuals have a right to be arrested. It is the program belief that in a situation where a "normal" offender would be arrested, a mentally retarded offender should also be arrested. Not arresting an offender in this situation simply teaches him or her that there are no consequences for their actions.

The Lancaster County model provides identification, realistic programming, goal setting, and training for all phases of the criminal justice system and provides for the habilitation of mentally retarded individuals, who become hardworking, law-abiding participants within their communities. These citizens have learned to live with their disability instead of attempting to hide from it.

# Appendix A: MRO Profile — Lancaster County, Pennsylvania.

| | September 1981 | April 1983 | December 1985 |
|---|---|---|---|
| Male | $-^a$ | $-^a$ | 83% |
| Caucasian | $-^a$ | $-^a$ | 91% |
| Single | $-^a$ | $-^a$ | 73% |
| Average age$^b$ | 23 | 25 | 26 |
| Average IQ$^c$ | 66 | 66 | 66 |
| Average highest grade completed | 10th | 9th | 10th |
| Prior MH/MR clients | 3% | 30% | 37% |
| Prior state MR institution residents | 15% | 11% | 12% |
| Dual diagnosis$^d$ | 22% | 20% | 47% |
| Living with parents | 50% | 60% | 55% |
| Unemployed at arrest | 70% | 95% | 71% |
| First offenders | 60% | 60% | 71% |
| Prior probation/parole clients | 40% | 40% | 29% |
| Most common offenses$^e$ | Arson and theft | Theft and burglary | Theft and criminal conspiracy |
| Presentence investigation ordered$^f$ | — | — | 17% |
| Average probation sentence | 31 months | 30 months | 26 months |
| Average parole sentence | 6–23 months | 6–23 months | 6–23 months |
| Felony offenses | 68% | 67% | 45% |
| Misdemeanor offenses | 32% | 33% | 55% |
| Court appearances, prior MRO$^g$ | 41 | 77 | 164 |
| Court appearances, after MRO$^g$ | 6 | 15 | 34 |
| Pre- or postcourt incarceration$^h$ | 50% | 60% | 56% |
| Recidivism$^i$ | 3% | 5% | 0% |

$^a$ Statistics on client's sex, race, marital status, and presentence investigations not kept before this date.
$^b$ Average age of clients at intake to the program.
$^c$ Full-scale IQ, as measured by the Wechsler Adult Intelligence Scale (WAIS) given just prior to client intake *or* IQ taken from available Psychological Evaluation performed within two years previously.
$^d$ Diagnosis of mild or moderate retardation combined with drug and alcohol abuse, personality disorders, antisocial behavior, or other MH diagnosis.
$^e$ Most common offenses at the time of disposition.
$^f$ Presentence investigation is a complete and total background check on a person.
$^g$ Court appearances (for commitment of a new offense or probation/parole violations — not including parole hearings, fines and costs hearings, or special condition hearings: Prior SOS is the total number of appearances by all clients before acceptance by the program. After SOS is the total number of appearances by all clients after intake to the program.
$^h$ Percentage of clients who have spent any time in jail (includes time awaiting hearing).
$^i$ Recidivism defined as recommitment of a crime during the period of probation/parole supervision.
*Note*: Developed by Hubert R. Wood and David L. White, codirectors, Office of Special Offenders Services.

# Appendix B: Eligibility and Review Cycle

| Criminal offense in Lancaster County | Arrest | Sentencing in criminal court | Police officer or investigator referral | MRO staff interview and appraisal | Psychological evaluation | MRO staffing | MRO Program or return to traditional supervision |
|---|---|---|---|---|---|---|---|
| 1. Incarceration | | PA state penitentiary | | | | | |
| 2. Incarceration | | Lancaster County prison | | | | | |

*Adjudication cycle*

PA state probation or parole

| Evaluation (1) MRO staff (2) Psychological | Preplanning for release | No MRO services |
| | | Probation/parole |
| | MRO program | MRO program |

| 3. Placed on Lancaster County probation |

*Treatment cycle*

| Evaluation (1) MRO staff (2) Psychological | MRO program |

| Probation commences | Intake interview | Unified treatment plan | Treatment individual/group and other agencies | Coordinated monitoring of client's progress |
|---|---|---|---|---|

## MRO Provides for Client

Specific referrals depending on client's needs
Personal counseling
Family counseling
Budgeting assistance
Housing assistance
Vocational testing
Job readiness
Employment counseling
Job placement
Coordination of services

## MRO Provides for Community

Training for criminal justice and social service professionals
Consultation for others requesting MRO information
Coordination of services to mentally retarded population
Prevention programs in schools and residential programs
Consultation with outside professionals concerning "potential" offenders

# 38
# Past, Present, and Future Roles for Institutional Settings in the Care of Mentally Retarded/Mentally Ill Persons

Richard C. Scheerenberger

Today, in the cyclical history of mental retardation, attention is once again being devoted to those individuals with mental retardation who also are considered to be mentally ill or emotionally disturbed. One of the service vehicles used throughout the course of history for such affected persons has been the institution, in one form or another.

## Early History

Although it is not the intent of this chapter to outline in any detail the historical development of institutional programs, it is known that institutions serving a combination of persons who are mentally retarded and/or mentally ill have existed at least from the days of the Roman Empire. In the beginning of the second century A.D., Seneca, for example, observed:

They [physicians] prescribe placing all patients in darkness without ascertaining whether the absence of light is in some cases irritating, without ascertaining whether or not this measure adds another burden to the affected head.... Rather than being themselves disposed to cure their patients, they seem to be in a state of delirium; they compared their patients to ferocious beasts whom they would subdue by the deprivation of food and by the torments of thirst. Misled without doubt by this error, they advise that patients be cruelly chained, forgetting that their limbs might be injured or broken, and that it is more suitable and much easier to restrain the sick by the hands of men than by the weights of often harmful iron. They even advise bodily violence, like the use of the whip, as if such measures could force a return to reason; such treatment is deplorable and only aggravates the patient's condition; it stains the body and limbs with blood—a sad spectacle indeed for the patient to contemplate when he regains his senses.... They have the patients fall asleep by the use of the poppy, but this provokes a drowsiness or morbid torpor instead of good sleep; they rub the patient's head with oil of rose, wild thyme, or castor oil, thus exciting the very organ which they are trying to quiet down; they use cold applications, ignorant of how often this acts as an exciting agent; often and with so little measure they use irritant clysters and by means of these more or less acid injections, they produce no other results than dysentery. (Scheerenberger, 1983, p. 18)

As will be noted, Seneca identified a number of the treatment procedures that resulted in repetitive attempts to reform institutions in both Europe and the United States during the eighteenth, nineteenth, and twentieth centuries.

The nature of the treatment and programming proferred in institutional settings varied significantly throughout the years, often reflecting the prevailing concept of mental retardation and its alleged social consequences, attitudes toward the deviant and the poor in general, and the underlying philosophy guiding each facility. At any given time in the history of institutional programming, both positive and negative systems were evident, although punishment, rather than programming, was more often the case, especially in public or state-supported facilities.

During the seventeenth century, for example, it was deemed most appropriate to house persons who were mentally retarded and/or mentally ill in cages stacked row on row in unheated buildings in the belief that they did not suffer from pain, cold, or other forms of neglect. Although attitudes improved over the following centuries, even during the latter years of the nineteenth century and the early years of the twentieth century, mildly mentally retarded persons in some community and institutional settings were viewed with suspicion because of "scientific" evidence indicating their inherent proclivity for crime. Thus, various forms of seclusion, including maximum-security type cells, straitjackets, and other forms of physical restraint were used with frequency. In later years, psychosurgery, chemical restraints, and aversive conditioning were added to the disciplinarian's armamentarium. Contrary to popular opinion, however, many facilities did not and do not rely on such forms of punishment or control to resolve problems associated with self-or social management.*

## Contemporary History

The past two decades have witnessed substantial changes in both the nature of the population served and treatment emphasis. First, following World War II, many mildly retarded persons were returned to the community, as were moderately mentally retarded individuals during the 1950s and 1960s. Thus, over the past 15 years, public institutions have tended to serve predominantly a multiply handicapped, severely and profoundly mentally retarded population gradually becoming older in age. In 1985, for example, of the approximately 105,000 persons served in public residential facilities, 85% were severely or profoundly mentally retarded, 83% were over age 21, 40% had more than one handicapping condition, and 39% were considered emotionally disturbed (Scheerenberger, 1986).

As illustrated by Figures 38.1, 38.2, and 38.3, four trends are clearly evident (Scheerenberger, 1986, pp. 19–20):

---

*Persons interested in a more extensive history of institutional programming are referred to Wolfensberger (1969) and Scheerenberger (1983, 1987a, 1987b).

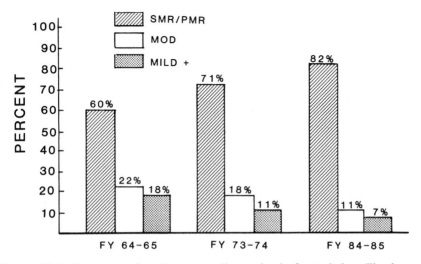

FIGURE 38.1. Percentage of residents according to level of retardation: Fiscal years 1964–1965, 1973–1974, and 1984–1985.

1. A decreasing resident population.
2. An increasing proportion of multiply handicapped, severely and profoundly mentally retarded individuals.
3. An increasing proportion of adults.
4. A diminished level of activity in terms of new admissions, readmissions, and discharges.

Second, a number of interrelated developments over the past 15 years required the abandonment of the dehumanizing techniques previously employed to control behavior. These included the widespread adoption of the principles of normalization and the developmental model, the impact of the civil rights movement,

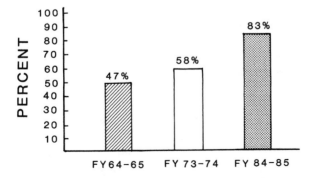

FIGURE 38.2. Percentage of residents 21 years of age or older: Fiscal years 1964–1965, 1973–1974, and 1984–1985.

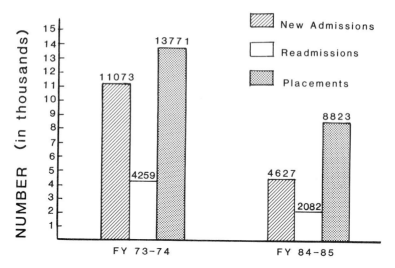

FIGURE 38.3. Number of persons newly admitted, readmitted, and placed: Fiscal years 1973–1974 and 1984–1985.

federal court decisions affecting institutional programs and procedures, and federally authorized programs such as P.L. 94-142 (The Education for All Handicapped Children Act).

As evidenced by the preceding comments, the current challenge in today's institutions is to promote and implement positive systems and approaches to assist even the most severely affected to attain sufficient social skills and personal confidence to facilitate community placement. As concerns behavior, research evidence involving both institutional and community experiences, continually report that the two primary behavioral reactions that reduce visibility for community placement or result in community failure are physical aggressiveness toward others or to property (Keys, Boroskin, & Ross, 1973; Scheerenberger, 1980).

Such undesirable behavior in institutional settings can be averted or modified only when four essential components are in place:

1. A driving philosophy that promotes greater independence among even the most severely affected in a manner consistent with the most humane of approaches.
2. A wide range of programs for all residents that not only foster skill acquisition but also take into consideration unique individual differences and interests. In many instances, much of the atypical behavior demonstrated by residents simply reflects boredom and a need for stimulation and activity. Adequate programming alone can significantly reduce such undesirable behaviorisms as stereotype movements and self-abuse.

3. A sufficient number of staff to deliver effective programming. Successful habilitation of the more severely affected requires not only a transdisciplinary approach but often a 1:1 staff–resident ratio.
4. An appropriately trained professional and paraprofessional staff, whose training is constantly upgraded. Unfortunately, staff training and development often do not receive sufficient emphasis or fiscal support; and in a day of budget cutting, both staffing levels and what little training does exist are both in jeopardy.

At the same time, there exists today a number of approaches for working with difficult-to-manage residents that are an outgrowth of research in the field of behavior modification. Two such approaches, positive in nature and respectful in concept, are described in Section IV. Briefly, "gentle teaching" (a system developed by John McGee and Frank Menolascino) has proved to be extremely effective with residents who are nonverbal and severely or profoundly mentally retarded. And, the "self-management" approach by William Gardner (also in Section IV) has proved equally beneficial with moderately and mildly mentally retarded individuals.

Many other techniques have been used with less severely affected individuals with reported success, including implosive therapy, film therapy, direct learning therapy, action therapy, music therapy, play therapy, art therapy, shadow therapy, and videotape and live modeling (Brier & Demb, 1980; Chess, 1962; Franzini, Litrownik, & Magy, 1980; Leland & Smith, 1965; Nordoff & Robbins, 1965; Ricker & Pinkard, 1964; Robertson, 1964; Ross, 1970; Roth & Barrett, 1977; Selan, 1976; Silvestri, 1977; Ucer, Goulden, & Mazzeo, 1968). These techniques are effective with children, adolescents, and adults in both group and individual therapy sessions (Chess, 1962; Szymanski, 1977).

All these approaches require greater visibility among institutional personnel. In essence, there is absolutely no need to rely on punitive, aversive measures.

## The Future Role of Institutions

As concerns the future role of institutions for those who are mentally retarded/mentally ill, there is no known answer. If the community becomes increasingly sensitive to the total needs of the developmentally disabled persons and is capable of providing the continuum of services required, then the role of institutions will continue to diminish. Yet, research has indicated that communities are often unable to provide those services desperately needed most by the current institutionalized population, including adult vocational/activity programs, behavioral therapy, and, all too often, appropriate medical attention (Scheerenberger, 1980).

Finally, a number of factors influence where a mentally retarded person (especially an adolescent or adult) will be institutionalized, including the nature or problem of the offense, availability of space, judicial predisposition, and cost. Thus, an adult, for example, may be placed in an institution for mentally retarded persons, a prison, or a mental institute even when the presenting difficulty and level of intellectual functioning may be identical or quite similar. Also, with today's emphasis on deinstitutionalization of public residential facilities for mentally retarded persons, the number of alternative institutional settings used have gradually expanded. Nursing homes, private institutions, correctional facilities, mental hospitals, and county homes all have been called on with increased frequency over the past 15 years. Sooner or later the mentally retarded/mentally ill population will have to be considered; in fact, several states, such as Virginia and New Mexico, have or are in the process of transferring emotionally troubled mentally retarded persons from their mental hospitals to their institutions. While a number of mental hospitals or institutes conduct excellent programs for mildly mentally retarded youngsters or adolescents with adjustment problems, the more severely affected, nonverbal individual with chronic aggressiveness often proves to present problems beyond staff experience and training or perceived treatment responsibilities.

In brief, the future of institutions is dependent on the future of community programming. Regardless of setting, however, each individual remains entitled to a full complement of services.

## Recommendations

1. Continued research into humane, effective treatment programs in both institutional and community environments.
2. Assurance that staffing levels in institutional settings will not only remain at their current levels but increase to meet the growing needs of residents and for facilitating community placement.
3. Increased use of positive behavioral programs and other therapeutic techniques in both institutional and community settings.
4. Substantially expanded staff development programs.
5. The term "dually diagnosed" should not be applied to individuals who are mentally retarded since it lacks precision and may further impede an individual's right to proper habilitation and community placement.

## References

Brier, N., & Demb, H. (1980). Psychotherapy with the developmentally disabled adolescent. *Developmental and Behavioral Pediatrics, 1*, 19–23.

Chess, S. (1962). Psychiatric treatment of the mentally retarded child with behavior problems. *American Journal of Orthopsychiatry, 32*, 863–869.

Franzini, L., Litrownik, A., & Magy, M. (1980). Training trainable mentally retarded adolescents in delay behavior. *Mental Retardation, 18*, 45–47.

Keys, V., Boroskin, A., & Ross, R. (1973). The revolving door in a MR hospital: A study of returns from leave. *Mental Retardation, 11*(1), 55–56.

Leland, H., & Smith, D. (1965). *Play therapy with mentally subnormal children*. New York: Grune & Stratton.

Nordoff, P., & Robbins, C. (1965). *Music therapy for handicapped children*. Blauvelt, NY: Rudolph Steiner Publications.

Richer, L., & Pinkard, C. (1964). Three approaches to group counseling involving motion pictures with mentally retarded adults. In J. Øster (Ed.), *Proceedings of the International Copenhagen Congress on the Scientific Study of Mental Retardation* (pp. 715–717). Copenhagen, Denmark: Det Berlingske Bogtrykkeri.

Robertson, M. (1964). Shadow therapy. In J. Øster (Ed.), *Proceedings of the International Copenhagen Congress of the Scientific Study of Mental Retardation* (pp. 661–664). Copenhagen, Denmark: Det Berlingske Bogtrykkeri.

Ross, D. (1970). Effect on learning of psychological attachment to a film model. *American Journal of Mental Deficiency, 74*, 701–707.

Roth, E., & Barrett, R. (1977). Parallels in art and play therapy with a disturbed retarded boy. *The Arts in Psychotherapy, 4*, 195–197.

Scheerenberger, R. (1980). *Community programs and services*. Madison, WI: National Association of Superintendents of Public Residential Facilities for the Mentally Retarded.

Scheerenberger, R. (1983). *A history of mental retardation*. Baltimore, MD: Paul H. Brookes Publishing Company.

Scheerenberger, R. (1986). *Public residential services for the mentally retarded*. Madison, WI: National Association of Superintendents of Public Residential Facilities for the Mentally Retarded.

Scheerenberger, R. (1987a). The historical development of institutional programming. In R. Kugel (Ed.), *Changing patterns in residential services for persons with mental retardation* (3rd ed.). Washington, DC: U.S. Government Printing Office.

Scheerenberger, R. (1987b). *A history of mental retardation: A quarter century of promise*. Baltimore, MD: Paul H. Brookes Publishing Company.

Selan, B. (1976). Psychotherapy with the developmentally disabled. *Health and Social Work, 1*, 73–85.

Silvestri, R. (1977). Implosive therapy treatment of emotionally disturbed retardates. *Journal of Consulting and Clinical Psychology, 45*, 14–22.

Symanski, L. (1977). Psychiatric diagnostic evaluation of mentally retarded individuals. *Journal of the American Academy of Child Psychiatry, 16*, 67–87.

Ucer, E., Goulden, G., & Mazzeo, A. (1968). Utilizing film therapy with emotionally disturbed retardates. *Mental Retardation, 6*(1), 35–38.

Wolfensberger, W. (1969). The origin and nature of our institutional models: In R. Kugel & W. Wolfensberger (Eds.), *Changing patterns in residential services for the mentally retarded* (pp. 59–177). Washington, DC: President's Committee on Mental Retardation.

# 39
# The North Carolina Willie M. Program: One Model for Services to Multiply Handicapped Children

LENORE BEHAR

Over the past 15 to 20 years, there has been a growing concern for the well-being of children among the professionals, parents, advocates, policymakers, and lawyers concerned with civil rights. There has been an increasing emphasis on deinstitutionalization, normalization, parent participation, and integration of the services of all agencies into a more systematic and comprehensive approach to the handicapped child. In comparison to earlier time periods, more positive change has taken place from the late 1960s to the present; however, given the concern and awareness that have emerged during that time period, change overall has been extremely slow.

This growing concern for the welfare of children has evolved into a major commitment to develop mainstream, community-based services, whether children are served from the perspective of mental retardation, juvenile justice, education, child welfare, or mental health systems. Although there have been common goals and common ideologies among those who care about and care for children, the separate efforts toward the apparent common goal of integrated community services have been only partially successful.

During the 1970s, major changes occurred in the area of special education or the education of handicapped children. In 1975, through the passage of significant legislation (P.L. 94-142), developmentally disabled children were guaranteed the right to a free and appropriate education. The focus on serving children in the least-restrictive setting and the emphasis on mainstreaming initially created turmoil within schools and communities, later resulting in more educational and related services and in more mainstreaming than initially seemed possible. Clearly, neither the federal nor the state funding that was needed to implement this law has been adequate, but P.L. 94-142 has represented the most significant legislative commitment to handicapped children to date. Although the services have not been sufficient to address their needs totally, this legislation has brought about a major change in thinking about the handicapped child and has brought about public awareness that handicapped children are indeed, and should be, a part of the mainstream of our society.

Only within the past five years has the federal agency responsible for mental health services, the National Institute of Mental Health, offered incentives for states to develop comprehensive and integrated planning processes for children with mental health needs, including developmentally disabled children. This new and tenuous initiative has been labeled the Child and Adolescent Service System Program (CASSP). Under the National Institute of Mental Health, the CASSP grants, totaling an extremely modest $4.7 million in fiscal year 1986–1987 are providing funds to 29 state mental health agencies: (1) to develop a focal point within a state agency for children's mental health services; (2) to stimulate a network or integrated approach across child-serving agencies to address the mental health needs of children; (3) to coordinate planning for integrated service delivery with case management/case advocacy services as the backbone; and (4) to foster a mechanism to improve technical assistance, training, and resource development capabilities at the state level (Lourie, Katz-Leavy, Kagan, & Forbes, 1984; Stockdill, 1983).

In their brief lifetime, the CASSP grants should have served to increase the focus on children with mental health needs and have fostered improved organization of planning and service delivery from the state level. These projects can serve as models for an integrated delivery system, particularly for developmentally disabled children.

In the 1980s, state governments have assumed a major role in the planning, organizing, and delivery of mental retardation and mental health services. This, in turn, has resulted in clearer policies regarding services to children. These policies have been derived from major changes in philosophy that occurred in the 1970s. These policies include commitments (1) to develop mainstream, integrated, community-based services, (2) to design services in the least-restrictive, most normalized environment that is appropriate, and (3) to include the family in the rehabilitative process.

Clearly, different states have progressed with the challenge of developing services to multiply handicapped children at different rates; in fact, there is wide discrepancy in the service systems focusing on only one disability. The Joint Commission on Mental Health of Children (1969) noted that "it is an undesirable fact that there is not a single community in this country which provides an acceptable standard of services for its mentally ill children, running a spectrum from early therapeutic intervention to social restoration in the home, in the school, and in the community" (pp. 6–7). Despite almost two decades of eloquent statements of need and the beginning of some service programs, a similar description applies to almost all communities and certainly to all states, particularly as it applies to the services to children whose needs cross more than one system.

Now that an emphasis has been placed on state agencies to develop a comprehensive, organized, and integrated service system, a clearer understanding of the barriers to implementation has evolved. A major barrier exists in the lack of priority or commitment that decisionmakers have placed on services to children and, particularly, to dually diagnosed children. Perhaps as an excuse for the lack of commitment to expanding such services for children, plans in some states have been stymied by the explanation that little is known about what is effective with these children. Admittedly, rigorous documentation of program effectiveness does not exist for many of the services considered by a consensus of professional opinion to be necessary. Certainly, further research is needed. However, even in 1969, the Joint Commission reported that "we have the knowledge and the riches to remedy many of the conditions which affect our young, yet we lack the genuine commitment to do so" (p. 7). In 1982, Knitzer similarly noted that "all the knowledge needed to diagnose and help children with serious emotional or behavioral difficulties is not available. But the ways in which mental health services are now funded, organized and delivered do not begin to reflect what we do know" (p. x).

In addition to the absence of priority placed on the development of services to dually diagnosed children, the fragmentation of all children's services represents another substantial barrier in planning, even when a commitment is attained. Most of the children to be served do not neatly divide themselves according to the way administrative agencies have been created. Many dually diagnosed children need the services of multiple agencies, including schools, child welfare agencies, vocational rehabilitative agencies, as well as mental retardation and mental health agencies for a "comprehensive" approach; yet most of the children are the responsibility of multiple agencies, each addressing a part of the children's needs.

Given the multiple needs of the child population in general and this population in particular, the challenge for the 1990s must include not only a programmatic aspect of developing a continuum of services but the challenge of organizing and coordinating the services and entitlements of many agencies.

As an example of how these concepts can be operationalized and of how such integration of services can be accomplished, the development of a well-funded, comprehensive community-based system of services is found in North Carolina, within the Division of Mental Health/Mental Retardation/Substance Abuse Services. The model service system is described in the following pages of this chapter. This complex effort represents one approach, or one model, of addressing the problems that have become the unanswered—or partially answered—challenge to meet the needs of multiply handicapped children. In this model, traditional methods of defining children's needs based on the agency that "owns" them have been ignored. Using an expansive definition, all children with serious behavior problems have been included in the service delivery network, regardless of the agency through which they have entered the service system(s). Although this approach is not necessarily the only model to addressing the needs of children, it does represent an approach that has shown promise.

A team of professionals reviewed the North Carolina system of services and reported in December 1983:

The State of North Carolina, under court order, has undertaken to do an enormously difficult task—the organization and implementation of an appropriate service program for about 1,000 of the most severely emotionally, neurologically, mentally handicapped and aggressive children in the State. In seeking to carry out this challenge, North Carolina is breaking new ground: there is no previous tradition that can be built upon; no other state has ever made such a substantial commitment of resources and staff to a group of children who typically are failed by not only mental health departments but other service systems as well; nor has any other state made a commitment to implement an integrated service delivery system to ensure that each child receives a full range of needed services in the least restrictive setting. (Knitzer, LaNeve, Pappanikou, Shore, & Steffek, 1983)

## Development of the Service System

Over the past seven years, the state of North Carolina has fostered the development of integrated systems of service in local communities for seriously emotionally, mentally, and neurologically handicapped children and adolescents who are also violent and assaultive. The integrated service system for this most difficult-to-serve population has been developed under the leadership of the Division of Mental Health/Mental Retardation/Substance Abuse Services within the Department of Human Resources as the lead agency in combination with all the child-serving agencies in the state.

The impetus for the development of these services came from the settlement of a class action lawsuit against the state, *Willie M. et al. v. James B. Hunt, Jr. et al.*, filed in 1979 in the United States Western District Court. The complaint stated that four minors, and "all others similarly situated," had been denied the appropriate treatment and education that were rightfully theirs under a series of federal and state statutes and the United States Constitution. At the time the lawsuit was filed, the four minors were in state institutions (three in training schools and one in a psychiatric hospital), further defining the class as children who "are or will be in the future involuntarily institutionalized or otherwise placed in residential programs."

Sufficient evidence was gathered in the year following the filing of the lawsuit to suggest that this particular subpopulation of children had significant unmet treatment and educational needs. Therefore, the state decided against the lengthy defense of their position and began negotiating a settlement in September 1980. The state agreed that a class of children under 18 has been denied their rights to treatment and education and thus were entitled to have these services developed for them in the least-restrictive setting. The state of North Carolina looked on this settlement as an opportunity to develop experimental systems of services and as a significant challenge.

A detailed process of identifying the population to be served was developed, with serious behavior problems being the primary consideration. Based on a thorough assessment of each child nominated by any person or agency, a determination was made as to whether or not the child met the following carefully and objectively defined criteria: (1) of being seriously emotionally, neurologically, or mentally handicapped; (2) with accompanying violent or assaultive behavior; (3) of receiving services inappropriate to his or her needs; and (4) at risk of being involuntarily institutionalized or otherwise placed in a residential program. The community mental health/mental retardation/substance abuse programs assumed responsibility as the lead agency in organizing the assessment process and eventually the service delivery process. An independent committee

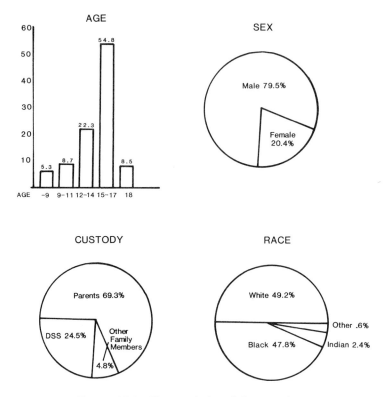

FIGURE 39.1. Characteristics of class members.

reviewed each diagnostic protocol and certified those who met the criteria listed above. Now, after seven years of an ongoing process to identify children, approximately 1,900 have been certified, with approximately 1,200 active cases at any given time.

Based on an analysis of the diagnostic materials collected on the first 1,000 cases at the time of their initial assessment, this group of children is described in Figure 39.1 and as follows:

1. *Age*: 78% of the children were age 12 through 17, with 55% age 15 through 17. Only 14% of the children identified were under age 12.
2. *Sex*: 80% were male and 20% were female.
3. *Race*: 49% were white, 48% were black, 2% were Indian, and 1% were "other."
4. *Custody*: At the time the diagnostic studies were completed for each member, 47% resided at home, 24% were in a detention facility or in a training school, and 16% were in a child care institution, a group home, or a hospital. Additionally, 5% were in foster care, and 9% were in other living arrangements.
5. *Family problems*: The large majority of families of these children (86%) had one or more family problems, which may have included family disintegration,

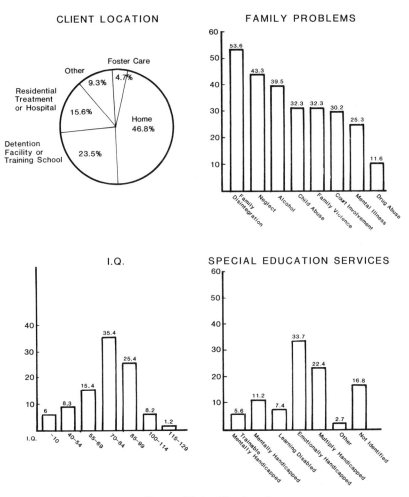

FIGURE 39.1. *(Continued)*.

child neglect, child abuse, mental illness, court involvement of the parents, or alcohol and/or drug abuse by the parents, as examples.

6. *Court involvement*: Over half the Willie M. children (51%) had been found guilty of a criminal act.
7. *Problem behaviors*: Of the 1,000 cases, more than 94% were indicated as demonstrating three or more problems on a 17-item problem behavior checklist. The most frequent problem behaviors included physical attacks without weapons, verbal aggression, uncontrollable temper tantrums, stealing, running away, physical attacks with weapons, and vandalism.
8. *Intellectual functioning*: As measured by standardized intelligence tests, 65.1% of this population were functioning below the range of 70 to 84, recog-

nizing that such measures may well be underestimations of intellectual potential.

9. *School placement*: Of the 1,000 cases, 651 (65%) attended school; of these, 56.1% were classified as seriously emotionally disturbed or multiply handicapped.

The agreement to provide services for this population of the most difficult-to-manage children in the least-restrictive, most-appropriate environment was taken very seriously and the expectation was that the majority of children could, and would, be served in community-based programs rather than in institutional settings. Based on the recognition that the mental health, mental retardation, substance abuse services system was, for the most part, well developed and organized with a strong base in local communities, the Division of Mental Health/Mental Retardation/Substance Abuse Services was designated to be the lead agency. The assumption of the lead agency role represented a significant expansion of responsibility for programs beyond the traditional position and especially broadened the concept of outreach far beyond the walls of the traditional local service system.

It was especially important to keep in focus that the needs of these multi-problem, very disturbed, and assaultive children cut across almost all agencies, and it was the role of the Division of Mental Health/Mental Retardation/Substance Abuse Services to provide leadership among all the other child-serving agencies in program development. In developing services for this population, it was recognized that the service problems of many of these children stemmed from (1) an absence of appropriately designed treatment and education programs to meet the individualized needs of these children, (2) the lack of link-ages, that is, the lack of planned, coordinated movement through the various agencies or service systems, and (3) the attitudes of professionals regarding the "treatability" of this population. A basic set of philosophical assumptions were developed that specified the characteristics of a responsive system of services for the identified population. These assumptions are as follows:

1. A complete system of services, ranging from highly restrictive settings to settings that approximate normal family living, is needed to rehabilitate these youngsters. To deal effectively with these children, the full continuum of care must be in place; discreet components whether of the more-intensive or the less-intensive variety, standing alone, will fail.
2. The system must provide for linkages among the various components within the system, as well as to services from other child-caring systems. There must be coordinated efforts between the human service providers—both public and private—educational systems, and courts.
3. There must be flexibility in funding and in decisionmaking to allow the movement of children through the system as their needs change, requiring less-restrictive or more-restrictive settings. There must be backup services and respite services available and readily accessible on a 24-hour basis.
4. There must be a management structure to the system so that shifts in funds and staff are possible, structured to allow for the movement of children dis-

cussed above; there can be no admissions criteria or admissions delayed to programmed components.

5. Children are best served close to their own communities to maximize the possibility of family involvement in services and to allow for reintegration of the child into his or her natural environment.

6. Individualized treatment and educational planning, with broadly defined case management as the backbone, are essential to the success of the service system. If a focus is maintained on the service needs of each client, the "administrative" labels such as juvenile delinquent, welfare client, mental health client, or special education student can be ignored, allowing each child broader access of services. Such needs-based planning should lead to utilization of appropriate services.

7. A "no eject/no reject" policy must be in place so that all children are served regardless of the perception of "treatability" or "nontreatability."

The development of systems of services on a statewide basis has been a large undertaking, calling for a need to reorganize service delivery patterns to bring about an integration of programs and services by *all* the child-serving agencies, with area mental health, mental retardation, substance abuse services programs as the lead agency. Services for children in North Carolina are organized, for the most part, within counties; however, the concept of area mental health, mental retardation, substance abuse services programs has brought about combinations of counties in order to provide a reasonable population base for the delivery of services. Using this approach, administrators developed the zone concept, with a zone representing a geographic unit with a substantial number of class members to support a complete system of services that was both geographically and economically feasible. By definition, a zone is a community, in the term "community based," and it has been expected that the children would be served by a continuum of care within their zone.

State funds for five zones were allocated in 1982; in 1983, the entire state, or 16 zones, were funded at a budget of $26 million per year to serve approximately 1,200 children, at an average cost of $21,700 per child served.

Each zone has developed the capacity to provide the following types of services, to be provided individually or more likely in combination, based on individual need.

1. Diagnostic and habilitation services to child and family support services.

2. In-home services to child and family as needed for support, crisis stabilization, or as a short-term alternative to other services.

3. Special education services within the local education agency and in an out-of-school setting for those clients needing a more restrictive setting.

4. Training in life skills, prevocational, or vocational preparation.

5. Residential services in small, home-type arrangements with individual families, or specialized foster care jointly with a foster care agency. The area program provides intensive training, weekly supervision, and consultation with families and 24-hour backup respite care.

6. Residential services in group living arrangements.

7. Supervised apartment living or monitored independent living for older class members ready to leave family-style living.
8. Emergency services in outpatient settings, medical and nonmedical residential settings for emergency treatment, crisis stabilization, and intensive diagnostic study.
9. Support services such as transportation for child and family, big brother/big sister programs, and recreation programs.
10. Respite services for children living with families, with foster parents, in therapeutic homes, or in group homes.
11. An integration of quality services by other agencies such as special education, protective, and probation services.
12. Last and most essential, expansive case management described in detail below.

Many of these services exist at several levels of intensity, totaling 39 program components; they are provided by a variety of public agencies or purchased from private providers. Zone plans also include components as part of the continuum, which are operated by the state, such as mental retardation centers, psychiatric hospitals, reeducation centers, or wilderness camps. The use of these out-of-zone services must include a plan agreed on by the zone and by the facility regarding admission, provision of services to the child's family, role and function of the case manager, and responsibility for discharge planning. In all out-of-zone services, active case management by the case manager employed by the area Mental Health/Mental Retardation/Substance Abuse services program is essential (1) to assess, on a monthly basis, the continued appropriateness of such placement and quality of services, (2) to develop transition and stepdown plans as the child's need for less-restrictive services emerges, (3) to assure that linkage to other essential parts of the child's ecological systems are maintained (i.e., parent(s) or guardian(s), family members, school, possible employers), and (4) to develop linkages to the adult service system if the child is approaching age 18.

The importance of maintaining these regular contacts is one of the reasons that out-of-state placements are considered to be inappropriate for most class members. The mechanism of case management is essential to assure that the appropriate services are identified, used, and coordinated across all relevant agencies and updated as needed. Because case management is provided in such an expanded manner and because this service is critical to the success of the system of services, it is described here in detail.

A case manager is assigned by the area program to each class member upon certification; each case manager is responsible for 12 to 15 cases. A "no eject/no reject" policy is in effect; each child must be served, regardless of perceived "treatability." It is the case manager's responsibility to review each diagnostic form and gather preliminary information on class members from agencies and individuals involved with the class member through personal contacts and records search, as well as from direct contacts with the class member. The case manager then summarizes all major diagnostic and habilitation issues, including a review of all strengths and deficits. Also, he or she indicates whether or not further diagnostic studies are needed and states the nature of any such evaluation. The case manager identifies the least-restrictive setting currently relevant for a client's needs. Using the concept of "needs-based" planning, services are tailor-made to the child rather than trying to find a program hole for him or her.

The case manager also schedules community habilitation planning conferences to which representatives of agencies who are, have been, or may be providing services and support are invited together with other individuals as appropriate, including the parents, parent substitutes, and the child. Some of the agencies may have legal responsibilities to the client and therefore have a significant stake in participating in service planning. The case manager should develop the habilitation plan and has responsibility to consider all relevant input gathered from record search, fact-finding, and the community habilitation planning conference. It is expected that the habilitation plan be developed and should not only involve input from other concerned agencies but should clearly state the role that each agency will play and how each agent and agencies should interact in the process. The habilitation plan should be coordinated with the education plan, which the child and his or her parents need to understand and to which they must agree.

The case manager reviews and updates the habilitation plan every 30 days. A comprehensive review is held with members of the community habilitation planning conference every 90 days. At this time, efforts and accomplishment are reviewed, and goals and strategies are reassessed and adjusted as needed.

It is also one of the case manager's responsibilities to advocate for the child, in court, in school, or in the intervention program to ensure that entitlements are granted and that the child's needs are understood.

## Indications of Effectiveness

Now, after a number of years of program development, there are several indices of the impact of such expansion and integration of services:

1. There are 75 additional children in secure settings, such as mental retardation centers, that are considered to be appropriate to their habilitation needs. This figure represents 6.3% of the Willie M. population being served out of the zone programs and in secure settings, or 0.01% of the total child population of North Carolina between the ages of 10 and 18.
2. Currently, there are approximately 1,200 certified class members and all are receiving services that they would not have received a few years ago. Well over half are receiving a complete and appropriate array of needed services; others are receiving partial services and are on their way to fully appropriate services.
3. The state training schools have not been considered appropriate placements for this population of children. Any child who becomes a class member while in a training school is to be moved to a community program within 60 days. In an 18-month period, 150 children were removed from training school, and equally as important, the tide has been turned, so to speak, and almost no class

members are sent to training schools. At this time, there are less than 30 of the most difficult children still remaining in state training schools and it appears that community-based treatment might be very risky for them.

4. As the service systems were developed, a data collection system was also put into place with the capacity to assess monthly movement of clients for most-restrictive to least-restrictive services, from a combination of many services to fewer services, and from expensive services to less-expensive services. An automated process for recording the habilitation plan has been developed, as has a monthly tracking of service utilization. Thus, on a case-by-case basis, a computerized system is available to flag cases where the habilitation plan and services are not compatible.

5. A unit cost system has been developed to cut across categorical funding by disability group.

## "Learnings" Thus Far

The most essential point to be made is that seriously behaviorally disturbed children, both those with and without retardation, *can* be served in community-based programs. Given the nature of the population in question—seriously behaviorally disturbed, assaultive children—there were initial misgivings among many professionals, decisionmakers, and citizens about whether community-based services could or should serve this population. Based on five years of experience, at this point, the response seems to be extremely positive; however, it should be understood that the North Carolina model works to the extent that (1) a wide continuum of services, many of which did not exist prior to 1980, is in place; (2) a management system is in place to keep the continuum flexible and responsive; (3) a case management system exists to develop the service plans and oversee the implementation of those plans for each client; and (4) a policy of "no eject/no reject" is in effect to ensure that no children are excluded from the system.

It is interesting to observe that the "no eject/no reject" policy does work and very difficult children can be served and do make progress. It would appear that our professional ability to predict outcomes for children, except at the very extremes, may be questionable; or possibly our tendencies to predict negative outcomes for many children result in a self-fulfilling prophecy. The concepts of least-restrictive and most-appropriate services are indeed realistic options for serving children well.

The second observation that can be made perhaps is the most obvious in the above discussion. Case management, which has been broadly defined in the North Carolina model, has been perhaps the most essential unifying factor in service delivery. Case management, in its most positive sense, has emerged as the element of planning and coordination that has held together the workings of all the agencies concerned with the child, as the energizing factor that has propelled the service plan into the reality of service delivery, as the case advocacy strength that has sustained a commitment to each child and an optimism about each child's capacity to change. The case managers have represented these strengths for the entire system of services and have kept the systems moving and honest. This type of case management appears to be a critical factor in bringing children and families into the service system, and in keeping them involved with the system and the system involved with them, as well. Most importantly, as discussed above regarding the individualized service plans, the case managers have been a strong force in designing and obtaining appropriate services for their clients. The key to the success of the case management component appears to be (1) the clearly defined roles and set of expectations for how case managers should function and (2) the administrative, fiscal, and psychological support provided to the case managers as employees of the area mental health, mental retardation, substance abuse program. Case managers cannot do their complex jobs without having a service system available; however, it would appear that the service system does not function maximally without the case manager. It should be mentioned that, initially, many clinicians responsible for the direct services to clients believed that the case managers represented threats to their relationships with their clients, and/or that they were capable of merging the case management function with the habilitation function. At this point, it appears that these staff generally do not see the case managers as threats to their role with the clients, but as people who augment and assist their functioning. Regarding the latter point, certainly some staff can and do merge these functions, but most believe that the functions are better separated.

A problem area emerged in the strong tendency to remove children from their natural environment with the belief that effective intervention for children with serious problems can only be accomplished in a residential setting. It is important to recognize that, for some children and families, this is true; however, the experience has been that residential services are overused for children and families who, in the long run, would do better not being separated. Historically, few programs have been in existence that would allow for intensive and extensive full-day programming, leaving the child to reside at home as a substitute for long-term residential services. Such intensive services, combined with intensive family services, a 24-hour on-call system for crises, and a respite care capacity, do seem effective for many children and families, avoiding the problems of separation, such as (1) reintegrating the child into the family and (2) the child's progress in the residential setting while sufficient change is not made in the home environment.

A second set of circumstances that has historically led to the separation of the child from his or her family is an intense family crisis where (1) a "cooling off period" seems indicated or (2) separation for a longer term seems appropriate to accomplish goals that cannot be addressed while the crisis continues. For some situations, the use of residential settings may be necessary; however, intensive in-home services similar to those provided by Homebuilders, Inc. of Tacoma, Washington (Kinney, Madsen, & Haapala, 1977) certainly have shown considerable promise in keeping children and families together. These services are provided from four to eight hours per day, or more, if needed for a time-limited period, usually up to two months. The focus of such services is to resolve the crisis, to improve communication, and to link the family and child to longer-term services, as needed. For some families, the addition of respite services may add to the effectiveness of such intervention. It is important as a new focus in the treatment of children to develop policies and programs that address more widespread use of in-home crisis services and intensive day services coupled with the belief that separation of child and family is usually not necessary.

A second major problem area in providing services to older adolescents is the importance of helping them to become employable, which is essential in helping them to become independent, as well as essential to their developing self-esteem. Many of these adolescents have a history of unsuccessful and unpleasant school experiences. They usually have no prevocational or vocational skills and developing such skills in community-based settings has been very difficult. In tight economic times, when jobs are hard to find in general, this population of youngsters is most likely to be the last considered for apprenticeship employment or for on-the-job training. Even when they are willing to continue in the public education system, they are apparently also the last considered for vocational education services when the teachers are not trained to work with retarded students or with emotionally/behaviorally disturbed, very difficult students. Nor are these adolescents viewed positively by vocational rehabilitation services, for they do not meet the criterion of showing promise for being employable.

Shore (1983) has noted the importance of addressing the vocational/employment needs of the delinquent population. His approach of "vocationally oriented psychotherapy" has shown much promise, as have less formalized approaches used in some North Carolina programs of (1) developing small training programs within the treatment program settings and/or (2) paying employers to hire and train one or two adolescents at a time. Even with tax benefits to employers who hire handicapped employees, the assaultive or explosive multihandicapped, unskilled adolescent is not well tolerated in the workplace. Working out such employment problems has taken a one-to-one approach, involving cajoling employers and running interference for the adolescents, as needed. The capacity to develop a prevocational and/or vocational services plan by a case manager independent of a specific program component has indeed led to a more appropriate definition of the adolescent's needs and interests and has therefore led to more tailor-made services, rather than trying to fit the youngster into an existing slot.

Nonetheless, a more systematic approach is needed; a public policy must be effected to add the important dimension of employment to the policies mandating special education and treatment for troubled adolescents.

At this point, six years hardly has seemed sufficient to implement a comprehensive service system, even given the breakneck pace that pervaded all aspects of program planning an program development. Substantive program evaluation any earlier, most likely, would not have yielded a sound picture of what stable and mature programs can provide for multiply handicapped, seriously impaired children and adolescents. Those evaluations are timely now. The value of the preceding years rests in the lessons learned about the problems and successes that occur in widescale program planning and development, including: (1) the attitudes that must change about children for community-based programs to succeed; (2) the range of services that must exist and be coordinated for children to be served well in communities; (3) recognition that individualized service plans can supersede the administrative classification of children as mentally retarded children, welfare children, juvenile justice children, or mental health children and can lead to appropriate services for them; and (4) the importance of broadly defined case management as the cohesive elements in a system of services.

## References

Joint Commission on Mental Health of Children. (1969). *Crisis in child mental health: Challenge for the 1970's.* New York: Harper & Row.

Kinney, J., Madsen, B., & Haapala, D. (1977). Homebuilders: Keeping families together. *Journal of Consulting and Clinical Psychology, 45*(2), 667–673.

Knitzer, J. (1982). *Unclaimed children: The failure of public responsibility to children and adolescents in view of mental health services.* Washington, DC: The Children's Defense Fund.

Knitzer, J., LaNeve, R., Pappanikou, A.J., Shore, M.F., & Steffek, J.R. (1983). *Report to the Division of Mental Health, Mental Retardation, Substance Abuse Services Regarding the Implementation of Willie M.* Internal Document, Raleigh, NC.

Lourie, J., Katz-Leavy, J., Kagan, E., & Forbes, M. (1984). *Status of current proposals for national initiatives for severely emotionally disturbed children and adolescents.* Presented at the National Council of Community Mental Health Centers Meeting, New Orleans, LA.

Shore, M.F. (1983). Juvenile delinquency in the United States: National issues and new directors for intervention. In *Juvenile delinquency: International perspective.* Montreal, Quebec: Boscoville Foundation. Unpublished manuscript.

Stockdill, J. (1983). *Child and adolescent service system program: Program announcement.* Washington, DC: National Institute of Mental Health.

*Willie M. et al. v. James B. Hunt, Jr. et al.*, Civil No. C-C 79-294-M (W.D.N.C. 1980).

# 40
# Developing a System of Services for the Dually Diagnosed Adult Population in North Carolina: After Willie M.

Donald Taylor

North Carolina is embarking on a major effort to develop services for mentally retarded adults who are also diagnosed as mentally ill. Although this effort is in the early stages, a description of the planning process and the issues and concerns that have been raised should be instructive to other states facing the problem of delivering services to dually diagnosed adult clients. Much of the planning is based on our experience with the Willie M. program for children (as discussed by Behar in Chapter 39) and represents an attempt to maximize the strengths as well as to avoid some of the problems experienced in that program, particularly in the planning phases of the program.

In 1985, the North Carolina Division of Mental Health/Mental Retardation/Substance Abuse Services adopted as one of the agency's major goals, the development of a plan to serve this population. Fortunately, both mental retardation services and mental health services are organized within a single state agency. Moreover, the local elements of the system, 41 area programs, made up of one or more of North Carolina's 100 counties, have a legal mandate to provide community-based services for both persons with mental illness and/or mental retardation. Therefore, the barrier of different agencies with separate service mandates was not a problem during the planning process. Additionally, these same local agencies have participated in the delivery of services to the Willie M.class— which is a multihandicapped population of minors, many of whom are both mentally retarded and mentally ill (see Behar, Chapter 39).

The initial step in the planning process was the creation of a central guidance group and four regional planning committees. Regional planning committees were composed of community program staff, psychiatric hospital and mental retardation staff, and regional office coordinators. Each planning committee represented a balance of mental retardation and mental health professionals, as well as a balance of institutional and community staff. The central guidance committee was made up of the chairpersons of each regional committee, key staff from the state offices of mental health and mental retardation, and other professionals selected such as the chief of statistical services and clinical staff from each disability area who were knowledgeable about diagnostic criteria, records content, and screening and assessment. In addition, the services of a consultant who had participated in a similar planning effort in another state were very help-ful. The role of the central committee was to develop a uniform process of client identification, needs assessment, and service planning. Regional chairpersons identified and brought to the central committee issues, problems, and concerns that surfaced throughout the planning process, and the central committee func-tioned as a problem-solving mechanism during the entire planning process.

As described by Behar, the planning for the Willie M. program had been done much more centrally, under the pressure of a timetable imposed by the federal court and resulted in initial resistance by local programs. However, our experi-ence with the Willie M. program, in part, had fostered attitudes of commitment to clients and a commitment to community-based services that facilitated the role of managers in planning for the mentally retarded and mentally ill adult population.

Several useful strategies emerged during the development of a statewide planning structure. First, it is extremely important to include in this process professionals from both disability groups and from all levels of the system: state, regional, and local. Involving clinicians, administrators, and data specialists early in the process provides instantaneous feedback from a variety of necessary perceptions and improves the power of the problem-solving role of the committees.

Developing and using a common data base, definitions, and procedures for identifying clients were also an important aid to uniform planning. Including the state system's chief data expert was of great help in identifying quickly what data were already available for planning and what questions could be answered by modifying the existing data system. In addition, clinicians, such as psychiatrists and psychologists, were able to assist the group in assimilating the implications of DSM-III-R diagnoses, AAMD criteria, and adaptive behavior scales.

Also, the active participation of top-level state administrators demonstrated the consistent commitment of the state's Mental Health/Mental Retardation/Substance Abuse Services agency. Moreover, decisions could be reached easily about such things as the use of consultants, scheduling training, and allocating available resources, especially during the screening and assessment phases.

The planning process was carried out in three distinct phases: screening, assessment, and service planning.

The screening phase began with a listing of all patients in the four regional psy-chiatric hospitals who were carried on the Division's Client Information System as having a diagnosis of mental retardation and mental illness. The lists generated were provided to ward staff of each hospital, and they were asked to nominate additional patients based on their direct knowledge of the patients' histories and behavior, and to delete patients whose placement on the list was erroneous. Hospital records of all the patients on the revised lists were reviewed in detail to determine the existence of a valid individual psychological evaluation and evi-dence that impairment occurred prior to age 22. Where valid current psychologi-cal evaluations were not available, an individual evaluation was performed by psychologists from the psychiatric hospital or nearby mental retardation centers.

Psychologists from the mental retardation centers were often called on to evaluate patients in the hospitals who were severely or profoundly retarded.

The second phase of the process involved the further assessment of all patients who were significantly intellectually impaired with evidence of a developmental origin of the impairment. The assessment included the administration of both an adaptive behavior scale and a maladaptive behavior scale. Altogether, the screening and assessment phases identified 380 patients with a diagnosis of mental illness who met all three components of the AAMD criteria for mental retardation: intellectual deficit, developmental origin, and impairment in adaptive behavior.

Levels of mental retardation among the mentally ill/mentally retarded population assessed in the psychiatric hospitals are as follows:

Profound mental retardation    17.4%
Severe mental retardation    15.6%
Moderate mental retardation    25.0%
Mild mental retardation    41.7%

The service planning phase began with a case-by-case review of each of these 380 dually diagnosed individuals. Following the case reviews of service needs conducted by local staff from both mental retardation and mental health services, decisions were made about the most appropriate service setting for each client and proposals for each area were developed. Although each regional committee was given discretion to use clinical and program judgment, certain basic principles were employed by each group in the service planning process.

1. The existing mental health and mental retardation service delivery structures are to be used rather than attempting to develop a third separate system for the dually diagnosed. Staff at all levels were concerned about adding additional labels to clients who were already suffering from stigmatization. Moreover, integrating these clients into the present systems would give them opportunities to interact with peers who can serve as positive models. Service costs can also be reduced by using "new" money to fill in the gaps for individual clients, rather than spending funds to start up new programs.
2. Clients are assigned to core programs on the basis of need rather than diagnosis. Having staff from both disability areas made this possible, in that personnel making the placement decisions were also those who would later be providing services.
3. Augmentation or enhancement of the core program with specific services, which would allow variations in core programs, was planned on a case-by-case basis. Thus, a client whose basic needs were found to be mental illness related, and who was therefore placed in a mental health program, might be provided with certain developmental services delivered by professionals in the field of mental retardation.
4. Intensive restrictive programs are to be developed last, and only after the need for such programs has actually been demonstrated. For example, the first year of the plan emphasizes residential services, such as placement in supported

private homes, and vocational services, such as supported work models. Recognizing that not all clients will make easy adjustments, itinerant crisis intervention teams, respite, and intensive case management are also part of the first year plan.

Persons, whose primary intervention needs were for developmental services, were targeted for transfer to the regional mental retardation center or for placement in the mental retardation service system in their home communities. In such cases, plans included enhancement or augmentations of the mental retardation service with appropriate mental health services. The clients, whose most significant disabilities were mental illness, were designated to be placed in a community mental health setting. Again, in either case, the setting is augmented by developmental services appropriate for persons with mental retardation. Clients designated to remain in the hospitals are those with severe mental illness for whom community placement is not feasible, at the time, and a few fragile, elderly patients felt to be at high risk for transfer trauma.

The summarized placement decisions made by regional committees are as follows:

1. Remaining in a psychiatric hospital — 159 — (43.8%)
   (a) Due to age/transfer trauma — 66 — (18.7%)
   (b) Due to need for continued hospitalization — 102 — (26.7%)
2. Transfer from psychiatric hospitals — 221 — (56.2%)
   (a) To mental retardation settings in the mental retardation centers — 64 — (16.8%)
   (b) To mental health or mental retardation settings in the community — 170 — (44.7%)

For those clients placed directly into community programs, the plans identify a full range of residential, day, and support services needed. The array of services planned for the community is extensive; over 25 different types of services are specified, all based on the individual needs of the clients.

Uniform cost levels for each service type have been established, based on existing similar services, line item projections, and other experience. The plans also incorporate continuous infrastructure needs, such as training, administration, and case management.

Already, two cross-training sessions have been conducted, attended by over 250 professionals from both disability groups and from community and institutional settings. Additional training is scheduled with training content awaiting the evaluation of the first two training events.

Although the planning phase has been completed with a high degree of success, several critical issues have been identified.

First, although in the case of North Carolina both disability groups are located in the same state and local agency, we do not yet have a common language or common base of understanding all across the system. For example, mental health professionals were, for the most part, unaware of the need for and value of adaptive behavior scales. On the other hand, mental retardation professionals were hard pressed to defend the relevancy of the developmental origin criteria contained in the AAMD definition. However, the good news is that already through collaboration on the planning effort and the cross training, which has been held, one can observe the beginning development of a greater shared vocabulary and understanding. It is interesting to note that these problems did not exist in the Willie M. program, most likely because those professionals who work with children, in either the mental retardation or the mental health area, have more of a common language and common understanding based on their common concern with developmental issues.

Second, the concept of enhancing or augmenting primary mental retardation or mental health services has not yet been tested with the adult population. We lack experience in integrating services and enhancement could become periphral and irrelevant to the real needs of clients.

Third, the funding bases for mental health and mental retardation are separate and categorical in North Carolina. Multiple funding bases tend to drive service delivery programs in different directions. Clients, who are initially misplaced, may have difficulty migrating to a more-appropriate service setting, unless funding is flexible.

Fourth, the kinds of collaborative efforts exhibited in the initial planning must continue at the local level. Case planning and management, provided at the individual client level, will need to be an ongoing process to ensure that clients with dual diagnosis are appropriately served in response to their mental retardation and mental health needs. Hopefully, the professionals delivering services to the adult population can learn from other counterparts in the children's area, particularly regarding joint case planning and case management (see Chapter 39).

Finally, one of the strengths of the plan thus far appears to be that we have avoided a preoccupation with system design, while focusing on the *functional role of the system*. What has been planned is not a separate system for people with a dual diagnosis. To the contrary, it builds on the present systems as they are, recognizes their strengths, and seeks to remedy their weaknesses through service enhancement. This was not a compromise based on the failure of either disability service area to negotiate; instead it was a deliberate attempt to achieve the appropriate integration for persons with differing degrees of mental retardation and mental illness.

# 41
# Families and the Developmental Needs of Dually Diagnosed Children

PAUL R. DOKECKI and CRAIG ANNE HEFLINGER

Dually diagnosed children represent a major psychoeducational and biomedical problem for the nation. All known prevalence research on the topic has shown that children with mental retardation have higher rates of psychopathology—perhaps as much as five to six times higher—than in the population as a whole (Matson & Frame, 1985). These findings are striking since intellectual impairment often diagnostically overshadows psychopathology in children with mental retardation. Despite the extensive prevalence of coexisting intellectual and emotional problems, however, the dually diagnosed are grossly underserved in the United States (Reiss, Levitan, & McNally, 1982). Although we accept the validity of the claimed high rates of mental retardation joined with psychopathology, and of attendant unmet developmental needs, we believe that a longstanding conceptual problem has impeded meaningful address to the issue.

## Toward Conceptual Clarification

Over the centuries, scholars have divided the whole human organism into parts, usually including a distinction between the intellect and the emotions. This distinction, however, is not inherent in the nature of the organism; rather, it is created for the conceptual and pragmatic purposes of those who make it. The distinction involves theoretical constructs devised to facilitate understanding. Constructs referring to intellect and emotions may or may not be useful and, if not useful, ought to be discarded. Regarding their application to dually diagnosed young children, we contend that their utility should be questioned and perhaps they should be discarded or their use significantly modified.

The question then is: How valid, reliable, and scientifically and socially useful is the distinction within a given child between mental retardation (intellectual disorder) and psychopathology (emotional disorder), especially for young children up to the age of 8 or 9? This chapter attempts to answer this question. Clearly, mental retardation and psychopathology have often been identified in the same children, intertwined in dynamic and complex behavioral patterns. This coexistence has been interpreted in several ways, including: the phenomenon reflects the observation that the emotional development of children with mental retardation is correlated more strongly with mental age than with chronological age; emotional disturbance may cause intellectual retardation, the issue of pseudoretardation; and psychosocial experience, perhaps interacting with constitutional factors, may produce multiple handicaps in the areas of intellect and emotion (Reiss et al., 1982). Another plausible alternative is that the coexisting phenomena in question may often be one in the same, or manifestations of the same process, but subject to different constructions—in effect, two sides of the same coin. On this view, what exists in nature is a developing child-in-transaction-with-an-environment (Sameroff & Chandler, 1975), who is judged at given times and in given contexts to be developmentally disabled or not. Those developmentally disabled children, identified as mentally retarded, manifest a variety of needs and behavior, some of which are diagnosable as psychopathology, often leading to a dual diagnosis. What these children require is that their needs be addressed—*all* their needs.

While developmental needs may be viewed as related to intellectual disorder at one time by mental retardation professionals, and to emotional disorder at another time by mental health professionals, what remains constant are children's needs requiring care and intervention. And regarding needs, Reiss et al. (1982) observed that "a sustained effort to address the mental health needs of mentally retarded people should have positive benefits for them as a group. The effort could reorient professional thinking about retarded people toward services for the 'whole' person; the more attention people give to the emotional dimensions of mental retardation, the more they should appreciate the humanity of mentally retarded people" (p. 366). Our position is that the humanity of a young child with mental retardation may best be served by a view of the "whole" child that recognizes the conceptual difficulties in distinguishing between mental health and mental retardation needs, and that calls for a plain and simple focus on developmental needs.

We are not arguing that coexisting intellectual and emotional disorders are always and everywhere identical or manifestations of the same process. In young children with mental retardation, however, the distinction is usually difficult to make and sustain, and it is less important that it be made than it is to recognize and deal with these children's developmental needs. In short, we are arguing for a developmental and needs-based perspective (Hobbs, 1975) on dual diagnosis. This perspective entails a focus on the whole child-in-environmental context, with intellectual or emotional constructs used only as necessary to enhance understanding and to make appropriate intervention decisions. The child's ecology is seen as influencing development, with the family as its most important element, both for the purposes of scientific understanding and of preventive and ameliorative interventions. The family, moreover, provides a useful vantage point for analyzing the often observed tension and lack of coordination between mental retardation and mental health professionals in dealing with dually diagnosed children, as we show in a later section.

# The Social Ecology of Families
# with Dually Diagnosed Children

A developmental and needs-based approach to dually diagnosed young children relies on a social ecological perspective, with a focus on the family as society's key human development enhancing system (Hobbs, 1975; Hobbs et al., 1984). Before explicating this perspective, a closer look at the phenomenon of psychopathology in mental retardation helps ground our understanding. In this regard, the Matson and Frame (1985) biosocial model provides a comprehensive framework.

Matson and Frame (1985) identified three factors in the dual diagnosis phenomenon: biological, social, and psychological and developmental processes. In the biological factor, they include: "1. Developmental Factor 2. Genetic Factors   3. Biochemistry   4. Physical Impairments   5. Neurological Impairments" (p. 29). The social factor entails: "1. Social Skills   2. Family Interactions   3. Personality Variables   4. Self-Help Skills   5. Prenatal, Perinatal, and Postnatal Factors   6. Normalization/Institutionalization   7. Work and School" (p. 29). And finally, the psychological and developmental processes factor includes: "1. Short and Long Term Memory   2. Cognitive Development 3. Perceptual and Motor Skill   4. Self-Control   5. Personality Variables" (p. 29). Although only specifically mentioned in the social factor, the family has been linked in research findings to elements in all three of these factors. But how should we understand the specifics of the family's functioning in the social ecology of the young dually diagnosed child? Recent work at Peabody's Kennedy Center is helpful in this regard.

The Peabody family development model has been useful in helping to understand a variety of phenomena, including the early childhood intervention process (Newbrough, Dokecki, Dunlop, Hogge, & Simpkins, 1979), child abuse and neglect (Simpkins, Newbrough, Dokecki, & Dunlop, 1979), and the management and control of childhood diabetes (Newbrough, Simpkins, & Maurer, 1985). It has obvious relevance for understanding the social ecology of families with dually diagnosed children. The Peabody model "is based on the family development assumptions that behavior is a function of the preceding as well as the current conditions of the social milieu and the individual, and that behavior cannot be understood apart from the developmental stage of the person. The model . . . has, at its core, a stress-support process. The model takes on a systems complexity that encompasses past experiences, present situations, and expectations for the future" (Newbrough et al., 1985, p. 87). The reader is referred to the primary sources for a detailed exposition of the model. We present here an outline of its components, in order to help identify fruitful research topics and possible approaches to intervention.

The Peabody family development model entails 11 factors contributing to an observed developmental phenomenon, such as that of a mentally retarded young child who manifests emotional problems. Factors from the past history of the child, understood as a functioning member of a community and family ecology, include: (1) each parent's history and developmental stage, (2) community and peer norms and culture, and (3) the child's history and developmental stage. Mediating the influence of the past on present functioning is (4) the family's developmental level or stage. Present regular functioning, in turn, entails the operation of (5) each parent's perception and knowledge of the child and his or her developmental problem, (6) the child's perception and knowledge of self and his or her problem, (7) each parent's psychological and physical state, (8) the life events and routines of the ongoing family situation, (9) the child's psychological and physical state, (10) each parent's instrumental and affective resources, and (11) the child's instrumental and affective resources. The child's ongoing behavior and the family's response to that behavior provide feedback to the child, the parents, and the entire system, and "the model is continuously dynamic. Each incident becomes a part of history and contributes to future events, functioning, and behavior" (Newbrough et al., 1985, p. 87).

In terms of the Cromwell, Blashfield, and Strauss (1975) analysis of the components entailed in classifying children's behavior disorders, the Peabody model suggests that the family may be implicated in the phenomenon of the dually diagnosed child at multiple levels: (a) etiology, (b) behavioral manifestation of the problem, (c) intervention, (d) prognosis and intervention outcome, (e) preventive intervention, and (f) outcome of preventive intervention. Given the Matson and Frame (1985) biosocial model, we do not claim that the family is the sole factor in dual diagnosis. Given the Peabody social ecological model, however, the family cannot be ignored in any serious address to the problem.

# Families of Dually Diagnosed Children and the Service System

The service delivery system for severely handicapped children has been described as inadequate, inaccessible, and inappropriate. Needed services are often unavailable, or they may be available only with limited access based on categorical or income restrictions. The services that do exist are in short supply, have been criticized as low in quality, and are often in highly restrictive settings (Gorham, Des Jardins, Page, Pettis, & Scheiber, 1975; Moroney, 1980; Paul & Beckman-Bell, 1981).

Families have experienced the service delivery system for severely handicapped children as both fragmented and dehumanizing (Gorham et al., 1975). Being "referred around" or "falling between the cracks" (McNett, 1980) often follows the parents' initial attempt to discover what is going on with their child and where appropriate services are available. Diagnosis is typically deficit oriented, rarely attending to the child's assets or including specific recommendations for intervention. Parents report they feel as if they are placed in a special category, given a label as is the case with their child (Paul & Beckman-Bell, 1981). Labeling the child, often as a substitute for entry to services, follows diagnosis. "Ironically, the help given by the service system works in direct reverse ratio to the help needed by parents. The more crisis laden the child and his family, the less likely they are to find help" (Gorham et al., 1975, p. 181). The many specialists to whom the family is referred are often in different settings or agencies, and little if any coordination or case management is available. Furthermore, parents are bombarded, sometimes subtly and sometimes directly, by the societal message that their child is not worthy of much investment.

Instead of promoting parents' involvement in the treatment of their severely handicapped child, the service system discourages their participation. Although regulatory mechanisms ensure parents' attendance at formal decisionmaking meetings, they are often excluded from meaningful participation in the evaluation process or in the premeeting conferences held to put all the information together. Professionals typically maintain the expert role, discounting parents' knowledge and ability to care for their handicapped child. This approach fosters the dependence of families instead of contributing to their enablement and independence. Services are often unavailable at less restrictive, supportive levels and often become available only when services "substitute" for family care.

Moroney (1986) conducted an extensive review of the literature to determine professional attitudes and found four views toward families with handicapped members:

1. The family as part of the problem: Family pathology—genetic, social, or both—is viewed as causing the problem and interfering with treatment.
2. The family as a resource to the handicapped person: Families are acknowledged as caregivers but not as having needs in their own right.
3. The family as team participant: The family is viewed as part of the caregiving team in treatment.
4. The family as needing resources: The focus here shifts from the individual handicapped member to the family as a unit in its own right, a unit that needs support.

The problem for families with dually diagnosed children is Moroney's finding that the two systems concerned with them tend to split on the views. The mental health system prefers the first and second; the mental retardation system prefers the third and fourth—leading to a number of problems.

In addition to fragmentation of services within the mental retardation and mental health systems, there is virtually no communication across the boundaries of these two systems. A primary diagnosis of either mental retardation or emotional disturbance is usually required, with one or the other system then assuming primary responsibility, even though services may be needed from the other system. This problem is exacerbated by the inherent differences of these two systems in conceptual approaches to the severely disabled child and family, as suggested by Moroney's findings. The mental retardation system uses an educational approach, treats the disability as a chronic condition, and provides a number of "hard" services to families, such as respite care and financial support. Mental retardation professionals also tend to view families as effective members of the treatment team and recognize the pressures associated with having a severely handicapped family member and the need for practical support. The mental health system, on the other hand, tends to apply the psychiatric model to severely handicapped children and their families, emphasizing pathology. Focus is on "cure" of the child, in an acute illness model, and families are viewed by professionals as part of the problem, with little emphasis on their participation in the treatment team. Imagine the frustration of the family experiencing both systems simultaneously.

## Value Considerations in Program Development and Public Policy

We have identified some of the many problems characterizing the interactions between families with young dually diagnosed children and the fragmented service system. It is now important to deal with value issues encountered in developing programs and public policies in this area. In this regard, we have recourse to a recently developed value analytic framework (Dokecki, 1983), which served to focus policy research on the family's role in child development reported in *Strengthening Families* (Hobbs et al., 1984).

To emphasize the social ecology of families with dually diagnosed children is to take on a commitment of promoting community and human development values. This value commitment can be expressed in two interrelated ways:

1. The aim of intervention should be to *enhance community* . . . so that individuals and their families may develop to their potential. Individuals and families have a legitimate claim on community resources and support in the performance of their developmental tasks.
2. The aim of intervention should be to *enhance human development* so that individuals and their families might be effective participants in the community. The community can legitimately expect individuals and families to master their developmental tasks. (Dokecki, 1983, pp. 115–116).

The pursuit of these values, relative to dually diagnosed young children, requires that we pose four general questions about possible programs and policies. Does a given program or policy (1) enhance the community of the dually diagnosed child and the family, (2) strengthen the families of dually diagnosed children, (3) enable the parents of dually diagnosed children to do their jobs well, and (4) enhance the individual development and protect the rights of individual members of the family of a dually diagnosed child? Brief elaboration is in order.

To assess a program's or a policy's capacity to *enhance the community of the dually diagnosed child and his or her family*, additional specific questions must be posed. Is the program or policy demeaning by devaluing and stigmatizing these children and their parents, causing them to lose self-esteem? Is it divisive by separating the dually diagnosed from their community and allowing, even encouraging, invidious social comparison? Does the program or policy bestow unwarranted advantage beyond meeting special needs that are socially important? On the positive side, does it increase shared heritage, mutual aid, and community building by bringing dually diagnosed children and their families together with other children and families, highlighting human commonalities and shared values?

A program's or a policy's capacity to *strengthen the families of dually diagnosed children* can be assessed, first, by asking about its ability to improve the capacity of these families to master a broad range of developmental tasks. This capacity is built through services that enhance parental knowledge, skill, and ability to make decisions about their children. Furthermore, does the program or policy improve the liaison or linkage functions that mobilize social resources and supports needed by these families? In this regard, families should be helped both to identify and to make use of formal human service agency networks and to look toward more primary kinds of social support, such as family members, kinship groups, neighbors, and voluntary associations. Finally, does it protect these families from unwarranted intrusion and allow parents choice by providing a variety of service options and adequate information about these options?

Assessment of a program's or a policy's capacity to *enable the parents of dually diagnosed children to do their jobs well* also requires posing additional questions. Does it minimize stress by making available to these parents essential resources, such as time and energy, knowledge, and resources — and consequent satisfaction in the form of positive affect and feelings of worth — in order to carry out their parental functions? Does the program or policy promote shared responsibility among parents and service providers; in other words, does it operate according to enablement and empowerment principles? Parents are enabled when they are treated as capable adults and helped by professionals to become even more capable. Empowerment occurs when parents are provided with resources and legal rights so they may negotiate effectively with societal institutions.

The final value element, *enhancing the individual development and protecting the rights of all the members of families with dually diagnosed children*, entails several questions. Does the program or policy enhance all individual family members' opportunities for the development of competence and self-realization by providing services that enhance physical, cognitive, affective, and interpersonal development? Does it protect individual members of the family from abuse and severe neglect?

The value framework articulated in this section suggests questions and criteria for making societal choices regarding dually diagnosed young children and their families. We now turn to recommendations for intervention and research flowing from the needs-based and developmental perspective we have developed thus far.

## Conclusions and Recommendations

We began this chapter by calling for a developmental, needs-based model for diagnosis and service delivery. Such an approach not only recognizes but values the role of the family, as shown in the previous section. A three-pronged approach, suggested by Moroney (1986), would be required to implement this model in the best interests of dually diagnosed children and their families: (1) restructuring the service delivery system, (2) increasing the flow of resources into the system, and (3) reorienting professional knowledge and attitudes.

First, the service system should ideally be restructured to include a wide range of services geared toward meeting the needs of children and their families. A separate system for dually diagnosed children and their families should not be developed; instead, the service system should adopt a comprehensive approach toward meeting the developmental needs of *all* children and families. Similarly, funding mechanisms allowing universal service eligibility based on developmental needs, instead of the present system of categorical and income eligibility, must be developed. In this model, needs would be defined functionally instead of by diagnostic category. Two broad functional needs of families are, first, support for their childrearing functions, instead of substitution of programs for family care, and second, periodic relief from the associated stress of childrearing (Moroney, 1981). Strategies to meet these needs of families include the provision of (1) hard services, such as income support, respite care, transportation, homemaker services, and home appliances; (2) process skills, to enhance parental capability to manage their family functioning; and (3) counseling, to include education, information, and therapy, for all members of the family who need it (Moroney, 1980, 1981).

Developing a range of community and residential services is but one step; organizing these services so that children and their families can move easily from one service to another depending on their needs, as well as coordinating multiple services, should also be integral to the system. Needed is a continuum-of-care, ranging from least- to most-restrictive levels of care, including prevention and early intervention, in addition to the more traditionally offered outpatient and residential services. A liaison component, linking elements throughout the continuum, would promote the coordination of services and transitions in the system.

Second, the need for additional resources is painfully obvious. The coordination of service delivery through a continuum-of-care model would tend to reduce redundancy in the system; however, service gaps will undoubtedly become much more obvious. Research defining the needs of families and children, including those identified as dually diagnosed, and describing presently available services, is needed to identify gaps in need of immediate address.

The third prong needed for developing a better service system is the reorientation through appropriate preservice and inservice training programs of professional knowledge and attitudes about the needs of children and their families. Misconceptions about children who are both mentally retarded and emotionally disturbed must be challenged (Matson & Frame, 1985). Conceptual barriers to integrating mental health and mental retardation systems must be overcome. It is crucial to recognize the needs of families in their own right and to acknowledge their value as intervention team members. Humanizing the fragmented and dehumanizing system is vital: "The sensitivity of the professional brings dignity and integrity to the moment for the family" (Paul & Beckman-Bell, 1981, p. 125).

Our recommendation for needed research is simply stated, but rich and complex in its specifics: *The phenomenon of dually diagnosed children should be studied from the perspective of the social ecology of the family.* Returning to material we have used to make our case, we would suggest that the family's relationship to the biological, social, and psychological and developmental processes factors identified by Matson and Frame (1985) be investigated. The particulars of this relationship might entail the Peabody family development model (Newbrough et al., 1985). In addition, the elements of the Cromwell et al. (1975) approach to classifying behavior disorders could serve to organize research programs encompassing a range of issues from etiology and prevention through symptomatology, prognosis, and intervention. Finally, the Dokecki (1983) and Hobbs et al. (1984) value framework suggests broad areas of intervention research, ranging from the community to the individual.

In summary, we have attempted to demonstrate that a needs-based and developmental approach to the phenomenon of dually diagnosed children, with an emphasis on the family as society's key human development enhancing system, is required for a comprehensive address to this major national problem.

## References

Cromwell, R.L., Blashfield, R.K., & Strauss, J.S. (1975). Criteria for classification systems. In N. Hobbs (Ed.), *Issues in the classification of children* (Vol. 1, pp. 4–25). San Francisco, CA: Jossey-Bass.

Dokecki, P.R. (1983). The place of values in the world of psychology and public policy. *Peabody Journal of Education, 60*(3), 108–125.

Gorham, K.A., Des Jardins, C., Page, R., Pettis, E., & Scheiber, G. (1975). Effect on parents. In N. Hobbs (Ed.), *Issues in the classification of children* (Vol. II, pp. 1548–1588). San Francisco, CA: Jossey-Bass.

Hobbs, N. (1975). *The futures of children.* San Francisco, CA: Jossey-Bass.

Hobbs, N., Dokecki, P.R., Hoover-Dempsey, K., Moroney, R.M., Shayne, M., & Weeks, K. (1984). *Strengthening families.* San Francisco, CA: Jossey-Bass.

Matson, J.L., & Frame, C.L. (1985). *Psychopathology among mentally retarded children and adolescents.* Beverly Hills, CA: Sage.

McNett, I. (1980). Part II: Mental health services for handicapped fall between agencies. *APA Monitor, 11*, 15.

Moroney, R.M. (1980). Mental disability: The role of the family. In J.J. Bevilacqua (Ed.), *Changing government policies for the mentally disabled* (pp. 209–230). Cambridge, MA: Ballinger.

Moroney, R.M. (1981). Public social policy: Impact on families with handicapped children. In J.L. Paul (Ed.), *Understanding and working with parents of children with special needs* (pp. 180–204). New York: Holt, Rinehart & Winston.

Moroney, R.M. (1986). *Shared responsibility: Families and social policy.* New York: Aldine.

Newbrough, J.R., Dokecki, P.R., Dunlop, K.H., Hogge, J.H., & Simpkins, C.G. (1979). *Families and family-institution transaction in child development: An analysis of the*

Family Research Program of HEW's Administration of Children, Youth, and Families. John F. Kennedy Center for Research on Education and Human Development, Vanderbilt University, Nashville, TN.

Newbrough, J.R., Simpkins, C.G., & Maurer, H. (1985). A family development approach to studying factors in the management and control of childhood diabetes. *Diabetes Care, 8,* 83–92.

Paul, J.L., & Beckman-Bell, P. (1981). Parent perspectives. In J.L. Paul (Ed.), *Understanding and working with parents of children with special needs* (pp. 119–153). New York: Holt, Rinehart & Winston.

Reiss, S., Levitan, G.W., & McNally, R.J. (1982). Emotionally disturbed mentally retarded people: An underserved population. *American Psychology, 37*(4), 361–367.

Sameroff, A.J., & Chandler, M.J. (1975). Reproductive risk and the continuum of caretaking casualty. In D. Horowitz, E.M. Hetherington, S. Scarr-Salaptek, & G.M. Siegel (Eds.), *Review of child development research* (Vol. 4). Chicago, IL: University of Chicago Press.

Simpkins, C.G., Newbrough, J.R., Dokecki, P.R., & Dunlop, K.H. (1979). *Child abuse and neglect in families.* Center for Community Studies, Vanderbilt University, Nashville, TN.

# Conclusion

DONALD TAYLOR and LENORE BEHAR

The eight chapters contained in this last section focused on the delivery of services to the mentally ill/mentally retarded population via model service systems. Based on these findings, the authors of these chapters offered the reader a number of recommendations to accomplish these goals:

1. Federal assistance through incentive grants to states should be given to encourage interagency collaboration and cooperation regarding the dually diagnosed. Such funding should itself emanate jointly from federal agencies such as NIMH, ADD, and MCH and might be similar in concept to the CASSP grants and would be directed at planning and implementation of state service systems for the dually diagnosed.
2. State agencies, with local participation, should ensure training of specialists in both fields regarding the need for joint service planning and service delivery on behalf of dually diagnosed clients.
3. Development of a consistent data base within and among states must be implemented to provide both diagnostic and behavioral data. Federal agencies could augment state efforts through technical assistance aimed at general use of common diagnostic criteria and terminology.
4. A national evaluation project, jointly sponsored by NIMH, ADD, and MCH, should be developed to determine the relative effectiveness of alternative administrative models and the efficacy of both existing and newly formulated strategies for providing mental health services to the mentally retarded.
5. We must ensure that state and local education agencies are aware of the special needs of children who are both mentally retarded and mentally ill and that the presence of both diagnoses has implications for learning.
6. And last, HCFA should consider modifying the definition of "conditions related to mental retardation" in the regulations relating to eligibility for Intermediate Care Facilities for the Mentally Retarded (ICF/MR). Included in the definition should be specific recognition of the dually diagnosed person's eligibility for ICF/MR.

# Author Index

# Subject Index